ADVANCES IN BIOENGINEERING

Advances in Bioengineerings

Editor:

Stephen Rego, Ph.D.

ArclerPress

www.arclerpress.com

Advances in Bioengineering
Editor: Stephen Rego, Ph.D.

© 2017 Arcler Press LLC
708 3rd Avenue, 6th Floor
New York
NY 10017
United States of America
www.arclerpress.com

ISBN: 978-1-68094-362-7

Library of Congress Control Number: 2016950946

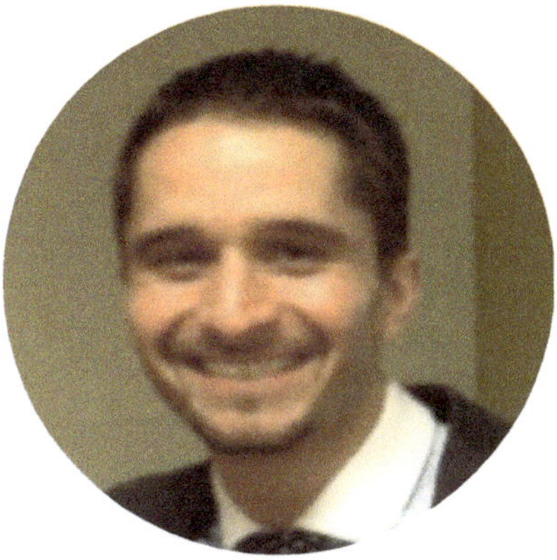

About the Editor

Stephen Rego, Ph.D.

Stephen obtained his PhD from the University of North Carolina at Charlotte in 2013 where his graduate research focused on cancer immunology and the tumor microenvironment. He received postdoctoral training in regenerative and translational medicine, specifically gastrointestinal tissue engineering, at the Wake Forest Institute of Regenerative Medicine. Currently, Stephen is an instructor for anatomy and physiology and biology at Forsyth Technical Community College.

Contents

List of Contributors xiii
Preface .... *xxi*
Introduction .... *xxiii*

Chapter 1 Scientific Advancements and Clinical Application 1
1. Introduction 1
2. Are We Speaking The Same Language? 2
3. Lifting the Silos 4
4. Training and Career Advancement 5
5. Death Valleys of Translational Progress 6
6. Catalysts for Translation 7
7. From the Bedside to the Bench and Back: Rethinking Translation 8
   Author Contributions 8
   Conflict of Interest Statement 8
   References 8

Chapter 2 Ex Vivo Dermis Mechanical Behavior in Relation to Decellularization Treatment Length 11
1. Background 11
2. Materials and Methods 12
3. Results and Discussion 15
   Conclusion 17
   References 18

Chapter 3 Biomaterials for Control of Stem Cell Behavior 21
1. Introduction 21
2. Stem Cell Characteristics 23
3. Cell–Surface Interaction 24
4. Chemically Controlling Stem Cell Fate 26
5. Cell Response to Topography 28
6. Alterations in Matrix Stiffness 31
7. How Do Cells Process this Materials Information? The Central Role of Adhesion 33
8. A Dynamic Future? 34
9. Summary 36
10. Author Contributions 36
11. Conflict of Interest Statement 36

Acknowledgments 37
References 37

Chapter 4 **Bone Defect Regeneration by a Combination of a β-Tricalcium Phosphate Scaffold and Bone Marrow Stromal Cells in A Non-Human Primate Model 49**
1. Introduction 49
2. Materials And Methods 51
3. Results 54
4. Discussion 56
Acknowledgements 59
References 59

Chapter 5 **Mesenchymal Stem Cell Morphology and Migration on Microtextured Titanium 63**
1. Introduction 63
2. Materials and Methods 65
3. Results 67
4. Discussion 73
Author Contributions 75
Conflict of Interest Statement 75
Funding 75
References 75

Chapter 6 **Modeling of Drug Delivery by a Pump Driven Micro-Needle Array System 79**
1. Introduction 79
2. Description of Mathematical Model 81
3. Calculation Results 85
4. Qualitative Experiments 91
5. Discussion 93
Conclusion 94
Acknowledgements 94
Disclosure 95
References 95

Chapter 7 **Recent Patents and Designs on HIP Replacement Prostheses 97**
1. Introduction 97
2. Background Art 100
Conclusion 114
References 115

Chapter 8 **Improved Estimation of the Cardiac Global Function Using Combined Long and Short Axis Mri Images of the Heart 119**

1. Background 119
2. Methods 120
3. Results and Discussion 127

Conclusion 133

Declarations 133

References 133

Chapter 9 **Neural Network Model of Vestibular Nuclei Reaction to Onset of Vestibular Prosthetic Stimulation 137**

1. Introduction 137
2. Materials and Methods 139
3. Results 146
4. Discussion 151
5. Author Contributions 152
6. Conflict of Interest Statement 152

Funding 153

References 153

Chapter 10 **Ultrasound Guided Double Injection of Blood Into Cisterna Magna: A Rabbit Model for Treatment of Cerebral Vasospasm 157**

1. Background 157
2. Methods 158
3. Results 161
4. Discussion 164

Conclusions 166

Declarations 166

References 166

Chapter 11 **Dynamic Expressions of Monocyte Chemo Attractant Protein-1 and Cc Chamomile Receptor 2 After Balloon Injury and Their Effects in Intimal Proliferation 171**

1. Introduction 171
2. Materials and Methods 172
3. Results 177
4. Discussions 181

Conclusion 184

Declarations 184

Authors' Contributions 184

References 184

Chapter 12 **Sub-Millimeter Diameter Poly(Vinyl Alcohol) Vascular Graft Patency in Rabbit Model 187**

1. Introduction 187
2. Materials and Methods 188
3. Results 192
4. Discussion 198
5. Author Contributions 200
6. Conflict of Interest Statement 200

Acknowledgments 200

References 201

Chapter 13 **Analytical Side-to-Side Related Anastomotic Strategies and Artery Patching 205**

1. Introduction 205
2. Methods 206
3. Results 218
4. Discussion 222
5. Conflict of Interest 223

Acknowledgements 223

Appendix 223

References 225

Chapter 14 **Relationship of Short-Term Blood Pressure Variability With Carotid Intima-Media Thickness in Hypertensive Patients 227**

1. Background 227
2. Methods 228
3. Results 229
4. Discussion 236

Conclusions 239

Declarations 239

References 240

Chapter 15 **Longitudinal Follow Up of Coiled Intracranial Aneurysms: The Impact of Contrast Enhanced Mra in Comparison to 3dtof Mra At 3t 243**

1. Background 243
2. Methods 244
3. Mra 244
4. Results 246
5. Discussion 248

Conclusions 250

Authors' Contributions 250

References 250

Chapter 16 Computational Fluid Dynamics of Computed Tomography Angiography to Detect the Hemodynamic Impact of Intracranial Atherosclerotic Stenosis 253

1. Background 253
2. Methods 254
3. Results 256
4. Discussion 258

Conclusions 261
Authors' Contributions 262
References 262

Chapter 17 Cyanobacteria as a Platform for Biofuel Production 265

1. Introduction 265
2. Improving Genetic Parts for Cyanobacteria 268
3. Improving CO_2 Fixation 268
4. Improving Metabolic Yield 269
5. Managing Inputs: Nutrient and Water Requirements 270
6. Photosynthetic Efficiency and Bioreactors 271
7. Final Thoughts 272

Conflict of Interest Statement 272
References 272

Chapter 18 Biodiesel Production by Aspergillus Niger Lipase Immobilized on Barium Ferrite Magnetic Nanoparticles 279

1. Introduction 279
2. Materials and Methods 281
3. Results and Discussion 283

Conclusions 293
Acknowledgments 294
Author Contributions 294
References 294

Index 299

List of Contributors

Joseph S. Fernandez-Moure
Department of Surgery, Houston Methodist Hospital, Houston, TX, USA
Surgical Advanced Technologies Laboratory, Department of Regenerative and Biomimetic Medicine, Houston Methodist Research Institute, Houston, TX, USA

Mara Terzini
Department of Mechanical and Aerospace Engineering, Politecnico di Torino, Torino, Italy

Cristina Bignardi
Department of Mechanical and Aerospace Engineering, Politecnico di Torino, Torino, Italy

Carlotta Castagnoli
Department of Engineering, University of Perugia, Perugia, Italy

Irene Cambieri
Skin Bank, AOU Città della Salute e della Scienza, Torino, Italy

Elisabetta M. Zanetti
Department of Engineering, University of Perugia, Perugia, Italy

Alberto L. Audenino
Department of Mechanical and Aerospace Engineering, Politecnico di Torino, Torino, Italy

Hilary J. Anderson
Centre for Cell Engineering, University of Glasgow, Glasgow, UK

Jugal Kishore Sahoo
Department of Pure and Applied Chemistry, Technology and Innovation Centre, University of Strathclyde, Glasgow, UK

Rein V. Ulijn
Department of Pure and Applied Chemistry, Technology and Innovation Centre, University of Strathclyde, Glasgow, UK
Advanced Science Research Centre (ASRC), Hunter College, City University of New York, New York, NY, USA

Matthew J. Dalby
Centre for Cell Engineering, University of Glasgow, Glasgow, UK

Tomokazu Masaoka
Department of Rehabilitation Medicine, Graduate School, Tokyo Medical and Dental University, Tokyo, Japan
Department of Orthopaedic and Spinal Surgery, Graduate School, Tokyo Medical and Dental University, Tokyo, Japan

Toshitaka Yoshii
Department of Orthopaedic and Spinal Surgery, Graduate School, Tokyo Medical and Dental University, Tokyo,
Japan

Masato Yuasa
Department of Orthopaedic and Spinal Surgery, Graduate School, Tokyo Medical and Dental University, Tokyo,
Japan

Tsuyoshi Yamada
Department of Orthopaedic and Spinal Surgery, Graduate School, Tokyo Medical and Dental University, Tokyo,
Japan
Global Center of Excellence (GCOE) Program, International Research Center for Molecular Science in Tooth and Bone Diseases, Tokyo Medical and Dental University, Tokyo, Japan

Takashi Taniyama
Department of Orthopaedic and Spinal Surgery, Graduate School, Tokyo Medical and Dental University, Tokyo,
Japan

Ichiro Torigoe
Department of Orthopaedic and Spinal Surgery, Graduate School, Tokyo Medical and Dental University, Tokyo,
Japan

Kenichi Shinomiya
Department of Orthopaedic and Spinal Surgery, Graduate School, Tokyo Medical and Dental University, Tokyo,
Japan

Atsushi Okawa
Department of Orthopaedic and Spinal Surgery, Graduate School, Tokyo Medical and Dental University, Tokyo,
Japan
Global Center of Excellence (GCOE) Program, International Research Center for Molecular Science in Tooth and Bone Diseases, Tokyo Medical and Dental University, Tokyo, Japan
Hard Tissue Genome Research Center, Tokyo Medical and Dental University, Tokyo, Japan

Sadao Morita
Department of Rehabilitation Medicine, Graduate School, Tokyo Medical and Dental University, Tokyo, Japan

Shinichi Sotome
Department of Orthopaedic and Spinal Surgery, Graduate School, Tokyo Medical and Dental University, Tokyo,
Japan
Department of Orthopaedic Research and Development, Graduate School, Tokyo Medical and Dental University, Tokyo, Japan

Brittany L. Banik
Musculoskeletal Regenerative Engineering Laboratory, Department of Biomedical Engineering, The Pennsylvania State University, University Park, PA, USA

Thomas R. Riley
Perelman School of Medicine, University of Pennsylvania, Philadelphia, PA, USA

Christina J. Platt
Department of Electrical Engineering, The Pennsylvania State University, University Park, PA, USA

Justin L. Brown
Musculoskeletal Regenerative Engineering Laboratory, Department of Biomedical Engineering, The Pennsylvania State University, University Park, PA, USA

Kai Chen
School of Mechanical Engineering, Hangzhou Dianzi University, Hangzhou, China

Min Pan
School of Mechanical Engineering, Hangzhou Dianzi University, Hangzhou, China

Zhi-Gang Feng[2]
Department of Mechanical Engineering, University of Texas, San Antonio, USA

H Derar
Department of Mechanical Engineering, University of Maine, Orono, ME, USA

M Shahinpoor
Department of Mechanical Engineering, University of Maine, Orono, ME, USA

Hossam ElRewaidy
Systems and Biomedical Engineering Department, Cairo University, Cairo 12613, Egypt

Ahmed S. Fahmy
Systems and Biomedical Engineering Department, Cairo University, Cairo 12613, Egypt
Center for Informatics Science, Nile University, Cairo 12588, Egypt

Jack DiGiovanna
Center for Neuroprosthetics, Bertarelli Foundation Chair in Translational Neuroengineering, École Polytechnique Fédérale de Lausanne, Lausanne, Switzerland

T. A. K. Nguyen
Center for Neuroprosthetics, Bertarelli Foundation Chair in Translational Neuroengineering, École Polytechnique Fédérale de Lausanne, Lausanne, Switzerland

Nils Guinand
Cochlear Implant Center for French Speaking Switzerland, Service of Otorhinolaryngology – Head and Neck Surgery, Geneva University Hospitals, Geneva, Switzerland

Angelica Pérez-Fornos
Cochlear Implant Center for French Speaking Switzerland, Service of Otorhinolaryngology – Head and Neck Surgery, Geneva University Hospitals, Geneva, Switzerland

Silvestro Micera
Center for Neuroprosthetics, Bertarelli Foundation Chair in Translational Neuroengineering, École Polytechnique Fédérale de Lausanne, Lausanne, Switzerland

Yongchao Chen
Ultrasound Center, The 105th Hospital of PLA, Hefei, China

Youzhi Zhu
Department of Radiology, The 105th Hospital of PLA, Hefei, China

Yu Zhang
Department of Radiology, The 105th Hospital of PLA, Hefei, China

Zixuan Zhang
Department of Anatomy, Anhui Medical University, Hefei, China

Juan Lian
Ultrasound Center, The 105th Hospital of PLA, Hefei, China

Fucheng Luo
Ultrasound Center, The 105th Hospital of PLA, Hefei, China

Xuefei Deng
Department of Anatomy, Anhui Medical University, Hefei, China

Kelvin KL Wong
School of Medicine, Western Sydney University, Sydney, Australia

Zhigang Huang
Emergency Department, Peking University Shenzhen Hospital, Shenzhen 518036, China

Yuebing Li
The Second Affiliated Hospital of Zhejiang Chinese Medical University, Hangzhou 310005, China

Lili Niu
Paul C. Lauterbur Research Center for Biomedical Imaging, Institute of Biomedical and Health Engineering, Shenzhen Institutes of Advanced Technology, Shenzhen 518055, China

Yang Xiao
Paul C. Lauterbur Research Center for Biomedical Imaging, Institute of Biomedical and Health Engineering, Shenzhen Institutes of Advanced Technology, Shenzhen 518055, China

Xiaodong Pu
The Second Affiliated Hospital of Zhejiang Chinese Medical University, Hangzhou 310005, China

Hairong Zheng
Paul C. Lauterbur Research Center for Biomedical Imaging, Institute of Biomedical and Health Engineering, Shenzhen Institutes of Advanced Technology, Shenzhen 518055, China

Ming Qian
Paul C. Lauterbur Research Center for Biomedical Imaging, Institute of Biomedical and Health Engineering, Shenzhen Institutes of Advanced Technology, Shenzhen 518055, China

Marie F. A. Cutiongco
Mechanobiology Institute, National University of Singapore, Singapore
Department of Biomedical Engineering, National University of Singapore, Singapore

Marek Kukumberg
Mechanobiology Institute, National University of Singapore, Singapore

Jonnathan L. Peneyra
Comparative Medicine, National University of Singapore, Singapore

Matthew S. Yeo
Division of Plastic, Reconstructive and Aesthetic Surgery, Department of Surgery, National University Health System, Singapore

Plastic, Reconstructive and Aesthetic Surgery Section, Department of General Surgery, Tan Tock Seng Hospital, Singapore

Jia Y. Yao
Department of Biomedical Engineering, National University of Singapore, Singapore

Abdul Jalil Rufaihah
Department of Surgery, Yong Loo Lin School of Medicine, National University of Singapore, Singapore

Catherine Le Visage
INSERM, U791, Center for OsteoArticular and Dental Tissue Engineering, Université de Nantes, Nantes, France

Jackie Pei Ho
Department of Surgery, Yong Loo Lin School of Medicine, National University of Singapore, Singapore
Department of Cardiovascular and Thoracic Surgery, National University Health System, Singapore

Evelyn K. F. Yim
Mechanobiology Institute, National University of Singapore, Singapore
Department of Biomedical Engineering, National University of Singapore, Singapore
Department of Surgery, Yong Loo Lin School of Medicine, National University of Singapore, Singapore
Department of Chemical Engineering, University of Waterloo, Waterloo, ON, Canada

P.C Roussis
Department of Civil & Environmental Engineering, University of Cyprus, Nicosia, Cyprus

A.E Giannakopoulos
Department of Civil Engineering, University of Thessaly, Volos, Greece

H.P Charalambous
Department of Civil & Environmental Engineering, University of Cyprus, Nicosia, Cyprus

Yujie Chen
Guangdong Provincial Key laboratory of Medical Biomechanics, Department of Anatomy, School of Basic Medical Science, Southern Medical University, Guangzhou 510515, China

Huahua Xiong
Department of Ultrasound, The Second People's Hospital of Shenzhen, Shenzhen 518029, China

Dan Wu
Key Laboratory for Health Informatics, Chinese Academy of Sciences, Shenzhen 518055, China
Shenzhen College of Advanced Technology, University of Chinese Academy of Sciences, Shenzhen, China
Institute of Biomedical and Health Engineering, Shenzhen Institutes of Advanced Technology, Chinese Academy of Sciences, Shenzhen 518055, China

Sandeep Pirbhulal
Key Laboratory for Health Informatics, Chinese Academy of Sciences, Shenzhen 518055, China
Shenzhen College of Advanced Technology, University of Chinese Academy of Sciences, Shenzhen, China
Institute of Biomedical and Health Engineering, Shenzhen Institutes of Advanced Technology, Chinese Academy of Sciences, Shenzhen 518055, China

Xiaohong Tian
Cardiac Electrocardiogram Room, The Second People's Hospital of Shenzhen, Shenzhen 518029, China

Ruiqin Zhang
National-Regional Key Technology Engineering Laboratory of China for Medical Ultrasound, Department of Biomedical Engineering, Health Science Center, Shenzhen University, Shenzhen 518060, China

Minhua Lu
National-Regional Key Technology Engineering Laboratory of China for Medical Ultrasound, Department of Biomedical Engineering, Health Science Center, Shenzhen University, Shenzhen 518060, China

Wanqing Wu
Key Laboratory for Health Informatics, Chinese Academy of Sciences, Shenzhen 518055, China
Shenzhen College of Advanced Technology, University of Chinese Academy of Sciences, Shenzhen, China
Institute of Biomedical and Health Engineering, Shenzhen Institutes of Advanced Technology, Chinese Academy of Sciences, Shenzhen 518055, China

Wenhua Huang
Guangdong Provincial Key laboratory of Medical Biomechanics, Department of Anatomy, School of Basic Medical Science, Southern Medical University, Guangzhou 510515, China

Nicoletta Anzalone
Neuroradiology Department, Biostatistic Department, S Raffaele Hospital, Milan, Italy

C. De Filippis
Neuroradiology Department, Biostatistic Department, S Raffaele Hospital, Milan, Italy

F. Scomazzoni
Neuroradiology Department, Biostatistic Department, S Raffaele Hospital, Milan, Italy

G. Calori
Neuroradiology Department, Biostatistic Department, S Raffaele Hospital, Milan, Italy

A. Iadanza,
Neuroradiology Department, Biostatistic Department, S Raffaele Hospital, Milan, Italy

F. Simionato
Neuroradiology Department, Biostatistic Department, S Raffaele Hospital, Milan, Italy

C. Righi
Neuroradiology Department, Biostatistic Department, S Raffaele Hospital, Milan, Italy

Xinyi Leng
Department of Medicine and Therapeutics, the Chinese University of Hong Kong, Prince of Wales Hospital, Shatin, Hong Kong SAR, China

Fabien Scalzo
UCLA Stroke Center, University of California, CA 90095 Los Angeles, USA

Albert K Fong
UCLA Stroke Center, University of California, CA 90095 Los Angeles, USA

Mark Johnson
UCLA Stroke Center, University of California, CA 90095 Los Angeles, USA

Hing Lung Ip
Department of Medicine and Therapeutics, the Chinese University of Hong Kong, Prince of Wales Hospital, Shatin, Hong Kong SAR, China

Yannie Soo
Department of Medicine and Therapeutics, the Chinese University of Hong Kong, Prince of Wales Hospital, Shatin, Hong Kong SAR, China

Thomas Leung
Department of Medicine and Therapeutics, the Chinese University of Hong Kong, Prince of Wales Hospital, Shatin, Hong Kong SAR, China

Liping Liu
Department of Neurology, Beijing Tiantan Hospital, Capital Medical University, Beijing 100050 China

Edward Feldmann
Department of Neurology, Tufts University, Boston MA 02111, USA

Ka Sing Wong
Department of Medicine and Therapeutics, the Chinese University of Hong Kong, Prince of Wales Hospital, Shatin, Hong Kong SAR, China

David S Liebeskind
UCLA Stroke Center, University of California, CA 90095 Los Angeles, USA
UCLA Department of Neurology, Neuroscience Research Building, Suite 225, Los Angeles, CA 90095-7334, USA

Nicole E. Nozzi,
Department of Chemistry, University of California Davis, Davis, CA, USA

JohnW. K. Oliver
Department of Chemistry, University of California Davis, Davis, CA, USA

Shota Atsumi
Department of Chemistry, University of California Davis, Davis, CA, USA

Ahmed I. El-Batal
Drug Radiation Research Department, National Center for Radiation Research and Technology (NCRRT), Atomic Energy Authority, Cairo 11371, Egypt

Ayman A. Farrag
Botany and Microbiology Department, Faculty of Science, Al-Azhar University, Cairo 11371, Egypt

Mohamed A. Elsayed
Chemical Engineering Department, Military Technical College, Cairo 11371, Egypt

Ahmed M. El-Khawaga
Chemical Engineering Department, Military Technical College, Cairo 11371, Egypt

Preface

Bioengineering is an exciting field that is rapidly advancing and has enormous potential to benefit humanity in numerous ways. Bioengineering is a subfield of regenerative medicine that aims to utilize regeneration to improve human health. Approaches to bioengineering may include building organs in vitro using cells and scaffolds or modifying the genetic material of an organism to achieve a desired phenotype. Currently, there is a huge push to advance some of the technologies being developed through bioengineering into clinical or environmental use. However, there are a number of barriers that scientist must overcome in order for this goal to be realized. This subject is discussed in detail in the first section of this book. The remaining content of this book focuses on the advances of specific ideas and technologies in the field of bioengineering. With regards to biomedical research the specific advances discussed in this book include the use of decellularized matrices, mesenchymal stem cells, biological scaffolds, drug delivery, prostheses, bone regeneration, cardiac regeneration, neural regeneration and vascular grafts and implantation techniques. Advances in the use of bioengineering to produce biofuels are also discussed.

Editor

Stephen Rego, Ph.D.

INTRODUCTION

The principle engineering applications involving the fields of biology and medicine are known as bioengineering. The field addresses various challenges that exist within the biological scientific community and also encompasses all aspects of biomedical engineering and biotechnology. Basically, anything that involves technology and engineering as well as living systems is considered bioengineering. A number of different methodologies have been developed and implemented in an effort to achieve the best results in biological engineering. Each of these methods can be applied to medical equipment, diagnostic devices, bio-materials and other medical and biological needs. The varieties of methodologies have supported the development of different types of job fields for bioengineers.

In the general field of life sciences, bioengineering is relevant with a number of disciplines. Molecular biology uses bioengineering to aid in the study of molecules in the sciences of chemistry and genetics. Biochemistry and cytology utilize the principles to assist with studies of a living organism's chemical processes including the cellular components and structure. The applications are also implemented in the study of microorganisms known as microbiology. The medical field uses bioengineering to identify drug interaction in the field of pharmacology. The biomedical science of immunology utilizes it to help analyze the immune system and disorders with physiology. Neuroscience also makes use of the processes in the study of the brain.

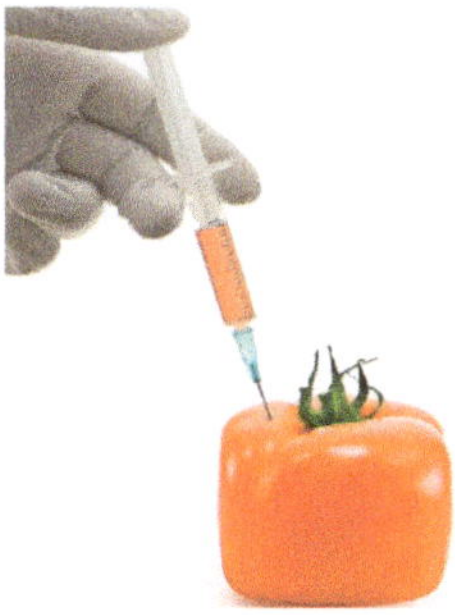

The concept of the science was coined by a British broadcaster named Heinze Wolff in 1954. Since that time, a number of advancements in the field have occurred and become commonplace in the world of human health care. Genetic engineering has made considerable progress in the understanding of the hereditary origins of many diseases. Also, the concept of artificial organs and limbs stems heavily from bioengineering.

An example of this is the artificial heart and prosthetic limbs, which are directly identified as being part of the field. Other applications for the field of science include the development of genetically modified foods. The simple adjustment of vegetation to produce more efficient and substantial yields has revolutionized the food industry. Other civil engineering construction also implement the engineering principles to assist with windbreaks, water runoff protection, surface soil protection and other ecological enhancements.

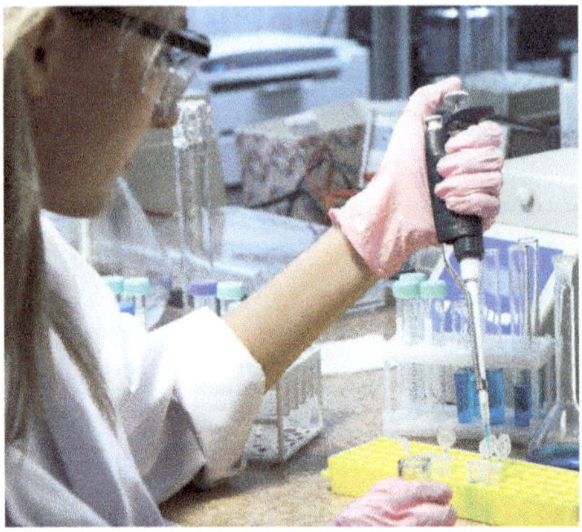

According to the National Institute of Health, bioengineering is one of the fastest-growing fields of science and medicine. The Federal Bureau of Labor Statistics estimates that bioengineering and biomedical engineering jobs with increase by approximately 7,600 each year until 2015. This is nearly a 32 percent increase each year. Various industries such as manufacturing, pharmaceuticals, health care and government are all estimated to have a larger need for people knowledgeable about this field.

Difference between Biotechnology and Bioengineering

The application of technology on living as well as nonliving organisms is known as Biotechnology. The developing, designing and transforming the technology that involves in biotechnology are called as Bioengineering. We can take a case in point. With the help of biotechnology we can create cells that will make hormones that will relive us of our stress, whilst Bioengineering will develop a system, that will manufacture those hormones much faster and in mass scale as to market that hormone as a product.

Key differentiators between Biotechnology and Bioengineering

Biotechnology and Bioengineering have their important roles in today's society. The key differentiators' between these two branches are given below:

- Whilst Biotechnology can be defined as the use of biological systems in the development of drugs or pertinent products, bioengineering is the use of the principles of engineering as well as its techniques to problems that arise in biology and medicine. We can take the design and manufacture of artificial limbs as well as organs as an example.

- Also Biotechnology is the application of aspects of living organisms in the arenas of medicine, agriculture, technology and business, Biological engineering is the use of the methods as well as concepts of science and mathematics to resolve problems that arise in life sciences.

One other major difference between the two is that, while biotechnology is mainly concerned with the genetic mutation as well as genetic machination of gene cells, Bioengineering encompasses two chief ideas - (i) the use of engineering sciences to examine and study how animals as well as plants function (ii) the use of engineering technologies as to create and design new devices.

Biotechnology vs Biomedical Engineering

Biotechnology and biomedical engineering are highly interdisciplinary subjects influenced by various other fields. As they share certain fundamentals of biology, sometimes, these two terms are used interchangeably. However, their scopes and applications differ considerably. Biotechnology covers a broader scope depending more on natural sciences, while biomedical engineering focuses mainly on medicine and engineering principles.

Biotechnology

Biotechnology is defined as "any technological application that uses biological systems, living organisms, or derivatives thereof, to make or modify products or processes for specific use." It is a broad and complex discipline mainly encompassing pure biological sciences such as genetics, microbiology, molecular and cell biology, biochemistry etc. and the fields outside biology, such as engineering and information technology. Although, the term 'biotechnology' is modern, it has been practiced since the dawn of civilization. The most common examples being making bread, beer, wine and cheese through fermentation and selective breeding of useful animal and plant species. Modern biotechnology uses new techniques that provide much more understanding and control over, living processes. Today, it has varied applications, predominantly in the areas of health care, agriculture, environment and industrial processes. Some common applications of biotechnology are production of disease resistant and nutritionally enhanced crops, gene therapy, genetic screening and enzymes that act as industrial catalysts. Biotechnology is also applied in the areas of pollution control, waste management, mining, energy production, forestry and aquaculture. However, biotechnology is not entirely free of risks. Huge controversies have arisen over the production of genetically modified organisms due to the alteration of their natural compositions which could damage the balance of nature, eventually leading to unknown consequences.

Biomedical Engineering

Biomedical engineering is defined as the application of engineering principles and design concepts to medicine and biology. It is involved in developing innovative biologies, materials, processes, implants, devices and informatics approaches for the prevention, diagnosis, and treatment of diseases, for patient rehabilitation, and for improving health. Biomedical engineering is a relatively new engineering discipline. It is an interdisciplinary subject, influenced by many other engineering and medical fields including biomedical electronics, biomaterials, bioinstrumentation, clinical engineering, cellular, tissue and genetic engineering. Some major biomedical engineering applications include the development of biocompatible prostheses, diagnostic and therapeutic medical devices ranging from clinical equipment to common imaging equipment such as MRIs and EEGs. Its biotechnology related applications include regenerative tissue growth and production of biopharmaceuticals. Examples of commonly used biomedical engineering products are prosthetic eye used in ophthalmology, breast implants and pacemakers.

Difference between Biotechnology and Biomedical Engineering

The scopes and applications of biotechnology and biomedical engineering overlap to some extent, but posses their own characteristics. Both are interdisciplinary areas influenced by various other fields. Biotechnology is more dependent on natural sciences, while biomedical engineering uses concepts and principles of physical science to solve problems. Further, biomedical engineering is more focused on medicine and healthcare applications while biotechnology addresses almost all forms of life sciences, hence covering a broader scope. The fundamental concepts of biotechnology have been practiced for centuries, but biomedical engineering has only recently emerged as its own discipline. Unlike the direct manipulation of biological materials in biotechnology, biomedical engineering emphasizes more on higher systems approaches when utilizing living things.

Biofuel Cell

A biofuel cell is a device that uses biological materials to generate electricity in a direct way through redox reactions. This contrasts with conventional use of biofuels to generate electricity from the heat provided by combustion of the material. The principle behind biofuel cell technology is to mimic various natural processes that are used to produce energy within living organisms. In some cases, bacteria may play a role in these fuel cells. As of 2011, biofuel cells show potential as an alternative energy source and in various medical and bioengineering applications.

Living organisms obtain energy from the oxidation of carbohydrates, which are generated by photosynthesis in plants and ingested as food by animals. Enzymes facilitate the reactions, in which carbohydrates are converted into carbon dioxide and water by the removal of electrons, which are then stored in adenosine triphosphate (ATP) molecules. In a biofuel cell, electrons produced by the oxidation of organic molecules — usually carbohydrates, as in living organisms — are used to generate an electrical current. The idea of using these biological processes to generate electricity has been around since the 1960s, but early attempts to construct a practical, working biofuel cell encountered difficulties.

A biofuel cell will typically consist of a container divided into two sections by a permeable barrier. In one section, the oxidation of a carbohydrate — for example, glucose — provides electrons. In the other section, a reduction reaction takes place, which uses these electrons. By connecting the two electrodes, a current can be made from the electrode in the oxidation section — the anode — to the electrode in the reduction section — the cathode.

One of the biggest practical problems hindering the development of biofuel cells has been finding an efficient way of getting the electrons released from the carbohydrate into the anode. The electrons are initially stored in the oxidizing enzyme and would, in the natural process, be chemically transferred into ATP molecules. There are two possible methods of extracting electrons from the enzyme into the anode in a biofuel cell.

In the Direct Electron Transfer (DET) method, the enzyme needs to be bonded onto the anode. This can be done chemically or by other methods, such as constructing the anode from a mesh of carbon nanotubes onto which the enzyme is adsorbed. These methods result in reduced activity in the enzyme and consequent loss of efficiency, but this is, at the time of writing, an area of ongoing research and improved techniques may be developed.

The other method of electron transfer is known as Mediated Electron Transfer (MET). This does not require the enzyme to be in contact with the anode; instead, the electrons are passed to another molecule wth a lower redox potential, which then gives up the electrons to the anode. This compound, known as a mediator, must also have a higher redox potential than the anode. This extra step involves a loss of energy and so the fuel cell is in practice less efficient than it could be in theory.

Biofuel cells are an area of active research and various possible solutions to these problems are being investigated. Among the possibilities is the use of bacteria in microbial fuel cells. Iron reducing bacteria that live in anaerobic conditions show particular promise as they naturally reduce iron in its +3 oxidation state to its +2 oxidation state. The iron can then give up an electron at the anode, returning to its +3 state and acting as a natural mediator molecule by transferring electrons from the bacteria to the anode.

The main advantages of biofuel cells are that they are non-polluting, do not require expensive catalysts and use common, inexpensive and easily renewable raw materials. The main disadvantages of biofuel cells is their inefficiency and low power output. As of 2011, however, there are hopes that these problems can be overcome, opening up a new range of possibilities. These include not only cheap, clean and renewable energy, but also the prospect of implanted biofuel cells, running on substances produced by the body, being used to power medical devices such as pacemakers.

Biomechanics

Biomechanics is a scientific discipline which applies principles studied in mechanics to the understanding of living organisms. This discipline incorporates researchers from fields such as biophysics, bioengineering, biology, and medicine, and covers organisms from plants to whales. A number of colleges and universities have biomechanics programs which offer training to students along with numerous research possibilities in this very broad field.

The study of biomechanics can take place on a range of scales and levels, from the molecular level of cell signaling to the study of entire organisms. Understanding how organisms move is an important aspect of this field, as is the understanding of mechanical systems in the body such as the circulatory system and the digestive tract. While people may not think of living organisms as machines, in many ways, they actually perform a lot like machines, and the concepts used in basic mechanics can also be applied to the body.

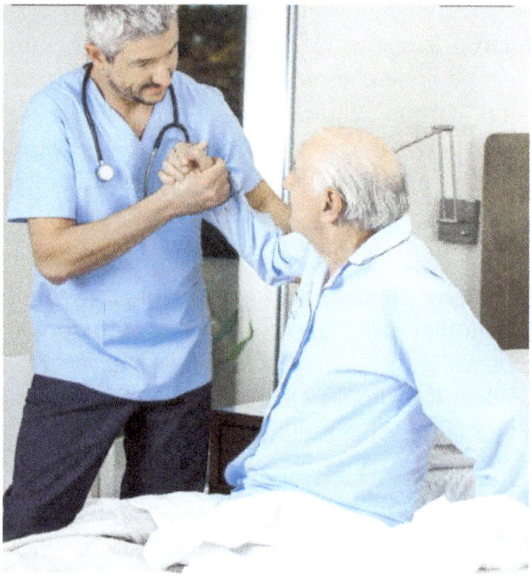

One field of interest in biomechanics is the study of injuries. Sports injuries in particular are compelling to some researchers, with people interested in learning about how athletes at the peak of their performance move and injure themselves in addition to studying injuries in people who are not as athletic. Biomechanics researchers also look at topics like how the loss of a limb can change movement patterns, how prosthetic devices can be better designed to move with the body, and how bodies respond to stress and strain ranging from depletion of bone mass in space to working as manual laborers.

On a clinical level, biomechanics is very important for understanding patterns of injury and for developing physical therapy programs which will increase strength. Biomechanics is also the science behind many ergonomics recommendations for everyone from massage therapists to office workers. Understanding how activities like using a computer, sitting in an uncomfortable chair, or lifting heavy objects strain the body is an important first step in finding ways to help people reduce strain. Biomechanics is also used to show people how to use their bodies more efficiently, as in the case of a massage therapist who uses the pressure of elbows instead of just the hands.

Researchers are also interested in how different kinds of organisms move and function, and how these variations confer advantages. For example, fish and marine mammals swim in a variety of different ways, while plants have developed a variety of creative ways to access nutrients and resources such as sunlight.

Types of Biomedical Technology

Biomedical technology refers to the application of technological and engineering advances to medical science. Biomedical research has made strides in a number of fields, such as pharmaceuticals, creating biopharmaceuticals, drugs produced by using biomedical technology that can treat a number of diseases. Genetic testing uses biotechnical methods to provide information about a person's genetic makeup. Gene therapy, where faulty genes are replaced using biomedical technology, can help cure genetic diseases. Medical teaching and information management also utilize advances in computer science.

Biopharmaceuticals are proteins or nucleic acids produced with biomedical technology. These types of drugs have been around since 1982, when biomedical engineers created synthetic insulin. Biopharmaceuticals can treat a variety of diseases, such as anemia, leukemia, multiple sclerosis, and some types of arthritis.

Genetic testing, another application of biomedical technology, can detect genetic diseases and mutations. Newborn screening is one of the most common genetic tests. Newborn screening uses biotechnical genetic testing techniques to test newborns for inherited disorders such as phenylketonuria, a disorder that can lead to mental illness if not treated.

When a person shows signs of a genetic disorder, diagnostic testing is used to determine if the cause is genetic. People who have a family history of a genetic disorder may also receive carrier testing to show if they are carrying faulty genes that could lead to the disease occurring in their children. Prenatal testing can detect genetic abnormalities such as Down's syndrome and inherited diseases.

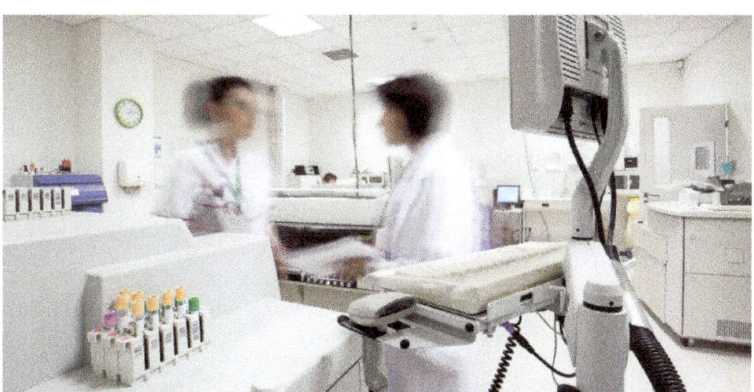

Often there is no cure for genetic diseases because they are caused by mutations or problems in the genetic code. A new branch of biomedical technology called gene therapy allows doctors to actually inject a new, functional gene into a person's cells to replace a faulty gene. Researchers have used bioengineering to modify certain types of bacteria or viruses so they can carry the replacement gene into the cells.

Biomedical informatics is another application of technology to medical problems. This branch of biomedical technology uses computer science to store and retrieve vital medical information in a virtual environment. For example, patient charts containing background and diagnostic information can be digitized, so a physician can simply pull them up on a computer for quick reference.

Biomedical technology has also been incorporated into medical teaching. Computer models are often used to demonstrate the functions of certain organs or show what the organs look like when they are diseased. Medical students can get experience working with virtual models before they treat an actual patient.

1
CHAPTER

SCIENTIFIC ADVANCEMENTS AND CLINICAL APPLICATION

Joseph S. Fernandez-Moure

Keywords: Translational research, bench to bedside, clinician-scientist, FDA, NCATS, translational medicine

INTRODUCTION

The "Knowledge Doubling Curve," coined by Buckminster Fuller, described that, by the end of World War II, the totality of human knowledge would double every 25 years (Fuller, 1982). As time has passed, this theory has become not only more evident but also more complex, with new scientific disciplines being created, each expanding at different rates. Medical knowledge, now, has a doubling time every 18 years, while newer disciplines, such as nanotechnology, double on the average of every 2 years (Densen, 2011). While the breath of knowledge in each subject varies greatly, these figures highlight the speed with which advancement now occurs.

The bench to bedside process is founded on the principle of translating findings in basic science into therapeutic interventions for patients. This "process" has been fundamental to the implementation of remarkable achievements, such as statins for dyslipidemia, targeted cancer therapy, and anti-hepatic medicines effective in HIV (Muss, 2006; Mora et al., 2010). Yet so many more bench-side success stories have found themselves stranded on the road to translation with negligible impact in the clinic. Bioengineering and biotechnology have seen a tremendous explosion of knowledge and innovation (Zucker and Darby, 1996), although these discoveries rarely materialize into FDA-approved devices or more rarely become commonly adopted by the medical community (Bagchi-Sen, 2007). The diversity of devices suffers as companies continue

Citation: Fernandez-Moure JS (2016) Scientific Advancements and Clinical Application. Front. Bioeng. Biotechnol. 4:43. doi: 10.3389/fbioe.2016.00043.

to recycle "old" materials to streamline the FDA approval process and meet their financial goals. New materials continue to be developed and vetted, yet the clinical impact is not felt as many clinicians rely on a handful of devices for tissue engineering and reconstruction.

Abdominal wall and orthopedic reconstruction are two of the most common surgical genres today. Over 350,000 hernia repairs are performed annually, and in 2011, ~25% of all operating room procedures performed were musculoskeletal procedures (Poulose et al., 2012; Weiss and Elixhauser, 2014). Polypropylene was invented over 60 years ago and still remains the most commonly used material in abdominal wall repair, although in use since the 1950s (Usher et al., 1958). Another example in the delay to market of bench-side materials' success is the use of biologic or functionalized biomaterials. Regenerative medicine has reached new heights of innovation with the addition of dynamic manufacturing processes and novel drug delivery capabilities (Dimmeler et al., 2014). At the bedside, though, the use of simple acellular matrices prevails in clinical implementation, and use of functionalized biomaterials is rare (Mariette et al., 2014; Majumder et al., 2015). The unavailability, lack of options, and prohibitive costs of biologic devices has made their implementation as standard of care impossible, although they have characteristics known to be extremely favorable for tissue repair (Cevasco and Itani, 2012). Similarly, the translation of functionalized devices, often categorized as drug–device combinations, through the tireless FDA-regulatory pathways, halts their progress and ultimately their clinical implementation (Meslin et al., 2013). As we move into an era where scientific discovery and advancement occur more rapidly every year, the question lingers: why aren't the advances at the bedside commensurate with the advances on the bench?

ARE WE SPEAKING THE SAME LANGUAGE?

"Bench to bedside" has more recently evolved into the relatively new area of investigation known as*translational research*. Translational research describes the iterative process of not only basic science discoveries being integrated into clinical applications but also clinical needs and observations driving the focus of basic science (Figure 1). Fundamental to the translation of scientific discoveries to clinical impact is the collaboration and integration of scientists with clinicians, as well as the integration of academia, health care, and industry. Herein lies the problem. The cultural and academic identities of both clinicians and basic scientists are different.

Over time, two cultures have evolved in the translational landscape: the preclinical and clinical researcher. In his influential 1959 Rede lecture, British scientist and novelist, Snow, described "The Two Cultures." The thesis of this lecture was that "the intellectual life of the whole of western society" was split into two cultures: the humanities and the sciences (Snow, 2012). While exaggerated, it draws attention to how intelligent people can differ greatly based on their perspective and backgrounds. Similarly, the culture of preclinical work and clinical work differs. Most basic scientists rarely step foot in hospitals while few physicians carry out any "wet" lab work past undergraduate or medical school, well before they have gained a true understanding of clinical needs. How hypotheses are generated, how they are tested, and how they are abandoned vary greatly between the two. One example of this lies in the current "bench to bedside" paradigm. Phase I clinical trials are the initial testing ground for novel treatments that have been found successful and potentially profitable. They provide great opportunity for groundbreaking bench work to truly prove useful, yet few rarely materialize as Phase II studies due to minimal clinical benefit demonstrated and loss of enthusiasm as the next wave of bench to bedside therapeutics hits the clinical shore.

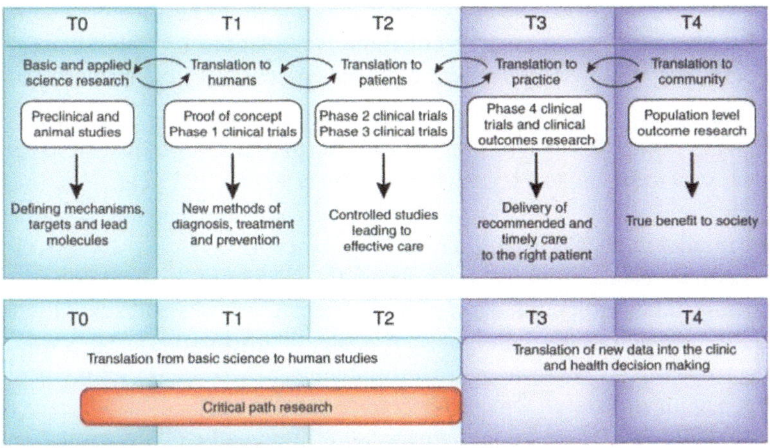

Figure 1: Operational challenges for translational research and medicine. Adapted from Blumberg et al. Harvard Catalyst Website (https://catalyst.harvard.edu/). Translational research is an iterative, dynamic, and layered process with several obstacles that must be negotiated (top). These layers include T0, identification of clinical problem followed by preclinical and optimization studies to define material candidates for compound synthesis or cellular mechanisms for intervention; T1, initial Phase I studies in humans that aim to demonstrate proof of concept and safety; T2, Phase II and III clinical trials that allowed for incremental and sequential evaluations and approvals prior to implementation; T3, post-marketing surveillance trials, conducted after the device has been in the market, are used to determine long term efficacy, impact on quality of life, and comparison to other similar devices; and T4, outcomes research to determine the impact of effectiveness intervening on patients in the general community, cost-effectiveness compared to equivalent technologies. Valley of death (red) comprises research related to the T0, T1, and T2 stages (Blumberg et al., 2012).

Another example of disconnection occurs at the Phase III level. In clinical research, if one of the two blinded randomized trials fails to show benefit or either fails the entire study, testing is abandoned. This concept of halting a study based on a final pivotal experiment is absent from preclinical work where it would be unheard of to stop an entire line of study because of one result. Again, we see where the current scientific environment fails us. In this scenario, one would be inclined to learn why Phase II or III failed and study the root cause of less than expected efficacy, yet there is no room, money, or time to pursue why things did not work as planned. Further, because the scientific literary community is not interested in publishing negative results, many of the finding never make it to paper to instruct and guide those on the next wave of trials.

LIFTING THE SILOS

The success of any translational research program lies in the elimination of silos segregating scientists, doctors, and industry professionals from each other. While this seems intuitive to those engaged in translational medicine, the reality is that in most nations, revenue streams are strictly separated between the "hospital" and "research institute." As the landscape of health care and reimbursement continues to evolve, clinicians will continue to be seen as earners with little to no incentive to spend any additional time pursuing innovative collaborative relationships in science. This has lead to a deficiency in the development of clinician-scientists and translational science collaboration.

The US has been a leader in the implementation of translational research partnerships for over 100 years. Since the Flexner Report was released, 105 years ago, the tradition of integrating university-owned hospitals in the research and teaching process has been a pillar to medical education and scientific advancement (Beck, 2004). As a model for this paradigm, Johns Hopkins exemplified the system of medical education where university hospitals were coupled to research-oriented schools and scientific institutes. This model is seen across the nation in such academic institutions as Harvard, Stanford, and Johns Hopkins, to name a few. Unfortunately a new breed of medical schools has emerged with a distinct separation between academia and health care, which is challenging the long-trusted academic paradigm. Frequently, clinicians are challenged to decide between "academic" and "private" clinical practice. This further widens the divide between the clinician and the scientist, a relationship crucial to success of translational medicine.

As the world embraces the need for more integrated relationships in health care and science, several initiatives have emerged to encourage partnerships. The National Institutes of Health (NIH) has led this charge with the development of the National Center for Translational Sciences (NCATS). With a focus on enabling and encouraging collaborative partnership between, not only, clinicians and scientists, but also, academia, health care, and pharmaceutical industries, NCAT focuses on bringing scientific innovation to the patient community. In 2016, the budget for Clinical and Translational Science Awards (CTSA) was $685.417 million (http://www.ncats.nih.gov/about/center/budget), indicating a substantial commitment toward the translational initiative. The international scientific community has also taken on this initiative. Germany has succeeded in promoting translational process with the Fraunhofer Institutes and combining training programs with industry partnerships. The Fraunhofer Institutes, one of the largest organizations for applied research in Europe, are strongly linked to industry with a focus on generating products for market. Similarly, in Germany, the Helmholtz Society and the Translational Centre for Regenerative Medicine (TRM) in Leipzig are designed to combine science and technology to translate science to health. Lifting the silos and promoting multidisciplinary, inter-institutional, and entrepreneurial collaboration will prove to overcome some of the current limitations, but a fundamental paradigm shift in education and academia must also occur.

TRAINING AND CAREER ADVANCEMENT

A key point of contention for the progression of translational research is the length of time and resources required to carry out these, often, multiyear projects. A truly translational study takes many steps during the preclinical stage before even making it to the clinical phase of study. How are those researchers undertaking translational efforts to be evaluated and supported? Translational study-support programs like those at MIT's Dashpande Center for Technological Innovation, University of Southern California's Stevens Center for Innovation, or Houston Methodist Hospital Research Institute's Translational Research Initiatives have evolved to support this work, understanding that translational work may not generate traditional career elevating metrics. Publication in high impact journal and NIH funding are often sacrificed for intellectual property and patents, without which, translation would never be achieved. The customary anti-entrepreneurial world of academia will need a culture shift if they are to embrace this new breed of researcher focused on solving clinical problems rather than asking more questions about them. This will involve rethinking current criteria for promotion, such as high impact publications, grants, and invited lectures.

While regulatory issues and capital generation remain hurdles to translational success, a new pipeline of hybrid researchers is needed to cultivate the translational landscape. As pressure to generate revenue overcomes many clinicians, and scientists find it ever more difficult to obtain NIH and equivalent funding, clinician-scientists and applied-scientists must be trained to undertake the challenges of navigating an already treacherous path. With this must come administrative understanding that translational projects take longer and are born out of large multi-institutional and multidisciplinary teams where a researchers contributions may not be adequately represented. Along this continuum from the bedside to bench to bedside live the applied-scientist and the clinician-scientist. There needs to be more crossover and integration between the "two cultures" Snow described over 50 years ago. Many times thought to have an identity crisis, emphasis on translational research by the NIH and large academic institutions has empowered these individuals and highlighted their need going forward. Multidisciplinary institutions are primed to carry this agenda to fruition.

Training of this new breed of researchers not only requires support and understanding but an infrastructure capable of providing a favorable and productive environment for success. Traditional training schemes continue to promote silos in both the basic scientific and clinical realms. These walls must be broken down to create the next wave of translational researchers. Already, translational research programs in the basic sciences are evolving out of the traditional schemes. From the clinical standpoint, more focus and institutional support must be given to attract physicians to engage in research previously thought to have no place in clinical work. The Mayo Clinic Graduate School Clinical and Translational Research Program and Brown's Masters in Clinical and Translational Research are two examples of multidisciplinary institutions incorporating translational research into their curriculums. So too has the American Board of Surgery embraced these initiative by offering flexible pathways capable of turning out a new generation of surgeon-scientists poised to engage in the translational initiatives of the institutions they serve. Alternatively, there needs to be tracks where scientists engage the clinic to truly understand the disease they are trying to impact. For transitional research to succeed and translational researchers to emerge from the traditional systems of education, there must be a paradigm shift in training and career development that lays the foundation for funding and commercialization of breakthroughs. Breakthroughs, though, are plagued by a sequential set of hurdles and valleys that must be navigated in order to bring a novel scientific breakthrough to the community.

DEATH VALLEYS OF TRANSLATIONAL PROGRESS

Novel breakthroughs capable of funding are exciting when they occur. They stir up enthusiasm, bring attention to institutions, and generate donor revenue (Heinze et al., 2009). For the relatively few advancements developed by researchers at institutions where one can out-license the intellectual property, two "valleys of death" await the inventors (Figure 2) (Roberts et al., 2012). The first valley of death is the time between the initial discovery and the actual out-licensing of the invention. The reason why inventions die in this valley is the same reason why many never occur in the first place, a lack of resources. While the researcher may have done due diligence to prove the *in vitro* and *in vivo* efficacy of the invention, the institution within which they work does not have the resources to efficiently perform the duties needed to protect the discovery. Conversely, often the research while in possession of a potential blockbuster product may not have the resources to execute the comprehensive *in vitro* and *in vivo* preclinical studies required to fully demonstrate efficacy (Meslin et al., 2013).

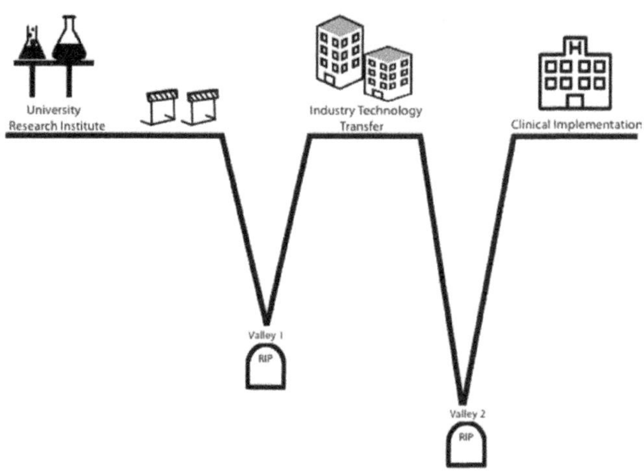

Figure 2: Valleys of death. The "valleys of death" concept is used to describe situations where technology failed to reach clinical implementation. Termination of studies in Valley 1 when a technology has shown efficacy, yet is unable to obtain financing to take it to commercialization and human trials. Termination of studies in Valley 2 is due to a rapid decline of funding during the costly human trial phase and occurs during the stage in-licensed technology becomes an actual revenue-generating product.

From the standpoint of industry, this period is seen in companies where initial trials drains funds to the point where prospect drugs or device never made it to market because they simply ran out of money to finish the trials (Murphy and Edwards, 2003). The second valley occurs, here, during the in-licensing and trials phase. There are few funding mechanisms specifically geared to support product-related translational efforts. US Small Business Innovation Research/Small Business Technology Transfer program is designed to support these efforts but is intended for small for-profit entities where the investigator is in the company not in an institution. Thus, most funding for novel biomedical tools originating at institutions must come from the private sector (Murphy and Edwards, 2003). Holders in private investment funds expect a return on their investment. They understand the risky nature of biomedical enterprise and thus, require substantial return to compensate for risk. This, again, leads to loss of funding when clinical outcomes do not reflect preclinical efficacy. Thus, we are again left with inconsistent support to move a potential life-saving therapy into clinical implementation.

CATALYSTS FOR TRANSLATION

Bioengineering has entered a transformational era where unprecedented breakthroughs and advances hold the promise of revolutionizing health-care practice and delivery. At the threshold stands the translational scientist poised to play the critical role in the bridging the gap of cultures and yet, as mentioned above, hurdles and "valleys of death" plague advancement. The NIH has played an integral role in facilitating these collaborations as early as the 1980s. Through the Bayh–Dole Act and the Stevenson–Wydler Act, they strengthened the incentives for academic and government institutions to engage with industry in research collaborations and partnerships (Schacht, 2000; Mowery et al., 2001). Through this legislation, public sector research institutions were allowed to own the intellectual property they generated using federal funding and license it for commercialization. Through this, institutions have been able to make effective partnerships with the private sector, leading to such advancements as the creation and patenting of biologic drug candidates and small molecules (Collins and Varmus, 2015).

As drug and device companies continue to cut research and development funding and the NIH budget continues to decline, the new hybrid of public–private entity relationships may be the backbone of translational research. Programs, such as the Defense Advanced Research Projects Agency's (DARPA) Armed Forces Institute of Regenerative Medicine (AFIRM), focus on translational initiative that will serve military clinical needs. With a focus on combat trauma and regenerative medicine solutions, DARPA has invested in research with a clear path from discovery to commercialization. The multimillion-dollar consortium collaborations born out of AFIRM are only considered for funding when a commercial entity willing to undertake the commercial manufacturing is partnered with the researchers. Launched in 2014, an emerging NIH-driven initiative is the accelerating medicine partnership (AMP). While not currently focused on materials development, the partnership, which is composed of the NIH, 10 biopharmaceutical companies, and several non-profit organizations, has raised over $180 million. A unique and groundbreaking element of this public–private partnership is the agreement to make all data analyses made during the collaboration publicly available for use by the broader health-care community. Under the current fiscal limitations of both sectors this relationship poises itself to be mutually beneficial for not only those involved but those in the medical community. As part of the greater medical knowledge explosion, collaborations such as these will rapidly accelerate the available data, leading to a greater exponential growth of scientific knowledge.

FROM THE BEDSIDE TO THE BENCH AND BACK: RETHINKING TRANSLATION

As we rethink the dogma of scientific research around the world, we must embrace the new paradigm of translational research and realize that the journey begins and ends at the bedside. As a health-care community, we must approach our practice honestly to admit and identify shortcomings of our care so that we may turn to our applied-scientist or clinician-scientist colleagues for solutions to these shortcomings. As a scientific community, we must open our labs to integrated inter-institutional, multidisciplinary collaborations where we acknowledge and reward those undertaking the brave task of developing solutions, rather than more questions. As administrators, teachers, and mentors, we must continue to invest in the new wave of researchers who may not fit into the traditional paradigm of academic advancement and support the long road of work they have before them. As government agencies, we must continue to build partnerships with the private sector to harness the strengths of all parties. Lastly, as a whole medical community, we must embrace each other with a solitary unifying goal: to act on behalf of our patients and provide solutions to their unsolved clinical needs.

AUTHOR CONTRIBUTIONS

The sole author, JF-M, wrote, edited, conceived the paper, and created the figures.

CONFLICT OF INTEREST STATEMENT

The author declares that the research was conducted in the absence of any commercial or financial relationships that could be construed as a potential conflict of interest.

REFERENCES

1. Bagchi-Sen, S. (2007). Strategic considerations for innovation and commercialization in the US biotechnology sector. *Eur. Plann. Stud.* 15, 753–766. doi: 10.1080/09654310701214226
2. Beck, A. H. (2004). The Flexner report and the standardization of American medical education. *JAMA* 291, 2139–2140. doi:10.1001/jama.291.17.2139
3. Blumberg, R. S., Dittel, B., Hafler, D., von Herrath, M., and Nestle, F. O. (2012). Unraveling the autoimmune translational research process layer by layer. *Nat. Med.* 18, 35–41. doi:10.1038/nm.2632
4. Cevasco, M., and Itani, K. M. (2012). Ventral hernia repair with synthetic, composite, and biologic mesh: characteristics, indications, and infection profile. *Surg. Infect. (Larchmt)* 13, 209–215. doi:10.1089/sur.2012.123

5. Collins, F. S., and Varmus, H. (2015). A new initiative on precision medicine. *N. Engl. J. Med.* 372, 793–795. doi:10.1056/NEJMp1500523

6. Densen, P. (2011). Challenges and opportunities facing medical education. *Trans. Am. Clin. Climatol. Assoc.* 122, 48–58.

7. Dimmeler, S., Ding, S., Rando, T. A., and Trounson, A. (2014). Translational strategies and challenges in regenerative medicine. *Nat. Med.* 20, 814–821. doi:10.1038/nm.3627

8. Fuller, R. B. (1982). *Critical Path*. New York City: Macmillan.

9. Heinze, T., Shapira, P., Rogers, J. D., and Senker, J. M. (2009). Organizational and institutional influences on creativity in scientific research. *Res. Policy* 38, 610–623. doi:10.1016/j.respol.2009.01.014

10. Majumder, A., Neupane, R., and Novitsky, Y. (2015). Antibiotic coating of hernia meshes: the next step toward preventing mesh infection. *Surg. Technol. Int.* 27, 147–153.

11. Mariette, C., Wind, P., Lupinacci, R. M., Tresallet, C., Adham, M., Arvieux, C., et al. (2014). Practice patterns in complex ventral hernia repair and place of biological grafts: a national survey among French digestive academic surgeons. *J Visc. Surg.* 151, 9–16. doi:10.1016/j.jviscsurg.2013.12.001

12. Meslin, E. M., Blasimme, A., and Cambon-Thomsen, A. (2013). Mapping the translational science policy 'valley of death'. *Clin. Transl. Med.* 2, 14. doi:10.1186/2001-1326-2-14

13. Mora, S., Glynn, R. J., Hsia, J., MacFadyen, J. G., Genest, J., and Ridker, P. M. (2010). Statins for the primary prevention of cardiovascular events in women with elevated high-sensitivity C-reactive protein or dyslipidemia: results from the Justification for the Use of Statins in Prevention: an Intervention Trial Evaluating Rosuvastatin (JUPITER) and meta-analysis of women from primary prevention trials. *Circulation* 121, 1069–1077. doi:10.1161/CIRCULATIONAHA.109.906479

14. Mowery, D. C., Nelson, R. R., Sampat, B. N., and Ziedonis, A. A. (2001). The growth of patenting and licensing by US universities: an assessment of the effects of the Bayh-Dole act of 1980. *Res. Policy* 30, 99–119. doi:10.1016/S0048-7333(99)00100-6

15. Murphy, L. M., and Edwards, P. L. (2003). *Bridging the Valley of Death: Transitioning from Public to Private Sector Financing*. Golden, CO: National Renewable Energy Laboratory.

16. Muss, H. B. (2006). Targeted therapy for metastatic breast cancer. *N. Engl. J. Med.* 355, 2783–2785. doi:10.1056/NEJMe068260

17. Poulose, B. K., Shelton, J., Phillips, S., Moore, D., Nealon, W., Penson, D., et al. (2012). Epidemiology and cost of ventral hernia repair: making the case for hernia research. *Hernia* 16, 179–183. doi:10.1007/s10029-011-0879-9

18. Roberts, S. F., Fischhoff, M. A., Sakowski, S. A., and Feldman, E. L. (2012). Perspective: transforming science into medicine: how clinician-scientists can

build bridges across research's "valley of death". *Acad. Med.* 87, 266–270. doi:10.1097/ACM.0b013e3182446fa3

19. Schacht, W. H. (2000). *Patent Ownership and Federal Research and Development (R & D): A Discussion on the Bayh-Dole Act and the Stevenson-Wydler Act.* Washington, DC: Congressional Research Service, Library of Congress.

20. Snow, C. P. (2012). *The Two Cultures.* Cambridge, UK: Cambridge University Press.

21. Usher, F. C., Ochsner, J., and Tuttle, L. L. Jr. (1958). Use of marlex mesh in the repair of incisional hernias. *Am. Surg.* 24, 969–974.

22. Weiss, A. J., and Elixhauser, A. (2014). "Trends in operating room procedures in U.S. hospitals, 2001–2011," in *HCUP Statistical Brief #171* (Rockville, MD: Agency for Healthcare Research and Quality). Available at: http://www.hcup-us.ahrq.gov/reports/statbriefs/sb171-Operating-Room-Procedure-Trends.pdf

23. Zucker, L. G., and Darby, M. R. (1996). Star scientists and institutional transformation: patterns of invention and innovation in the formation of the biotechnology industry. *Proc. Natl. Acad. Sci. U.S.A.* 93, 12709–12716. doi:10.1073/pnas.93.23.12709

2

CHAPTER

EX VIVO DERMIS MECHANICAL BEHAVIOR IN RELATION TO DECELLULARIZATION TREATMENT LENGTH

Mara Terzini, Cristina Bignardi, Carlotta Castagnoli, Irene Cambieri, Elisabetta M. Zanetti, Alberto L. Audenino

Keywords: Acellularized dermis, allografts, decellularization treatment, elastic modulus, extracellular matrix, human dermis, tensile tests, ultimate stress.

BACKGROUND

So far, artificial scaffold-based constructs are unable to closely mimic the properties of the respective native tissues in terms of biocompatibility, function, structure, and so on. On the other hand, human-derived biomaterials preserve the natural architecture from the native tissue; however, allogenic biomaterials would solicit an adverse immune response [1, 2]. The solution is making use of decellularized allogenic material, where cells have been removed to produce a tissue as free as possible of potentially immunogenic antigens. The optimal decellularization treatment should minimize cellular and nuclear materials in the matrix, without affecting the integrity of the tissue structure, and consequently its mechanical properties [2, 3]. Generally speaking, the duration of the decellularization treatment has to counterbalance two benefits: on the one hand, a longer duration gives more chance to eliminate all cellular and nuclear components; on the other hand, it could adversely influence collagen, elastin, and extracellular components.

This work focuses on acellular dermal allografts; these grafts were initially used as wound cover in burns and other large wounds [4]; however, they are now also finding numerous other clinical applications as a scaffold allowing for new tissue ingrowth: it is the case of wound healing (diabetic ulcers or burns), tendon and ligament repair [5], soft-tissue supplementation [6], and joint resurfacing [7]. Methods of decellularization

Citation: Mara Terzini, Cristina Bignardi, Carlotta Castagnoli, Irene Cambieri, Elisabetta M. Zanetti, Alberto L. Audenino, Ex Vivo Dermis Mechanical Behavior in Relation to Decellularization Treatment Length, DOI: 10.2174/1874120701610010034.

can have different processing times and they can employ different means, eventually producing alterations of the matrix structure; the most common processes include a combination of physical, chemical, and enzymatic agents. The use of NaOH medium for the decellularization of human skin has been reported in the literature as an effective low-cost method, which is able to remove donor cells and hairs [8]. The dermal tissue requires a more extensive biochemical exposure and longer rinse times, like other laminated thicker tissues (*e.g.*cardiac muscle tissue) [3]. However, bases run the risk of decreasing the extracellular matrix (ECM) mechanical properties due to the cleavage of collagen fibrils and disruption of collagen crosslinks [1]. The authors herein have tried to elucidate to what extent this process of decellularization affects the mechanical behavior of the dermal tissue, in relation to its duration. Apposite tensile tests have been planned both along Langer lines orientation and perpendicularly, and decellularized tissue properties have been compared with the native tissue ones. As a result, indications about the optimal decellularization treatment length have been given. In literature, the tensile properties of *ex vivo* native skin samples have been studied by Nì Annaidh *et al.* [8] who calculated engineering stresses and strains, and the elastic modulus for different back areas and different orientations. They demonstrated the variability of tissue properties in relation to specimen orientation (referred to Langer lines), body area, and among different donors; therefore, the influence of the decellularization treatment length has been tested on groups of specimens coming from the same donor, with the same orientation, and belonging to the same body area. Yoder and Elliott performed tensile tests on various graft materials used in soft-tissue applications, having outlined the relevance of mechanical properties of these tissues for a successful surgical reconstruction [9]. All these authors reported ultimate engineering stresses and this might be a limit since the specimen section undergoes a significant striction during tensile tests up to rupture; therefore, true stresses have also been calculated in this work, measuring specimen section in real time.

MATERIALS AND METHODS

Specimens

Human reticular dermal grafts have been harvested from human donors back: the strips have been dissected, and they have been decellularized through incubation in NaOH 0.06 N culture medium for 1-7 weeks, at room temperature in continuous tilting, changing the medium once a week. Grafts have been finally neutralized by means of incubation in HCl 0.1 N, obtaining human decellularized dermal matrices (HADM). HADM have been preserved at 85% glycerol in a 4°C refrigerator [8], at the Turin Skin Bank. They have been used for these experiments after the approval of the Regional Transplant Centre Ethical Committee (protocol number 0006730; January 23, 2012), having obtained the written informed consent from all the study participants. Before use, HADM have been dipped for at least 3 min, and thrice in saline solution (0.9%) at 37°C, to eliminate all the glycerol from skin samples. The specimens have been cut parallel (0°) and orthogonal (90°) to Langer lines by means of a custom-made die cutter. The cutter has been appositely designed to prevent notches and defects, which could bias mechanical tests. On the whole, there were 3-4 specimens for each decellularization treatment length; the final specimen sizes, measured by photogrammetry, were equal to 4.33±0.57 mm (average ± std width), 2.21±0.32 mm (average ± std thickness), and 10.10±0.38 mm (average ± std length).

Up to the instant preceding the tensile test, all samples have been kept in saline solution; during tests, they have not been hydrated since tensile tests lasted only for a few seconds.

Photogrammetry Setup

The size of the specimens prior to testing has been assessed through photogrammetry. A full-frame digital camera (Canon EOS 5D Mark II), with an autofocus lens for macro photography (Canon EF 100 mm f/2.8 Macro USM) has been used for this aim, together with a camera stand, and two light stands. Two pictures have been taken for each specimen: the top view and the side view; the respective 21.0 MP digitized images have been analyzed by means of ImageJ software. The resolution was equal to 0.01 mm/pixel. During mechanical tests, one more camera with its tripod (Canon EOS 400D) has been added to obtain both specimen width and thickness in real time; thanks to apposite capture software (DSLR Remote Pro).

Mechanical Tests

Specimens have been clamped to the Bose Electroforce® testing machine; some preliminary tests have been performed to optimize the gripping force, avoiding specimen slippage without damaging the tissue integrity. Rupture tensile tests have been performed for all samples in displacement control at a strain rate equal to 0.032 s^{-1}. The initial gap between machine clamps was equal to 5 mm. None of the specimens was ruptured near the clamps.

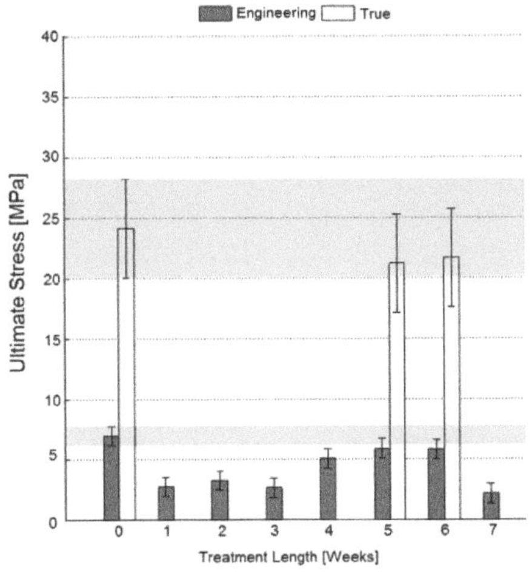

Figure 1: Ultimate stress for specimens perpendicular to Langer lines; error bars refer to Tukey-

Kramer test intervals. According to this test, overlapping intervals are not significantly different; therefore, specimens decellularized for 5-6 weeks have an ultimate stress close to the native dermis ones considering both engineering and true stresses ($p<0.05$).

Elaboration Data

The ultimate tensile stresses have been reported in different forms to allow making comparisons with other data in the literature. Engineering stresses have been calculated by dividing the load with the initial specimen area A_0 [9], while true stresses have been calculated by dividing the load with the current specimen area A_i [10]. Specimen images (frontal and lateral views) have been sampled every 3 s by the aforementioned digital cameras to calculate the actual specimen section. The true specimen area has been calculated for untreated specimens and for specimens treated for 5-6 weeks since the results obtained on these specimens justified performing more detailed inquiries, as detailed in the following.

Young's modulus (E) has been calculated from the linear portion of the stress-strain curve [11]: curve data have been locally derived with a moving average linear regression, and the constant trend of the derived curve has been considered.

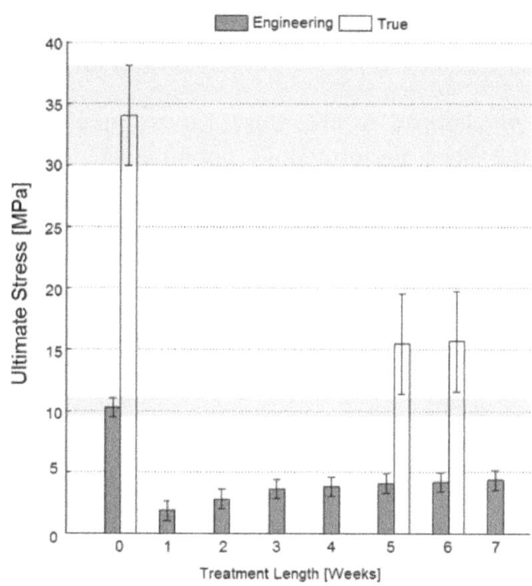

Figure 2: Ultimate stress for specimens parallel to Langer lines; error bars refer to Tukey-Kramer test intervals. According to this test, none of the specimens has an ultimate stress as high as the native dermis ones ($p<0.05$).

Statistical Analysis of Data

The mechanical properties of the dermis have been reported in relation to the duration of the decellularization treatment (from 0 to 7 weeks with a step size of 1 week, called

T0, T1, ..., T7 in the following) for both sample orientations (0° and 90° with reference to Langer lines).

The normality of the statistical distribution of all parameters has been preventively checked by lillie-test function. Tukey-Kramer post hoc test has been used to compare properties obtained for different durations of the decellularization treatment *versus* the initial tissue properties (T0-0° and T0-90°, respectively). The significance level has been set equal to 0.05 for all tests.

RESULTS AND DISCUSSION

Results concerning the ultimate tensile stress have been reported in Fig. (1) and Fig. (2), respectively, for specimens cut parallel and perpendicular to Langer lines, while results concerning the elastic modulus have been reported in Fig. (3) and Fig. (4), respectively, for 0° and 90° specimens. The comparison of mechanical properties measured on specimens parallel or perpendicular to the Langer lines is in accordance with the well-known dermal tissue anisotropy, and is related to the prevalent orientation of collagen fibers [9, 11]: with reference to data preceding decellularization treatment ("T0"), specimens cut along Langer lines have exhibited a higher ultimate stress (33.95 MPa true stresses, and 10.28 MPa engineering stress) and a higher elastic modulus (21.8 MPa) when compared with specimens cut perpendicularly to Langer lines (24.11 MPa ultimate true stresses, 7.01 MPa ultimate engineering stress, and 12.31 MPa elastic modulus)

(Figs. 1 and 2) testify that referring to engineering stress would lead to a considerable underestimation of the ultimate stress for tests like those performed here (white columns are always higher than grey columns), due to the significant specimen striction taking place before specimen rupture, and to the small section of the specimens tested here (the thickness of dermal tissue is lower than 3 mm). Nevertheless, the patterns of ultimate stress *versus* decellularization treatment length have been found to be consistent between engineering and true stress formulations for the tensile tests (5-6 weeks values are similar and are smaller than 'T0' values both in Figs. 1 and 2).

All pictures testify that the decellularization treatment set up with sodium hydroxide has weakened the mechanical properties of the tissue ('T0' values remain the highest for whatever treatment length both in Figs. (1) and (2)), and its effect is more deleterious for specimens cut along Langer line orientation where collagen fiber bundles are stressed more closely to their axes (the difference between 'T0' values and all treated specimens is higher in Fig. (2) compared with Fig. (1)). Effectively, it is known that alkaline bases are able to degrade the structural components of the matrix including collagen to some extent: Sheridan *et al.* [12] used sonication and 0.5 M NaOH to controllably degrade small collagen fibrils of decellularized pig arterial tissue; in more detail, bases reduce the mechanical properties due to the cleavage of collagen fibrils and disruption of collagen nonreducible crosslinks [13].

However, all results have demonstrated a partial recovery of mechanical properties for longer treatment lengths (with specific reference to the decellularization treatment performed here through incubation in NaOH 0.06 N culture medium at room temperature, in continuous tilting): according to Fig. (1), the ultimate engineering tensile stress of untreated tissues cut perpendicular to Langer lines is not significantly different from those of specimens treated for 5 weeks (Tukey-Kramer test, $p<0.05$), or for 6 weeks (Tukey-Kramer test, $p<0.05$). These observations have induced one to perform more detailed analyses where real-time specimen width and thickness have been acquired to calculate true stresses. These tests have further confirmed the similarity between untreated specimens and specimens treated for 5-6 weeks through incubation in NaOH 0.06 N in continuous tilting (Fig. 1, 'T0' and 'T5-6' white columns). On the contrary, the ultimate tensile stress of tissues cut along Langer line orientation has got significantly lower, for whatever treatment duration (Fig. 2, 'T0' and 'T5-6' grey columns), and this observation has also been confirmed referring to true stresses (Fig. 2, 'T0' and 'T5-6' white columns). The observation of results concerning the elastic modulus (and consequently to physiologic stress levels) has led to similar conclusions: with reference to 90° orientation (Fig. 3), the performance of specimens treated for 5-6 weeks in NaOH 0.06 N culture medium is again similar to the performance of untreated specimens ('T5-6' *vs.* 'T0', Fig. 3); however, specimens treated for 4 weeks ('T4' in Fig. 3) are most similar to untreated specimens. With reference to Langer line orientation (Fig. 4), whatever treatment length has degraded the tissue mechanical properties ('T0' column is the highest in Fig. 4), 5 and 7 week treatments in NaOH 0.06 N culture medium are slightly more conservative ('T5' and 'T7' in Fig.4). In summary, the experiments have demonstrated that there is an improvement in the mechanical properties mainly along 90° orientation for decellularization treatments in sodium hydroxide lasting 5-6 weeks (Fig. 3): this result can be explained assuming the recovery of intermolecular interactions between low-order collagen structures, resulting in fiber reassembly (the reversible dissociation of collagen has been clearly demonstrated [14]).

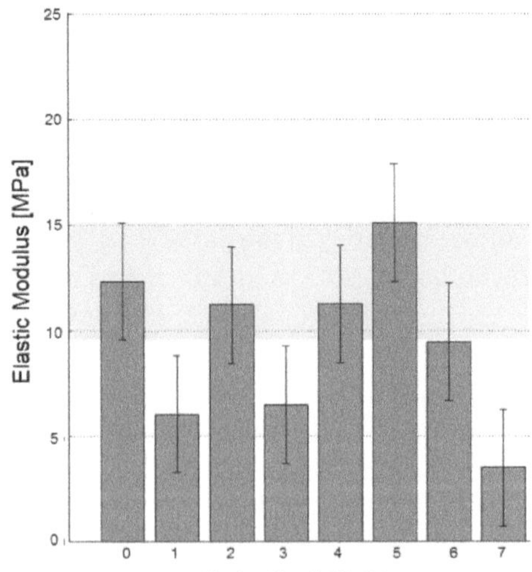

Figure 3: Elastic modulus for specimens perpendicular to Langer lines; error bars refer to Tukey-Kramer test intervals. According to this test, specimens decellularized for 2, 4-6 weeks have an elastic modulus close to the native dermis one ($p<0.05$).

Other authors agree with the final findings of the present experimental work: they evaluated a cost-effective method based on low concentrations of NaOH for the decellularization of human donor skin preserved in 85% glycerol [10] and found that a 6-week incubation period was optimal. It should be stressed how decellularization through chemical agents is commonly considered to be a cost-effective method [10, 15]; nevertheless, its long duration could have inherent problems from a commercialization standpoint.

Differences of behaviors between 0° and 90° orientation samples (Fig. 1 *vs.* Fig. 2, and Fig. 3 *vs.* Fig. 4) can be explained considering that 0° samples are stressed along the main collagen fibers orientation, and are therefore more sensitive to collagen molecules denaturation, cleavage, or partial disruption, which can take place during treatments in alkaline culture media.

The obtained results refer to "*ex vivo*" tests on pre-implant specimens; when these grafts are implanted, remodeling processes take place, and tensile mechanical properties are likely to undergo significant variations; some clues can be gained from the functional tests performed in a rat subcutaneous implant model and in a porcine transplantation model by Richters *et al.* [10]. In future, it would be very interesting to perform *in vivo* tensile tests [16, 17] on implanted dermal substitutes.

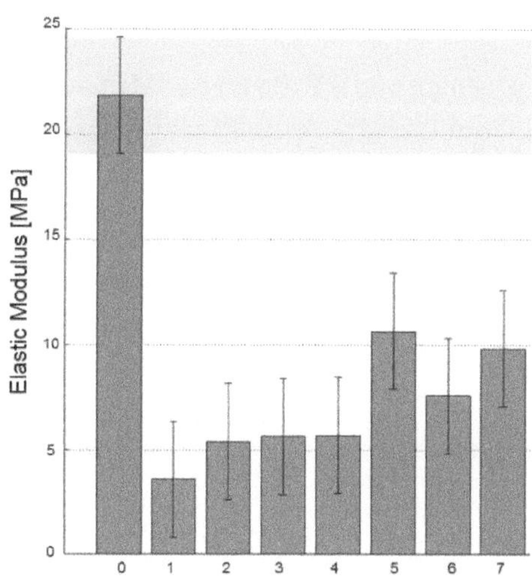

Figure 4: Elastic modulus for specimens parallel to Langer lines; error bars refer to Tukey-Kramer test intervals. According to this test, none of the specimens has an elastic modulus as high as the native dermis one ($p<0.05$).

CONCLUSION

This work has focused on the study of the consequences of an alkaline decellularization process (incubation in NaOH 0.06 N culture medium for 1-7 weeks, at room temperature in continuous tilting) on the structural function of dermal tissue, referring to the tissue strength (that is the ultimate stress measured during tensile tests at 3.2%/s strain rate), and to the tissue behavior at physiologic stress levels (elastic modulus of the linear portion of stress/strain curve).

The mechanical properties of the decellularized tissue have been compared with those of the native tissue, and considering two orthogonal orientations (parallel or perpendicular to the main orientation of collagen fibers), for different lengths of the decellularization treatment.

According to the results, the optimal duration of the decellularization treatment in NaOH is 5-6 weeks, since these treatment lengths have produced the most similar results to the native tissue.

The reliable quantitative measurement of structural properties of dermal tissue up to rupture requires an experimental setup able to capture specimen geometry variations in real time, while engineering stress and strain data have resulted in providing significant indication for comparative analyses among different decellularization treatment lengths.

REFERENCES

1. P.M. Crapo, T.W. Gilbert, and S.F. Badylak, "An overview of tissue and whole organ decellularization processes", Biomaterials, vol. 32, no. 12, pp. 3233-3243, 2011.
2. T.J. Keane, I.T. Swinehart, and S.F. Badylak, "Methods of tissue decellularization used for preparation of biologic scaffolds and in vivo relevance", Methods, vol. 84, pp. 25-34, 2015.
3. T.W. Gilbert, T.L. Sellaro, and S.F. Badylak, "Decellularization of tissues and organs", Biomaterials, vol. 27, no. 19, pp. 3675-3683, 2006.
4. M.L. Iorio, J. Shuck, and C.E. Attinger, "Wound healing in the upper and lower extremities: a systematic review on the use of acellular dermal matrices", Plast. Reconstr. Surg., vol. 130, no. 5, suppl. 2, pp. 232S-241S, 2012.
5. D.C. Acevedo, B. Shore, and R. Mirzayan, "Orthopedic applications of acellular human dermal allograft for shoulder and elbow surgery", Orthop. Clin. North Am., vol. 46, no. 3, pp. 377-388, x, 2015.
6. S.L. de Souza, A.B. Novaes Jr, D.C. Grisi, M. Taba Jr, M.F. Grisi, and P.F. de Andrade, "Comparative clinical study of a subepithelial connective tissue graft and acellular dermal matrix graft for the treatment of gingival recessions: six- to 12-month changes", J. Int. Acad. Periodontol., vol. 10, no. 3, pp. 87-94, 2008.
7. U.G. Longo, A. Berton, S. Alexander, N. Maffulli, A.L. Wallace, and V. Denaro, "Biological resurfacing for early osteoarthritis of the shoulder", Sports Med. Arthrosc. Rev., vol. 19, no. 4, pp. 380-394, 2011.
8. A. Ní Annaidh, K. Bruyère, M. Destrade, M.D. Gilchrist, and M. Otténio, "Characterization of the anisotropic mechanical properties of excised human skin", J. Mech. Behav. Biomed. Mater., vol. 5, no. 1, pp. 139-148, 2012.
9. J.H. Yoder, and D.M. Elliott, "Nonlinear and anisotropic tensile properties of graft materials used in soft tissue applications", Clin. Biomech. (Bristol, Avon),

vol. 25, no. 4, pp. 378-382, 2010.

10. C.D. Richters, A. Pirayesh, H. Hoeksema, E.W. Kamperdijk, R.W. Kreis, R.P. Dutrieux, S. Monstrey, and M.J. Hoekstra, "Development of a dermal matrix from glycerol preserved allogeneic skin", Cell Tissue Bank., vol. 9, no. 4, pp. 309-315, 2008.
11. A. Ní Annaidh, K. Bruyère, M. Destrade, M.D. Gilchrist, C. Maurini, M. Otténio, and G. Saccomandi, "Automated estimation of collagen fibre dispersion in the dermis and its contribution to the anisotropic behaviour of skin", Ann. Biomed. Eng., vol. 40, no. 8, pp. 1666-1678, 2012.
12. W.S. Sheridan, G.P. Duffy, and B.P. Murphy, "Mechanical characterization of a customized decellularized scaffold for vascular tissue engineering", J. Mech. Behav. Biomed. Mater., vol. 8, pp. 58-70, 2012.
13. J.S. Cartmell, and M.G. Dunn, "Effect of chemical treatments on tendon cellularity and mechanical properties", J. Biomed. Mater. Res., vol. 49, no. 1, pp. 134-140, 2000.
14. A.T. Yeh, B. Choi, J.S. Nelson, and B.J. Tromberg, "Reversible dissociation of collagen in tissues", J. Invest. Dermatol., vol. 121, no. 6, pp. 1332-1335, 2003.
15. T.H. Petersen, E.A. Calle, M.B. Colehour, and L.E. Niklason, "Matrix composition and mechanics of decellularized lung scaffolds", Cells Tissues Organs (Print), vol. 195, no. 3, pp. 222-231, 2012.
16. C. Flynn, A. Taberner, and P. Nielsen, "Modeling the mechanical response of in vivo human skin under a rich set of deformations", Ann. Biomed. Eng., vol. 39, no. 7, pp. 1935-1946, 2011.
17. F. Khatyr, C. Imberdis, P. Vescovo, D. Varchon, and J-M. Lagarde, "Model of the viscoelastic behaviour of skin in vivo and study of anisotropy", Skin Res. Technol., vol. 10, no. 2, pp. 96-103, 2004.

3

CHAPTER

BIOMATERIALS FOR CONTROL OF STEM CELL BEHAVIOR

Hilary J. Anderson, Jugal Kishore Sahoo, Rein V. Ulijn and Matthew J. Dalby

Keywords: Mesenchymal stem cells, bioengineering, materials synthesis, nanotopography, stimuli-responsive material

INTRODUCTION

The materials engineering field encompasses various techniques allowing the application of smart materials to tissue engineering (TE). TE can utilize these materials as either a scaffold to support cells *in vivo* or as an enabling technology to improve cell growth and differentiation *in vitro* (Murphy and Atala, 2013). TE has been applied to a range of organs, including the bladder (Atala et al., 2006) and trachea (Macchiarini et al., 2004), which have been used clinically. The knowledge and experience gained from these studies will enable the construction of organs of greater complexity and higher order architecture, e.g., the heart (Hoerstrup et al., 2000; Ott et al., 2008). In the future, the synthesis of organs in the lab potentially allows for the creation of "off the shelf" constructs that may alleviate the need for donors and complex surgeries (Kode et al., 2009). However, there are some limitations to the progress of this field, including the ability to precisely control growth and differentiation of stem cells. Stem cells are well placed to underpin TE due to their unique characteristics of self-renewal and differentiation. This feature of stem cells can address the requirement of complexity in TE, i.e., multiple tissue organs from a single cell source. It would, however, require precise organization of directive cues throughout a scaffold and ideally these cues should be presented only when required (i.e., introducing space-time control). In other words, producing man-made mimics that copy key features of extracellular matrix (ECM) and more specifically the stem cell niche is a worthwhile, albeit challenging endeavor

Citation: Anderson HJ, Sahoo JK, Ulijn RV and Dalby MJ (2016) Biomaterials for Control of Stem Cell Behavior. Front. Bioeng. Biotechnol. 4:38. doi: 10.3389/fbioe.2016.00038.

with potential clinical and socioeconomic benefits (Oreffo et al., 2005). Stem cells are non-specialized cells with the ability to differentiate (become other cell types) or self-renew (replicate without differentiating). To exploit the cells *in vivo*, scaffolds must be made from materials that are ideally bioactive, biodegradable, and biocompatible in order to replicate key features of the ECM. Polymers, such as polyglycolic acid (PGA), polylactic acid (PLA), and polyethylene glycol (PEG) make ideal scaffolds as they are biocompatible and FDA (Food and Drug Administration) approved (Koh and Atala, 2004). The first event of key importance upon stem cell interaction with materials is adhesion. Adhesion to the substrate is imperative as stem cells are anchorage-dependent meaning that those unable to adhere will apoptose via anoikis ("homelessness") (Dalby et al., 2014). Initial control of stem cell adhesion to biocompatible scaffolds ensures cell survival, then a differentiation cue can be provided to generate a desired cell population.

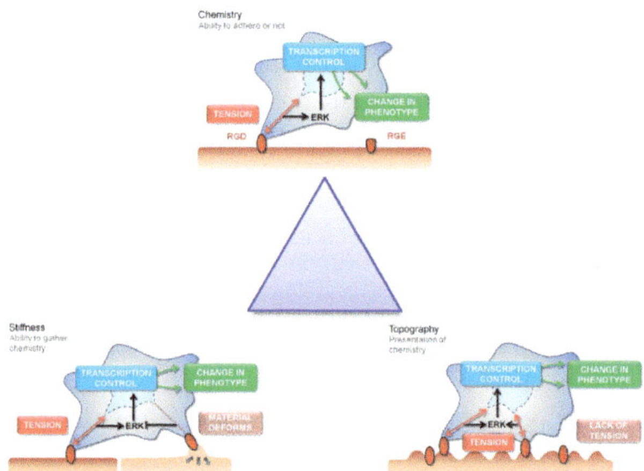

Figure 1: The "Triangle" of material/surface interface. The "triangle" of materials refers to variations in chemistry, stiffness, and nanotopography to control the interactions with MSC focal adhesions. The three cartoon panels show MSC adhesion to chemical, stiffness, and topographically modified surfaces and how this influences stem cell tension and signaling and, hence, subsequent differentiation and phenotype (as will be discussed). The cells are shown to extend filopodia to "find" adhesion ligands (shown in red). Binding of the cell through focal adhesions to these ligands creates tension and activates signaling. Chemical functionality can be used to fabricate areas of high adhesion (red) or low adhesion (capped in green) for the cells to respond to (the cell is shown in a 3D scaffold). Stiffness will affect the cells ability to produce tension through focal adhesions formation (the cell is shown on a planar surface). Topography will present the adhesion ligands to the cells in either a favorable or unfavorable manner, again affecting adhesion and subsequent tension and signaling (the cell is shown on a 2D surface).

Biomaterials have evolved rapidly over the last 30 years. Originally, first-generation materials purposed for biocompatibility and mechanical integrity gained popularity. This progressed to understanding that materials could be bioactive, eliciting desired cell response and could also be biodegradable with the aim of being replaced with native tissue after the support and templating role was complete; second-generation biomaterials included hydroxyapatite and bioglasses. There is a drive toward third-generation materials where reproducible molecular control of cells is targeted, activating the genome to regenerate the tissue (Hench and Polak, 2002). Such materials could be powerful tools for stem cell bioengineering as we start to manipulate biochemical control of stem cell fate and function (Oreffo et al., 2005). It is necessary to create and enhance existing technologies due to the limitations of existing culture methods. For example, tissue culture plastic, which has served well for somatic cells, is far from ideal to expand the stem cell population as niche cues that regulate self-renewal are missing. Therefore, there is a need to introduce new technologies that provide a stimulus to direct stem cell behavior in a user-defined manner (Lutolf and Blau, 2009; Lutolf et al., 2009). Attempts to improve cell culture methods have centered on the manipulation of three key materials features: topography, stiffness, and surface chemistry (Figure 1). Each example has provided more information on the nature of mesenchymal stem cell (MSC) adherence, growth, and differentiation.

STEM CELL CHARACTERISTICS

Stem cell self-renewal can be symmetrical where two stem cells are produced to enrich the stem cell population or asymmetrical where a stem cell and a progenitor cell is produced, hence responding to regenerative demand and maintaining stem cell number. Progenitor cells migrate from the niche expanding in number (transit amplification) and become more specialized as they progress from stem cell to progenitor cell to differentiated cell (Watt and Hogan, 2000). Stem cells have an extended capacity for self-renewal due to constitutive telomerase activity whereas terminally differentiated cells are subject to senescence. Furthermore, adult stem cells often use quiescence as a tactic to avoid DNA damage when they are not active (Watt and Hogan, 2000).

Adult stem cells, while able to self-renew, have a defined differentiation potential and only form cell types within a lineage range – usually to replenish cells in the area local to the niche that controls the stem cells (Heissig et al., 2002). For example, MSCs are derived from the mesenchyme layer in the developing embryo and form tissues derived from that layer, including bone and fat (Pittenger, 2008). MSCs are attractive as an autologous therapy source as they are ethically sourced and it is simple to obtain the cells from bone marrow, i.e., removal of bone marrow from hip replacement surgery for lab use or use of iliac crest aspiration or lipoaspiration. There is also evidence that MSCs are immune-modulatory as they lack the major histocompatibility complex (MHC) Class II, indicative of evasion of the immune system. Furthermore, they can reduce expression of inflammatory dendritic cells and suppress effector T cells making MSCs a candidate for allogeneic as well as autologous treatments (Kode et al., 2009).

Currently, the exact factors that stem cells require to differentiate *in vivo* are unknown. What is recognized is that the stem cell environment, the niche, is an important factor for the regulation of behavior. The niche is a 3D microarchitecture that incorporates many cell types supported by an ECM made of proteins, including collagen and fibronectin (Ehninger and Trumpp, 2011). It is not only the niche microenvironment that influences the cells but secreted factors of other cell types also have regulatory effects (Hartmann, 2006). The ECM is required not only for structural support but also provides substrate-specific ligands for migration, adhesion, proliferation, and function in addition to chemical and physical signals to regulate many aspects of the body's physiology (Visse and Nagase, 2003). The niche is dynamic and complex and it is, thus, unsurprising that the cells lose control of self-renewal and spontaneously differentiate when plated on tissue culture plastic (Lutolf and Blau, 2009). It is possible that learning from nature, replicating an aspect of the native system that is robust enough to be engineered and synthesized, could help us not only to develop scaffolds that direct differentiation as desired but also surfaces that could control growth of quality stem cells.

CELL–SURFACE INTERACTION

To interact with the ECM, cells use receptors such as integrins that ligate to specific peptide motifs within the ECM (Geiger et al., 2001). Each ECM protein has characteristic motifs within its sequence, for fibronectin; RGD and LDV (Yamada, 1991), for laminin; IKLLI, IKVAV, PDSGR, and YIGSR (Weber et al., 2007), for collagen; DGEA (Weber et al., 2007). Each sequence is recognizable by different cell receptors, namely integrins. Integrins are the principal family of receptors that mediate cell adhesion. Consisting of α and β subunits, forming a dimer to interact with the dynamic presentation of ECM proteins. The differing combination of α and β subunits allows ligand specificity for a particular motif (Hersel et al., 2003), for example, $\alpha_5\beta_1$ integrin binds to an RGD ligand, in addition, other integrin motifs that bind (although not limited to) RGD include most α_v combinations, $\alpha_8\beta_1$ and $\alpha_{IIb}\beta_3$ (Humphries et al., 2006). With the diversity of ECM motifs and the possibility of a number of integrin conformations to interact with, this has a direct impact on the type of cell–ECM interaction and subsequent cell behavior. Undoubtedly, the most characterized feature of the ECM is the sequence arginine, glycine, and aspartic acid (RGD) (sometimes lengthened with a serine residue to RGDS) often described as the cell adhesive peptide (Ruoslahti and Pierschbacher, 1987). This sequence is not limited to fibronectin and is incorporated into various ECM proteins, such as collagen, vitronectin, and osteopontin. We have chosen RGD as the focus of this review due to the preferential use in the biomaterials engineering. The aforementioned ECM motifs, while an intrinsic part of ECM interactions, are beyond the scope of this article.

Ligand-occupied integrins stimulate formation of focal adhesions (FAs) whereby integrin receptors cluster and recruit other proteins, including cytoskeletal elements to establish a connection between the cell and the ECM. It has been shown that FA formation is determined and limited by spacing between integrins driven by ECM ligand availability. Cavalcanti-Adam demonstrated this by tethering RGD to gold nanoparticles at pre-determined distances of either 58 or 108 nm, at 58 nm the cells spread and adhere to the particles after 3 h. In comparison, at 108 nm cell morphology remains rounded after 24 h. The spacing of 108 nm was beyond the optimal spacing for integrin gathering; therefore, adhesion, FA formation, and cell spreading were prevented (Cavalcanti-Adam et al., 2007). Structurally, the FAs act as an internal scaffold, their size is dependent on the number of actin fibers available to gather together (a direct result of binding ECM).

Direct mechanotransduction is the process by which cells turn adherent stimuli into a cellular response (creation of FA and maintenance of stress fibers) capable of directly manipulating chromatin, altering gene expression and, therefore, cell behavior (Tsimbouri et al., 2013). Indirect mechanotransduction describes biochemical cascades that are the result of cellular adhesion *via* activation of focal adhesion kinase (FAK) and mitogen-activated protein kinase (MAPK) mediated by G-proteins, such as Rac, Cdc42, and Rho (Figure 2). Rho belongs to the Ras superfamily and is responsible for the regulation of FA and stress fibers. Other G-proteins involved in cytoskeleton arrangement and spreading are Rac to control lamellipodia and cdc42 to control filopodia (Burridge and Chrzanowska-Wodnicka, 1996). Indirect mechanotransduction is also able to alter cell fate. Extracellular signal-regulated kinase (ERK)/MAPK signaling can be a key modulator for both osteogenic and adipogenic phenotypes. Osteogenic topographies alter expression of ERK at both the genomic (Dalby et al., 2008) and proteomic (Xiao et al., 2002) levels in MSCs. ERK signaling controls nuclear transcription factors. One such transcription factor that has been linked to ERK is RUNX2 (Prusty et al., 2002), the osteogenic master gene that is essential for osteoblastic differentiation (Figure 2). ERK signaling also links into PPARγ, important for adipogenesis (Yang et al., 2008), stat1 and 3 implicated in induction/reduction of osteogenesis (Petersen et al., 2008).

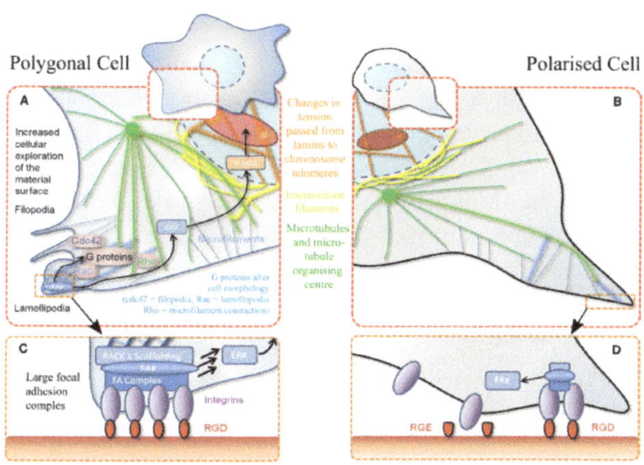

Figure 2: Schematic of MSC adhesion. (A) Binding to material surface by lamellipodia stimulates a signaling cascade. This results in transcription factor expression (RUNX2) that stimulates differentiation via other G-proteins and effectors. Polygonal cells adhere to a material at various positions encouraging cell spreading and decreasing motility. (B) Polarized cells refer to adhesion at a single point through the same mechanisms described in (A). (C) Increased magnification of adhesion event described in (A) whereby a favorable adhesion motif (RGD) is found in high density. (D) Magnification of adhesion event described in (B) whereby adhesion motif (RGD) is found in isolation. Also demonstrates non-adhesiveness of a closely related RGE (aspartic acid replaced with glutamic acid) peptide.

For cells to adhere to a synthetic surface, the material has to replicate an ECM motif or absorb ECM proteins to promote cell attachment, therefore, cell survival, and subsequent function.

CHEMICALLY CONTROLLING STEM CELL FATE

Cells respond to chemical information on a surface in various ways. Most generally, cell adhesion depends on the hydrophobicity of the chemical structures on the surface. Surface hydrophobicity controls and directs the adhesion of serum proteins on the surface and, hence, the presentation of these proteins chemical groups can influence cell behavior. Simple surface functionality (inclusion of alcohols, amines, acids, for example) has been shown to influence stem cell fate (Curran et al., 2005, 2006). Remarkably simple chemical groups incorporated into a polymer hydrogel have been demonstrated to influence stem cell differentiation (Benoit et al., 2008) as discussed in more detail below. Surface functionalization with single amino acids (Rawsterne et al., 2007) showed systematic control of adhesion and spreading of fibroblasts that correlated directly with the logP of the surface bond amino acids. Since it is still not possible to rationally design polymers with chemical functionalities that control stem cell behavior, large arrays of polymers onto glass slides have been used to identify polymers with differentiation inducing potential (Tourniaire et al., 2006; Mei et al., 2010). The most effective ways to control cell–surface interactions involves bioconjugation with bioactive elements, such as short peptides or cell adhesive proteins (typically fibronectin) through techniques, such as soft lithography.

Soft lithography includes printing, molding, and embossing. It is advantageous as it results in defined and controllable surface chemistries (Qin et al., 2010), over a range of substrates, in an inexpensive manner (Kane et al., 1999). It has been an important step in the miniaturization process to create novel technology for both health care and biotechnology, e.g., lab on a chip and microfluidics. Microcontact printing is particularly relevant to biological systems (Gates et al., 2005), where it is possible to create adhesive and non-adhesive areas within a substrate to study cell–surface interaction (Kane et al., 1999). This technique achieves spatiotemporal control that allows creation of defined patterns of polymers, for example, synthetic polymers or natural proteins, such as fibronectin, and has not only been employed to study cell survival (Chen et al., 1997) but also cell differentiation. McBeath et al. employed this method to pattern fibronectin of differing areas (1024 and 10,000 μm^2) stamped onto non-adhesive background. Confining cells to these adhesive areas showed that morphology and cell spreading was instrumental to differentiation. Specifically, MSC spreading on large areas of fibronectin aided osteoblastic differentiation, whereas smaller stamps facilitated a rounded morphology, encouraging lipid storage, and adipogenic phenotype (McBeath et al., 2004). Using this system, they demonstrated that osteogenic phenotype is tension dependent and mediated by the RhoA downstream effecter ROCK (McBeath et al., 2004). An eloquent update of this study using similar sized microcontact printed fibronectin stars and flowers illustrated that geometrical features control cell ability to form adhesions and, hence, control tension. Specifically, they illustrated sharp points to be more osteogenic that rounded curves (Kilian et al., 2010).

Dip pen nanolithography (DPN) is a method by which surface chemistry can be applied to a substrate on the nanometer scale with precision. Essentially, it involves the use of (an array of) very fine atomic force microscopy (AFM) tips, which can be inked with a suitable biomolecule, and then brought into contact with a surface where the ink is transferred to a nanoscale feature on the surface (Ginger et al., 2004). Surface chemistry can be defined by the user and encompasses organic molecules (thiols, amines, peptides, and oligonucleotides), polymers, and metal ions. DPN can be used in biomaterials engineering whereby functional molecules are printed in such an arrangement that stem cells can react and respond to. It has been shown that certain functional molecules can illicit distinct responses in MSC behavior (Curran et al., 2005, 2006). Curran et al. set out to optimize the spacing and presentation of dots of "chemistry" to manipulate MSC behavior by creating patterns of $–CH_3$, $–NH_2$, –CO, and $–CO_2H$ of 70 nm width in square or hexagonal array with varying distance of pitch. They found that functionalized $–CH_3$surface maintained stem cell markers in comparison to tissue culture plastic and gold surfaces. They also showed that NH_2 dots can increase adhesion and osteogenesis (Curran et al., 2010).

Polymer pen nanolithography (PPL) is a "direct write" technique that uses soft elastomeric tip arrays to deliver inks/materials to the surface. PPL effectively combines the feature size control of DPN with large area capability of contact printing. The feature size also can be regulated by the amount of force applied to the elastomeric pen arrays and tip-substrate contact time. Mirkin et al. (Giam et al., 2012) aimed to define the relationship between feature size of a fibronectin coated area and stem cell fate. Fibronectin, patterned onto the substrate via PPL, direct the MSC differentiation toward an osteogenic pathway. In addition, Fibronectin substrate with nanoscale features (300 nm) are more effective in inducing osteogenic behavior than microscale feature size (1 μm).

An alternative method to incorporate a chemical component to a material is through the use of nanofibers. Nanofibers can be created in a variety of methods; phase separation, electrospinning, and self assembly, each with their own advantages and disadvantages depending on the application (Rim et al., 2013). The fibers can be made from a myriad of polymers or natural proteins and can be further modified by the addition of bioactive molecules. For example, Frith et al. conjugated RGD peptides to self-assembled poly(ethylene oxide) copolymers (PS-PEO) (Frith et al., 2012). Changing the ratio of the copolymer and polystyrene homopolymer creates defined spacing between PEO domains (34, 44, 50, and 62 nm) to which the functional group are tethered to, then seeded with MSCs. They found that spacing of 34 and 44 nm encouraged cell spreading, the cells formed larger (super mature) adhesions and when cultured in osteogenic media, promoted increase in alkaline phosphatase (ALP) expression. In comparison at 50 and 62 nm, cells remained rounded and under adipogenic conditions, oil red O staining was observed (Frith et al., 2012). That cells remained rounded until spacing was reduced to 44 nm might be that a critical size was needed to switch from adipogenic to osteogenic differentiation (i.e., a certain number of integrin need to gather) or from differences in affinity of RGD group used (e.g., low affinity linear RGD compared to high affinity cyclic RGD) (Kilian and Mrksich, 2012).

Using the electrospinning technique, it is possible to create composite fibers, i.e., polymer and bioactive compounds, such as gelatin (Zhang et al., 2005), hydroxyapatite (Lee et al., 2010), and demineralized bone powder (Ko et al., 2008). Ko et al. utilized the material not only as an *in vitro* culture method but also an *in vivo* scaffold that remained in a mouse model for 12 weeks (Ko et al., 2008). While capable of acting as a scaffold, cell infiltration is a concern. Bone formation was limited to the periphery of the construct, while the center was subject to hypoxic conditions. Porosity, therefore, remains an issue which, for future applications, must be balanced with the load-bearing properties.

The discovery of using simple chemical functional groups that direct MSC behavior by effectively controlling their differentiation potentials could lead to production of simple, cheap biomaterials for applications in regenerative medicine. Anseth et al., reported in 2008, the introduction of a small set of functional groups (with different charges, hydrophobicity) into PEG hydrogels and showed that they could induce MSC differentiation to different lineages (Benoit et al., 2008). These functional groups included $–NH_2$, t-butyl, phosphate, –F, and –COOH. Depending on their charge and hydrophobicity, different MSC differentiation potential was observed, i.e., hydrophobic functional group like t-butyl induced adipogenic phenotype, while charged functional group (phosphate) promote osteogenic lineage and acid functionalized hydrogels demonstrated chondrogenesis.

Simple chemical groups are sufficient to influence MSC differentiation. Most likely these groups recruit and bind serum proteins in different ways thereby controlling presentation of adhesive groups. It will be of tremendous use if chemical functionality could be introduced in 3D scaffolds with precise spatial control. Ongoing developments in nanofabrication (both top down and bottom up) are likely to contribute significantly in the next decades.

CELL RESPONSE TO TOPOGRAPHY

Cell interactions with topography were first noted by Harrison in 1911. The term contact guidance was later coined in the 1950s when it was reported that altering the appearance of a cell's surroundings, in this case, density of fibrin networks resulted in changes in morphology of heart fibroblasts (Harrison, 1911;Weiss and Garber, 1952). Research in the area was popularized by Curtis and Wilkinson who applied development in microelectronics miniaturization to cell cultures through the 1980s and onwards (Wilkinson, 2004; Anderson, 2015). Thus, the term has long been employed to describe conformation to topography (Dalby, 2007). *In vivo*, the ECM topographical features are native to matrix infrastructure, their conformation provides the cells with behavioral cues. *In vitro*, it has been proven that the topographical cues influence stem cell behavior [altering gene expression that results in changes to adhesion, proliferation, and cytoskeletal conformation (Putnam et al., 2001; Dalby, 2007)], and it has been the work of many scientists to manipulate this interaction.

It has only recently been established that cells interact with their nanoscale environment, i.e., features much smaller than the cells themselves (Curtis et al., 2001; Dalby et al., 2002a; Gallagher et al., 2002). With the evolution of top-down lithography techniques, such as electron beam lithography (EBL) and aforementioned DPN (Curran et al., 2010), it is now possible to pattern areas large enough for cell experimentation (mm^2–cm^2) with features down to 10 nm in size (Gadegaard et al., 2003a). For a number of years, two separate approaches have dominated in topographical surface patterning: highly ordered patterns with sub-nm positioning error and random sub-μm roughened substrates. Ordered materials, typically generated by EBL, produce surfaces with low cell adhesion. By contrast, random sub-μm roughening can modify MSC differentiation relative to planar controls (Leven et al., 2004). Other topographical fabrication techniques include photolithography (Clark et al., 1987, 1990) and polymer demixing (Dalby et al., 2002b).

Highly controlled-disorder patterns have been generated with EBL. In these systems, random and highly ordered cell environments were mimicked using 120 nm diameter (100 nm deep) pits with random placement of the features or fixed 300 nm centre–centre spacing in a square pattern. MSC growth substrates were also fabricated with deliberately disordered pits in a square arrangement (±20 and ±50 nm offset). While planar control, true square, and random substrates produced only negligible differentiation, bone differentiation was observed on the disordered patterns (Figure 3A) (Dalby et al., 2007) with similar efficiency to that obtained following soluble chemical (dexamethasone and ascorbate) treatment. Disordered systems can also be applied to other materials, such as titanium substrates that are of value clinically due to load-bearing properties (Sjöström et al., 2009, 2013). Anodising titanium using through mask templating with Ps-b-P4VP allows precision patterning in bulk for both 2D and 3D designs. Patterning pillars to a height of 15 nm is one such design that was found to be osteoinductive (Figure 3B) (McNamara et al., 2011).

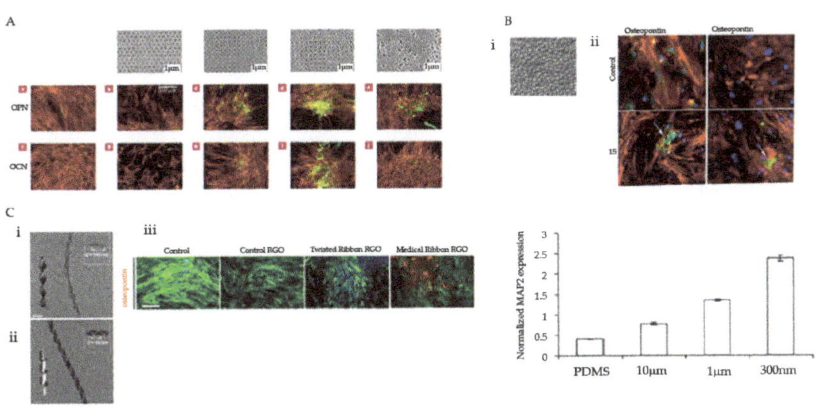

Figure 3: MSC response to topographical features. (A) EBL nanopatterned structures result in changes in gene expression. Those that exhibited “disorder” were found to stimulate osteogenesis. Reprinted (adapted) from Nature, copyright (2007) (Dalby et al., 2007). (B) i. Titanium was anodized to create a topography of 15 nm pillars. ii. These pillars were found to be osteoinductive by immunostaining for osteopontin and osteocalcin (green). Reprinted (adapted) from *Acta Biomaterilia*, copyright (2009) (Sjöström et al., 2009). (C) Creation of twisted nanoribbons at a periodicity similar to that of collagen (ii) resulted in osteogenic phenotype. (iii) Reprinted (adapted) from *ACS Nano*, copyright (2013) (Das et al., 2013). (D)MSCs can be differentiated toward a neural lineage using nanoscale channels, characterized by increasing MAP2 expression. Reprinted (adapted) from *Experimental Cell Research*, copyright (2007) (Yim et al., 2007).

Until recently, it has been considered that high precision manufacture (the top-down approach) is a requirement to gain precise control of the MSCs at the nanolevel. Nanofabrication engineers constantly strive to increase the complexity of designs that will be important for enhanced understanding of cell behavior at the nanoscale. Such criteria are readily met by EBL although the demand for scalability from current research level to that necessary in a clinical device (tens of square centimenter) may be a limitation of EBL due to the serial manner in which the patterns are produced.

Improving levels of order and disorder are becoming achievable with bottom-up methods, such as polymer phase separation (Affrossman et al., 2000), colloidal lithography (Denis et al., 2002), block copolymer lithography (Hur and Kim, 2002), and micelle lithography (Huang et al., 2009), where larger areas can be fabricated more simply. Block co-polymer micelles can, in fact, be generated with similar scale and level of order to the ±50 nm error EBL-fabricated pits (Krishnamoorthy et al., 2006) and have been shown to have osteogenic effects (Sjöström et al., 2009, 2012, 2013; McNamara et al., 2011;Maclaine et al., 2012). Furthermore, control of order to reduce any offset (rigid order of pitted features) has been shown to provide enhanced MSC growth that could be important, for example, provision of large numbers of high-quality stem cells (McMurray et al., 2011; Tsimbouri et al., 2012). The technology also appears to apply to other stem cell types, notably with ESCs where control of differentiation and growth have also been noted (Chen et al., 2012; Ji et al., 2012; Kingham et al., 2013; Kong et al., 2013).

One of the most attractive features of nanostructured surfaces as a tool for cell engineering is simplicity of mass production. Use of nickel shims (negative copies of the master structures made via electroplating) for embossing and injection molding allows high-throughput (incorporated within existing production lines) manufacture, with down to 5 nm fidelity, in a wide range of thermoplastics that could be used directly for cell culture (Gadegaard et al., 2003b).

Fabrication methods are ever evolving and engineering with complexity, creativity and replicating an aspect of nature. Das et al., inspired by the natural conformation of collagen, synthetically created Silica nanoribbons to mimic the *in vivo* cell–surface interaction to differentiate MSCs. The nanoribbons were synthesized using Gemini type amphiphiles to create two chiral nanoribbons with differing periodicities (measured as D) with either helical $D = 100$ nm (Figure 3C i) or twisted $D = 63$ nm confirmation (Figure3C ii). MSC osteoblastic differentiation was upregulated when seeded on the twisted fibrils (Figure 3C iii) (Das et al., 2013). Notably, 63 nm periodicity is close to the 67 nm repeat pattern of collagen and, thus, is more representative of the natural bone environment noting that bone is >90% collagen (Dalby et al., 2014).

There are further illustrations that topography has been utilized to tune MSC differentiation beyond the conventional lineage repertoire – toward a neural lineage. The creation of channels prevents cell spreading and provides directionality. MSC expression of neuronal marker microtubule-associated protein 2 (MAP2) increased in response to nanoscale channels in comparison to microscale (Figure 3D) (Yim et al., 2007). Exploring the transition from microscale to nanoscale reveals the differential behavior of cells in response to scale of their environment.

ALTERATIONS IN MATRIX STIFFNESS

Stiffness of the cell's environment is relevant to all stages of development, from embryogenesis (Pouille et al., 2009) to terminal cell differentiation (DuFort et al., 2011). Changes in tissue stiffness can be indicative in certain disease states. For example, breast cancer tumors are more rigid than the surrounding tissue due to clusters of collagen fibrils, which increases matrix stiffness. As shown experimentally, mammary epithelial cells that have been cultured on compliant matrices behave normally whereas those cultured on stiffer materials invade the basement membrane disrupting tissue formation and promoting malignancy (Paszek et al., 2005; Wei et al., 2015). Therefore, alterations in stiffness have a direct result on phenotype (as discussed in *Cell–Surface Interaction*).

Hydrogels are the principal tool for investigating cell response to stiffness *in vitro*. They can be synthesized from an array of polymers (including biological polymers and peptides) where the degree of crosslinking can be tailored to alter stiffness properties as desired by the user. Due to their properties of compliance and high hydration, they can be utilized to mimic natural tissues. Mimicking the stiffness of a particular tissue type can guide cellular behavior toward a particular phenotype (Discher et al., 2005,2009). It is further advantageous as hydrogels can be utilized as a delivery system for functional molecules. For example, using hydrogels for delivery of dexamethasone (Nuttelman et al., 2006), a synthetic corticosteroid that increases ALP secretion and bone morphogenetic protein (BMP), a signaling cytokine has been shown to drive osteoblast differentiation (Kim et al., 2007; Rahman et al., 2015). Furthermore, it is now possible to create hydrogel arrays that can test cell response to mechanical changes in a high-throughput manner (Gobaa et al., 2011).

In 2006, Engler and Discher produced a seminal study utilizing hydrogels to demonstrate that MSCs were responsive to a range of substrate stiffness, which in turn influenced differentiation. Three different substrate stiffnesses measuring 0.1–1, 8–17, and 25–40 kPa that represent E_{brain}, E_{muscle}, and E_{bone}, respectively (where E is the elastic modulus), were compared. It was noted that cell morphology was altered in response to these different moduli and cells began to take the phenotype of the native cells of those tissues (Figure 4A) (Engler et al., 2006).

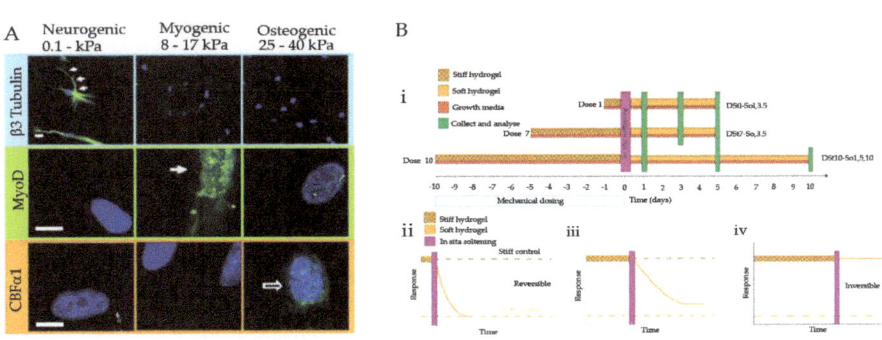

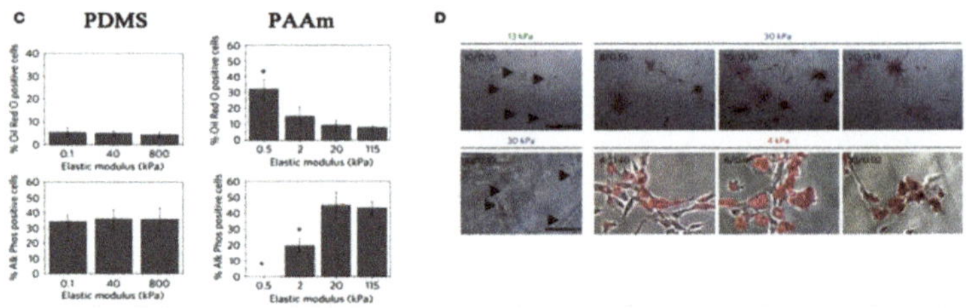

Figure 4: Effects of stiffness. (A) Altering stiffness results in differentiation into specified lineages, soft, intermediate, and hard matrices induce the differentiation of neuronal, myogenic, and osteogenic phenotypes, respectively. Reprinted (adapted) from *Cell*, copyright (2006) (Engler et al., 2006). (B) The effects of preculturing hMSCs on stiff substrates prior to seeding. ii. 1 day, iii. 7 days, iv. 10 days, where long-term pre-treatment resulted in maintenance of phenotype. Reprinted (adapted) from *Nature*, copyright (2013) (Gilbert et al., 2010). (C) Altering the elastic modulus resulted in same trend as (A) for PAAm substrates but not PDMS. Reprinted (adapted) from *Nature*ref copyright (2012) (Trappmann et al., 2012). (D) Altering the pore size of substrates does not result in changes in differentiation for that stiffness. Reprinted (adapted) from *Nature*, copyright (2014) (Wen et al., 2014).

In 2010, Gilbert showed that a pre-culture of muscle stem cells (MuSC) on pliant materials aided self-renewal of MuSC *in vivo* (Gilbert et al., 2010); therefore, *in vitro* culture conditions are central to cell behavior *in vivo*. This has been described as "mechanical memory" and has recently been tested by Yang et al. MSCs were cultured on stiff substrates for differing times prior to seeding on a soft substrate (Figure4B i), it was shown that there is a correlation between duration of pre-treatment and osteogenic phenotype. Those cells cultured the longest on stiff surface prior to transfer to a soft surface had a larger proportion of ALP positive cells and increase in Runx2 expression. With 10 days pre-treatment, osteogenic phenotype was maintained without the need for constant mechanical stimulation (Figure 4B ii–iv). Furthermore, this can be done *in situ* by culturing on light responsive hydrogels, after irradiation at 365 nm for 360 s the hydrogel changes from stiff (~10 kPa) to soft (~2 kPa) (Yang et al., 2014).

It is known that cell spreading and morphology is important for differentiation (Matsuoka et al., 2013). Khetan et al. investigated this using either permissive (degradable) or inhibitory (undegradable) hydrogels. These gels are phototunable, when exposed to light the gels are degraded allowing cells to remodel and deform the matrix. Degradable hydrogels encouraged spreading of MSCs and, therefore, osteogenesis, whereas restriction of spreading by crosslinked hydrogels maintained cellular circularity and, therefore, stimulated adipogenesis (Khetan et al., 2013). But is morphology the defining factor? Huebsch et al. confined murine MSC to pores in RGD modified hydrogels and, therefore, morphology was maintained rounded, traditionally a prerequisite for adipogenesis. Encapsulated cells still responded to matrix elasticity as 22 kPa stimulated osteogenesis even with rounded morphology. This was related to traction (the force generated by cytoskeletal pulling on the substrate) the cells were able to deform the substrate to gather RGD ligands, creating traction or high intracellular adhesion. Taken together, the results show that the presentation of ligands to the cell is crucial for creation of adhesion and subsequent traction generated by matrix reorganization is central to driving the osteogenic phenotype (Huebsch et al., 2010).

Stiffness is assumed to define the bulk properties of a material. However, different materials of comparable Young's Moduli can illicit differing responses in MSCs, for example, PDMS and PAAm gels as depicted in a study by Trappmann et al. (2012). Here, MSCs were seeded on PAAm at a range of elasticities similar to that Engler et al. demonstrated in 2006 (Engler et al., 2006). PAAm also followed the same trend, i.e., osteogenic phenotype at a high elastic moduli (stiff), adipogenic phenotype at low elastic moduli (soft). Conversely, PDMS at the same range of moduli showed no trend (Figure 4C). Further experimentation revealed that both materials had a comparable bulk stiffness, however, topography (pore size) was altered. They argue that ECM adsorption differed with topography as the ECM dictated the number of anchoring points available to the ECM. Cells, therefore, respond to the mechanical properties of the ECM rather than the bulk stiffness of the substrate. However, in a more recent study, Wen et al. argue that differentiation occurs regardless of protein tethering and that stiffness is the deciding factor. Adjusting the crosslinking density of their hydrogels to alter pore size for each stiffness, suggested that pore size had no effect on the differentiation of cells; as pore size varies, phenotype is maintained (Figure 4D). In short, it is cell deformation of the material that is driving the process (Wen et al., 2014).

HOW DO CELLS PROCESS THIS MATERIALS INFORMATION? THE CENTRAL ROLE OF ADHESION

In his 2005 commentary, Ingber discusses that tissue organization must be controlled by other factors in addition to soluble morphogens and local tissue factors. He explains how biochemical reductionism tends to overlook factors, such as tension, and instead focuses on genes and gene products (Ingber, 2005). While we consider his ideas of tensegrity (Ingber, 1993) to be beyond the scope of this article, Ingber's tensegrity model shows that the adhesions are the "tent-pegs" to which the cellular guy ropes (the cytoskeleton) are attached to give the cell the pre-stress required for stability, development of tension and possibly tensegrity. Through this mechanism, tension directly links to cell proliferation, functionalities, and differentiation.

Changing environmental factors culminate in relatively similar cellular detection, integrin binding, and response. However, there is differing cellular response to the microscale in comparison to the nanoscale. At the microscale, it is easy to envisage how cells are forced to contact guide (align) by features of a similar height to themselves. At the nanoscale, the cell will be guided one adhesion at a time. As adhesive proteins encounter a nanoscale cue (e.g., a nanogroove), the cells adhesions will remodel along the cue, reorganizing the cytoskeleton and direction of tension applied to the adhesion (Teixeira et al., 2006). Adhesion to a material begins with the rearrangement of actin filament to form microspikes, or filopodia, that have been shown to interact with features as small as 10 nm (Dalby et al., 2004). This contracture will gather integrins forming a large adhesion and will group actin filaments into stress fibers, a cell activity important for cell survival and exquisitely modulated by force (Riveline et al., 2001; Jiang et al.,

2003). Changes in chemistry, stiffness, and topography influence the size and number of cell adhesions. Furthermore, it seems likely that there are critical adhesion sizes for cells to be able to gather spatial information through filopodial extension (Arnold et al., 2008). Adhesions can be classified by size and include focal complexes (<2 μm long, transient, involved in motility) FAs (>2 μm long, stable, formed during cell maturation and ECM production) and super mature adhesions (SMAs that are very large >5 μm long). The currently used classification of SMAs is really an evolution of the classical "dot" and "dash" adhesions described by Bershadsky et al. (1985).

The study of FAs appears to demonstrate that alterations in the size and number of adhesions are important for MSC differentiation. As has been discussed, MSCs differentiate to bone efficiently on a disordered nanoscale pattern (Dalby et al., 2007). Investigation of adhesion size has demonstrated that on the osteogenic pattern much larger adhesions were generated by the MSCs (Dalby et al., 2007). It was postulated by the Spatz group that the disordered nature allowed adhesive points to group closer together [within the critical 70 nm range described by Cavalcanti-Adam (Albelda and Buck, 1990; Cavalcanti-Adam et al., 2008)] and, thus, facilitate integrin gathering (Kingham et al., 2013) and the formation of SMAs (Biggs et al., 2008, 2009) (> 5 μm long). It is likely that these larger adhesions are stabilised by scaffolding proteins such as RACK1 (Buensuceso et al., 2001; Dalby et al., 2008), decreasing cell motility, but allowing formation of cytoskeletal tension (Balaban et al., 2001; Shemesh et al., 2005) important to MSC fate culminating in large morphology and osteogenic phenotype (Curtis et al., 2001; Putnam et al., 2001; Wen et al., 2014).

There is a variation in size of mature cell types generated from MSCs (small, round adipocyte to large orthogonal appearance of the osteoblast). We can postulate a role for the natural environment of the stem cell in defining cell morphology. This environmental regulation of adhesion size, cytoskeletal tension, and overall cell morphology will have important roles in the induction of cell differentiation, which importantly can be dictated by designing the material interface. The ability to control cell fate through presentation of chemical functionality (i.e., promoting the binding of transmembrane integrins to ECM proteins or peptide ligands) is well understood. The roles of stiffness and topographical interventions are less intuitive. With regard to material stiffness, it has been observed that FA size is increased on materials of higher stiffness, which enhances the ability of a cell to form a contractile cytoskeleton (Wen et al., 2014;Yang et al., 2014). These cytoskeletal changes determine cell tension, morphology, and fate.

A DYNAMIC FUTURE?

All the examples that have been discussed thus far have been "static" in nature, i.e., a single topography or chemical functionality is used to perform a specific role (self-renewal or differentiation). However, the stem cell niche is dynamic, regulating growth and differentiation on demand. Thus, it makes sense that next-generation materials should also have dynamic aspects, in particular to support self-renewal *and*differentiation with spatiotemporal control. Indeed, stimuli-responsive surfaces have attracted significant scientific interest in recent years in this context. Stimuli, such as light (Ohmuro-Matsuyama and Tatsu, 2008; Petersen et al., 2008; Liu et al., 2009; Wirkner et al.,

2011a), enzymes (Todd et al., 2007; Zelzer et al., 2012), temperature (Yamato et al., 2002), and electric fields (Yeo et al., 2003), have been investigated. These external stimuli should ideally be cytocompatible and bioorthogonal in order for them to be utilized in a cellular context.

Light has been applied to control cell adhesion, typically by changing the chemical functionality or presentation of RGD molecules. In 2008, Del Campo et al. demonstrated the modification of RGD with a photoresponsive caging group on the carboxylic acid side chain of aspartic acid. Prior to irradiation, the photocaging group prevents integrin recognition and consequent adhesion. In response to light, the caging group is released allowing for on-demand adhesion. They concluded that this system had many applications and suggested developing patterned areas of photoactivity (Petersen et al., 2008). In a follow-up study, they modified the photoliable element to include a 4,5-dialkoxy 1-(2-nitrophenyl) ethyl that was incorporated in between the amine terminated surfaces and RGD peptide. The photoliable element could be irradiated to allow adhesion and in addition they also patterned the substrate demonstrating specific area of HUVEC (human umbilical vein endothelial cell) attachment (Wirkner et al., 2011b). One of the main advantages of using light as a method of controlling adhesion is that it can be applied locally, e.g., using photomasks. This has enabled patterning of a cell culture dish with spatiotemporal control permitting adhesion in defined areas on demand. The examples that have been discussed so far relate to activation/deactivation by making use of one-off breaking of chemical bonds. In order to produce a reversible system, Jiang et al. used azobenzene as a conformational switch to alter the presentation of RGD ligands. Irradiation at 340–380 or 450–490 nm resulted in trans-cis or cis-trans isomerization, respectively, either promoting adhesion or preventing cell adhesion to substrate (Liu et al., 2009).

Photochemical control can also be applied in three-dimensional systems. In 2009, Anseth et al. utilized copper free click chemistry to synthesize hydrogels with thiol-ene groups that could be photocoupled in order to pattern biochemical functionalities at user-defined locations. They showed the surface to maintain a population of 3T3 fibroblast cells (DeForest et al., 2009). Later, DeForest and Tirrell improved such a system creating reversible patterning of bioactive ECM protein (i.e., vitronectin) inside a three-dimensional polymeric hydrogel scaffold. In doing so, they succeeded in differentiating hMSCs to osteoblasts.

Mosiewicz et al. employed both light and enzymatic control of substrate. Caged FXIIIa (transglutaminase factor XIII) was covalently incorporated into a PEG hydrogel. FXIIIa enzyme catalyzes reactions between ε-amine of lysine with γ-carboxamide residue of glutamine. Upon exposure to light, the caged substrate in the hydrogel activated and FXIIIa catalyzed reaction of the substrate with counter-reactive substrate of biomolecule in a covalent fashion within the hydrogel matrix. Through this photopatterning of hydrogel with desired biomolecules 3D manipulation of MSCs within hydrogel matrix can be achieved spatiotemporarily (Mosiewicz et al., 2013).

Electric field has been used as a stimulus by Mrksich et al. Incorporating an electroactive moiety, *O*-silyl hydroquinone on the surface with RGD at a defined electric field (550 mV), *O*-silyl hydroquinone undergoes electrochemical oxidation to form benzoquinone, thereby hydrolyzing the silyl ether that causes the selective release of RGD ligand from the surface (Yeo et al., 2003).

Stimuli such as light and electric field are unsuitable for some biological applications. Enzymes, however, provide an alternative. Enzymes act as a benign physiological trigger with the potential advantage of selectivity, specificity, biocompatibility, and dynamicity, and perform under physiological environment (Hedstrom, 2010). Enzymes are potentially an effective alternative to trigger a chemical change in the surface that can affect MSC behavior. Until now, there are very few examples of enzyme responsive surfaces in the literature. To create such a platform, Todd et al. utilized solid phase peptide synthesis (SPPS) to tether amino acids to a glass coverslip. The advantage of SPPS is that any sequence can be synthesized depending on the application. Todd et al. developed a sequence Fmoc-A↓ARGD-Glass that is cleavable by the enzyme elastase. The full sequence, Fmoc capped, prevents cell adhesion to RGD. Application of the enzyme cleaves the sequence at the dialanine linker allowing attachment to RGD. This system is biocompatible and easily controlled (Todd et al., 2007; Zelzer et al., 2012).

SUMMARY

At present, these materials approaches have characterized the nature of MSC adhesion and subsequent behavior. What is lacking is an optimal system that provides the quantity of stem cells required for a TE construct. Furthermore, material use as *in vivo* scaffolds is still not fully exploitable due to limited invasion, porosity, vascularization, and load-bearing properties that are all challenges that have still to be optimally addressed. The key to delivery of regenerative therapies lies in the development of stem cell culture platforms where stem cells can grow and differentiate into different phenotypes for incorporation into TE scaffolds supported by biomaterials. Materials have been used to demonstrate basic niche functions. However, the current materials strategies, although providing new insights into stem cell biology, especially, MSC behavior, are static technologies and have certain limitations. The materials available to date that target continued self-renewal are useful for promoting growth but they are poor in differentiation and *vice versa*. The immediate challenge is to fabricate niche-mimicking biomaterials, i.e., a material system where MSCs will be cultured as a growing stem cell population and when triggered (either user induced or autonomously, by cell secreted factors), will switch to a phenotype of choice, on demand.

AUTHOR CONTRIBUTIONS

All authors were involved in writing the review: HA, Univeristy of Glasgow. MD, University of Glasgow. JS, University of Strathclyde. RU, CUNY.

CONFLICT OF INTEREST STATEMENT

The authors declare that the research was conducted in the absence of any commercial or financial relationships that could be construed as a potential conflict of interest.

ACKNOWLEDGMENTS

HA is funded by DTC/ESPRC (EP/F500424/1), MD is funded by BBSRC (BK/K006908/1). JS and RU are funded by BBSRC (BB/K007513/1). We thank Rob Mart, Cardiff University, for Figures 1 and 2.

REFERENCES

1. Affrossman, S., Jerome, R., O'Neill, S. A., Schmitt, T., and Stamm, M. (2000). Surface structure of thin film blends of polystyrene and poly(n-butyl methacrylate). *Colloid Polym. Sci.* 278, 993–999. doi:10.1007/s003960000358
2. Albelda, S. M., and Buck, C. A. (1990). Integrins and other cell adhesion molecules. *FASEB J.* 4, 2868–2880.
3. Anderson, H. J. (2015). *An Interview with Adam Curtis | Centre for Cell Engineering Glasgow*. Available at:http://www.cceuog.co.uk/#!An-Interview-with-Adam-Curtis/cmbz/5617e0ec0cf2c3576e558247
4. Arnold, M., Hirschfeld-Warneken, V. C., Lohmüller, T., Heil, P., Blümmel, J., Cavalcanti-Adam, E. A., et al. (2008). Induction of cell polarization and migration by a gradient of nanoscale variations in adhesive ligand spacing. *Nano Lett.* 8, 2063–2069. doi:10.1021/nl801483w
5. Atala, A., Bauer, S. B., Soker, S., Yoo, J. J., and Retik, A. B. (2006). Tissue-engineered autologous bladders for patients needing cystoplasty. *Lancet* 367, 1241–1246. doi:10.1016/S0140-6736(06)68438-9
6. Balaban, N. Q., Schwarz, U. S., Riveline, D., Goichberg, P., Tzur, G., Sabanay, I., et al. (2001). Force and focal adhesion assembly: a close relationship studied using elastic micropatterned substrates. *Nat. Cell Biol.* 3, 466–472. doi:10.1038/35074532
7. Benoit, D. S. W., Schwartz, M. P., Durney, A. R., and Anseth, K. S. (2008). Small functional groups for controlled differentiation of hydrogel-encapsulated human mesenchymal stem cells. *Nat. Mater.* 7, 816–823. doi:10.1038/nmat2269
8. Bershadsky, A. D., Tint, I. S., Neyfakh, A. A., and Vasiliev, J. M. (1985). Focal contacts of normal and RSV-transformed quail cells. Hypothesis of the transformation-induced deficient maturation of focal contacts. *Exp. Cell Res.* 158, 433–444. doi:10.1016/0014-4827(85)90467-7
9. Biggs, M. J., Richards, R. G., Gadegaard, N., Wilkinson, C. D., Oreffo, R. O., and Dalby, M. J. (2009). The use of nanoscale topography to modulate the dynamics of adhesion formation in primary osteoblasts and ERK/MAPK signalling in STRO-1+ enriched skeletal stem cells.*Biomaterials* 30, 5094–5103. doi:10.1016/j.biomaterials.2009.05.049
10. Biggs, M. J., Richards, R. G., McFarlane, S., Wilkinson, C. D., Oreffo, R. O., and Dalby, M. J. (2008). Adhesion formation of primary human osteoblasts and the functional response of mesenchymal stem cells to 330nm deep microgrooves. *J. R. Soc. Interface* 5, 1231–1242. doi:10.1098/rsif.2008.0035
11. Buensuceso, C. S., Woodside, D., Huff, J. L., Plopper, G. E., and O'Toole, T. E.

(2001). The WD protein Rack1 mediates protein kinase C and integrin-dependent cell migration. *J. Cell Sci.* 114, 1691–1698.

12. Burridge, K., and Chrzanowska-Wodnicka, M. (1996). Focal adhesions, contractility, and signaling. *Annu. Rev. Cell Dev. Biol.* 12, 463–518. doi:10.1146/annurev.cellbio.12.1.463
13. Cavalcanti-Adam, E. A., Aydin, D., Hirschfeld-Warneken, V. C., and Spatz, J. P. (2008). Cell adhesion and response to synthetic nanopatterned environments by steering receptor clustering and spatial location. *HFSP J.* 2, 276–285. doi:10.2976/1.2976662
14. Cavalcanti-Adam, E. A., Volberg, T., Micoulet, A., Kessler, H., Geiger, B., and Spatz, J. P. (2007). Cell spreading and focal adhesion dynamics are regulated by spacing of integrin ligands. *Biophys. J.* 92, 2964–2974. doi:10.1529/biophysj.106.089730
15. Chen, C. S., Mrksich, M., Huang, S., Whitesides, G. M., and Ingber, D. E. (1997). Geometric control of cell life and death. *Science* 276, 1425–1428. doi:10.1126/science.276.5317.1425
16. Chen, W., Villa-Diaz, L. G., Sun, Y., Weng, S., Kim, J. K., Lam, R. H., et al. (2012). Nanotopography influences adhesion, spreading, and self-renewal of human embryonic stem cells. *ACS Nano* 6, 4094–4103. doi:10.1021/nn3004923
17. Clark, P., Connolly, P., Curtis, A. S., Dow, J. A., and Wilkinson, C. D. (1987). Topographical control of cell behaviour. I. Simple step cues.*Development* 99, 439–448.
18. Clark, P., Connolly, P., Curtis, A. S., Dow, J. A., and Wilkinson, C. D. (1990). Topographical control of cell behaviour: II. Multiple grooved substrata. *Development* 108, 635–644.
19. Curran, J. M., Chen, R., and Hunt, J. A. (2005). Controlling the phenotype and function of mesenchymal stem cells in vitro by adhesion to silane-modified clean glass surfaces. *Biomaterials* 26, 7057–7067. doi:10.1016/j.biomaterials.2005.05.008
20. Curran, J. M., Chen, R., and Hunt, J. A. (2006). The guidance of human mesenchymal stem cell differentiation in vitro by controlled modifications to the cell substrate. *Biomaterials* 27, 4783–4793. doi:10.1016/j.biomaterials.2006.05.001
21. Curran, J. M., Stokes, R., Irvine, E., Graham, D., Amro, N. A., Sanedrin, R. G., et al. (2010). Introducing dip pen nanolithography as a tool for controlling stem cell behaviour: unlocking the potential of the next generation of smart materials in regenerative medicine. *Lab. Chip* 10, 1662–1670. doi:10.1039/c004149a
22. Curtis, A. S., Casey, B., Gallagher, J. O., Pasqui, D., Wood, M. A., and Wilkinson, C. D. (2001). Substratum nanotopography and the adhesion of biological cells. Are symmetry or regularity of nanotopography important? *Biophys. Chem.* 94, 275–283. doi:10.1016/S0301-4622(01)00247-2
23. Dalby, M., Gadegaard, N., Tare, R., Andar, A., Riehle, M. O., Herzyk, P., et al. (2007). The control of human mesenchymal cell differentiation using nanoscale

symmetry and disorder. *Nat. Mater.* 6, 997–1003. doi:10.1038/nmat2013

24. Dalby, M. J. (2007). Cellular response to low adhesion nanotopographies. *Int. J. Nanomedicine* 2, 373–381.
25. Dalby, M. J., Gadegaard, N., and Oreffo, R. O. (2014). Harnessing nanotopography and integrin-matrix interactions to influence stem cell fate. *Nat. Mater.* 13, 558–569. doi:10.1038/nmat3980
26. Dalby, M. J., Hart, A., and Yarwood, S. J. (2008). The effect of the RACK1 signalling protein on the regulation of cell adhesion and cell contact guidance on nanometric grooves. *Biomaterials* 29, 282–289. doi:10.1016/j.biomaterials.2007.09.030
27. Dalby, M. J., Riehle, M. O., Johnstone, H., Affrossman, S., and Curtis, A. S. (2002a). In vitro reaction of endothelial cells to polymer demixed nanotopography. *Biomaterials* 23, 2945–2954. doi:10.1016/S0142-9612(01)00424-0
28. Dalby, M. J., Yarwood, S. J., Riehle, M. O., Johnstone, H. J., Affrossman, S., and Curtis, A. S. (2002b). Increasing fibroblast response to materials using nanotopography: morphological and genetic measurements of cell response to 13-nm-high polymer demixed islands.*Exp. Cell Res.* 276, 1–9. doi:10.1006/excr.2002.5498
29. Dalby, M. J., Riehle, M. O., Johnstone, H., Affrossman, S., and Curtis, A. S. G. (2004). Investigating the limits of filopodial sensing: a brief report using SEM to image the interaction between 10 nm high nano-topography and fibroblast filopodia. *Cell Biol. Int.* 28, 229–236. doi:10.1016/j.cellbi.2003.12.004
30. Das, R. K., Zouani, O. F., Labrugere, C., Oda, R., and Durrieu, M. C. (2013). Influence of nanohelical shape and periodicity on stem cell fate. *ACS Nano* 7, 3351–3361. doi:10.1021/nn4001325
31. DeForest, C. A., Polizzotti, B. D., and Anseth, K. S. (2009). Sequential click reactions for synthesizing and patterning three-dimensional cell microenvironments. *Nat. Mater.* 8, 659–664. doi:10.1038/nmat2473
32. Denis, F. A., Hanarp, P., Sutherland, D. S., and Dufrene, Y. F. (2002). Fabrication of nanostructured polymer surfaces using colloidal lithography and spin-coating. *Nano Lett.* 2, 1419–1425. doi:10.1021/nl025750g
33. Discher, D. E., Janmey, P., and Wang, Y.-L. (2005). Tissue cells feel and respond to the stiffness of their substrate. *Science* 310, 1139–1143. doi:10.1126/science.1116995
34. Discher, D. E., Mooney, D. J., and Zandstra, P. W. (2009). Growth factors, matrices, and forces combine and control stem cells. *Science*324, 1673–1677. doi:10.1126/science.1171643
35. DuFort, C. C., Paszek, M. J., and Weaver, V. M. (2011). Balancing forces: architectural control of mechanotransduction. *Nat. Rev. Mol. Cell Biol.* 12, 308–319. doi:10.1038/nrm3112
36. Ehninger, A., and Trumpp, A. (2011). The bone marrow stem cell niche grows up: mesenchymal stem cells and macrophages move in. *J. Exp. Med.* 208, 421–428.

doi:10.1084/jem.20110132

37. Engler, A. J., Sen, S., Sweeney, H. L., and Discher, D. E. (2006). Matrix elasticity directs stem cell lineage specification. *Cell* 126, 677–689. doi:10.1016/j.cell.2006.06.044
38. Frith, J. E., Mills, R. J., and Cooper-White, J. J. (2012). Lateral spacing of adhesion peptides influences human mesenchymal stem cell behaviour. *J. Cell Sci.* 125, 317–327. doi:10.1242/jcs.087916
39. Gadegaard, N., Thoms, S., Macintyre, D. S., McGhee, K., Gallagher, J., Casey, B., et al. (2003a). Arrays of nano-dots for cellular engineering. *Microelectron. Eng.* 67, 162–168. doi:10.1016/S0167-9317(03)00067-4
40. Gadegaard, N., Mosler, S., and Larsen, N. B. (2003b). Biomimetic polymer nanostructures by injection molding. *Macromol. Mater. Eng.*288, 76–83. doi:10.1002/mame.200290037
41. Gallagher, J. O., McGhee, K. F., Wilkinson, C. D., and Riehle, M. O. (2002). Interaction of animal cells with ordered nanotopography.*IEEE Trans. Nanobioscience* 1, 24–28. doi:10.1109/TNB.2002.806918
42. Gates, B. D., Xu, Q., Stewart, M., Ryan, D., Willson, C. G., and Whitesides, G. M. (2005). New approaches to nanofabrication: molding, printing, and other techniques. *Chem. Rev.* 105, 1171–1196. doi:10.1021/cr030076o
43. Geiger, B., Bershadsky, A., Pankov, R., and Yamada, K. M., (2001). Transmembrane extracellular matrix – cytoskeleton crosstalk. *Nat. Rev. Mol. Cell Biol.* 2, 793–805. doi:10.1038/35099066
44. Giam, L. R., Massich, M. D., Hao, L., Shin Wong, L., Mader, C. C., and Mirkin, C. A. (2012). Scanning probe-enabled nanocombinatorics define the relationship between fibronectin feature size and stem cell fate. *Proc. Natl. Acad. Sci. U.S.A.* 109, 4377–4382. doi:10.1073/pnas.1201086109
45. Gilbert, P. M., Havenstrite, K. L., Magnusson, K. E., Sacco, A., Leonardi, N. A., Kraft, P., et al. (2010). Substrate elasticity regulates skeletal muscle stem cell self-renewal in culture. *Science* 329, 1078–1081. doi:10.1126/science.1191035
46. Ginger, D. S., Zhang, H., and Mirkin, C. A. (2004). The evolution of dip-pen nanolithography. *Angew. Chem. Int. Ed. Engl.* 43, 30–45. doi:10.1002/ange.200300608
47. Gobaa, S., Hoehnel, S., Roccio, M., Negro, A., Kobel, S., and Lutolf, M. P. (2011). Artificial niche microarrays for probing single stem cell fate in high throughput. *Nat. Methods* 8, 949–955. doi:10.1038/nmeth.1732
48. Harrison, R. G. (1911). On the stereotropism of embryonic cells. *Science* 34, 279–281. doi:10.1126/science.34.870.279
49. Hartmann, C. A. (2006). Wnt canon orchestrating osteoblastogenesis. *Trends Cell Biol.* 16, 151–158. doi:10.1016/j.tcb.2006.01.001
50. Hedstrom, L. (2010). *Enzyme Specificity and Selectivity*. Massachusetts: John Wiley & Sons, Ltd.
51. Heissig, B., Hattori, K., Dias, S., Friedrich, M., Ferris, B., Hackett, N. R., et al.

(2002). Recruitment of stem and progenitor cells from the bone marrow niche requires MMP-9 mediated release of kit-ligand. *Cell* 109, 625–637. doi:10.1016/S0092-8674(02)00754-7

52. Hench, L. L., and Polak, J. M. (2002). Third-generation biomedical materials. *Science* 295, 1014–1017. doi:10.1126/science.1067404

53. Hersel, U., Dahmen, C., and Kessler, H. (2003). RGD modified polymers : biomaterials for stimulated cell adhesion and beyond.*Biomaterials* 24, 4385–4415. doi:10.1016/S0142-9612(03)00343-0

54. Hoerstrup, S. P., Sodian, R., Daebritz, S., Wang, J., Bacha, E. A., Martin, D. P., et al. (2000). Functional living trileaflet heart valves grown in vitro. *Circulation* 102, III44–III49. doi:10.1161/01.CIR.102.suppl_3.III-44

55. Huang, J., Grater, S. V., Corbellini, F., Rinck, S., Bock, E., Kemkemer, R., et al. (2009). Impact of order and disorder in RGD nanopatterns on cell adhesion. *Nano Lett.* 9, 1111–1116. doi:10.1021/nl803548b

56. Huebsch, N., Arany, P. R., Mao, A. S., Shvartsman, D., Ali, O. A., Bencherif, S. A., et al. (2010). Harnessing traction-mediated manipulation of the cell/matrix interface to control stem-cell fate. *Nat. Mater.* 9, 518–526. doi:10.1038/nmat2732

57. Humphries, J. D., Byron, A., and Humphries, M. J. (2006). Integrin ligands at a glance. *J. Cell Sci.* 119, 3901–3903. doi:10.1242/jcs.03098

58. Hur, E. M., and Kim, K. T. (2002). G protein-coupled receptor signalling and cross-talk: achieving rapidity and specificity. *Cell. Signal.*14, 397–405. doi:10.1016/S0898-6568(01)00258-3

59. Ingber, D. (1993). Cellular tensegrity: defining new rules of biological design that govern the cytoskeleton. *J. Cell*

60. Ingber, D. E. (2005). Mechanical control of tissue growth: function follows form. *Proc. Natl. Acad. Sci. U.S.A.* 102, 11571–11572. doi:10.1073/pnas.0505939102

61. Ji, L., LaPointe, V. L. S., Evans, N. D., and Stevens, M. M. (2012). Changes in embryonic stem cell colony morphology and early differentiation markers driven by colloidal crystal topographical cues. *Eur. Cell. Mater.* 23, 135–146.

62. Jiang, G., Giannone, G., Critchley, D. R., Fukumoto, E., and Sheetz, M. P. (2003). Two-piconewton slip bond between fibronectin and the cytoskeleton depends on talin. *Nature* 424, 334–337. doi:10.1038/nature01805

63. Kane, R. S., Takayama, S., Ostuni, E., Ingber, D. E., and Whitesides, G. M. (1999). Patterning proteins and cells using soft lithography.*Biomaterials* 20, 2363–2376. doi:10.1016/S0142-9612(99)00165-9

64. Khetan, S., Guvendiren, M., Legant, W. R., Cohen, D. M., Chen, C. S., and Burdick, J. A. (2013). Degradation-mediated cellular traction directs stem cell fate in covalently crosslinked three-dimensional hydrogels. *Nat. Mater.* 12, 458–465. doi:10.1038/nmat3586

65. Kilian, K. A., Bugarija, B., Lahn, B. T., and Mrksich, M. (2010). Geometric cues for directing the differentiation of mesenchymal stem cells. *Proc. Natl. Acad. Sci.*

U.S.A. 107, 4872–4877. doi:10.1073/pnas.0903269107

66. Kilian, K. A., and Mrksich, M. (2012). Directing stem cell fate by controlling the affinity and density of ligand-receptor interactions at the biomaterials interface. *Angew. Chem. Int. Ed. Engl.* 124, 4975–4979. doi:10.1002/anie.201108746
67. Kim, J., Kim, I. S., Cho, T. H., Lee, K. B., Hwang, S. J., Tae, G., et al. (2007). Bone regeneration using hyaluronic acid-based hydrogel with bone morphogenic protein-2 and human mesenchymal stem cells. *Biomaterials* 28, 1830–1837. doi:10.1016/j.biomaterials.2006.11.050
68. Kingham, E., White, K., Gadegaard, N., Dalby, M. J., and Oreffo, R. O. C. (2013). Nanotopographical cues augment mesenchymal differentiation of human embryonic stem cells. *Small* 9, 2140–2151. doi:10.1002/smll.201202340
69. Ko, E. K., Jeong, S. I., Rim, N. G., Lee, Y. M., Shin, H., and Lee, B. K. (2008). In vitro osteogenic differentiation of human mesenchymal stem cells and in vivo bone formation in composite nanofiber meshes. *Tissue Eng. Part A* 14, 2105–2119. doi:10.1089/ten.tea.2008.0057
70. Kode, J. A., Mukherjee, S., Joglekar, M. V., and Hardikar, A. A. (2009). Mesenchymal stem cells: immunobiology and role in immunomodulation and tissue regeneration. *Cytotherapy* 11, 377–391. doi:10.1080/14653240903080367
71. Koh, C. J., and Atala, A. (2004). Tissue engineering, stem cells, and cloning: opportunities for regenerative medicine. *J. Am. Soc. Nephrol.* 15, 1113–1125. doi:10.1097/01.ASN.0000119683.59068.F0
72. Kong, Y. P., Tu, C. H., Donovan, P. J., and Yee, A. F. (2013). Expression of Oct4 in human embryonic stem cells is dependent on nanotopographical configuration. *Acta Biomater.* 9, 6369–6380. doi:10.1016/j.actbio.2013.01.036
73. Krishnamoorthy, S., Pugin, R., Brugger, J., Heinzelmann, H., Hoogerwerf, A. C., and Hinderling, C. (2006). Block copolymer micelles as switchable templates for nanofabrication. *Langmuir* 22, 3450–3452. doi:10.1021/la052299a
74. Lee, J. H., Rim, N. G., Jung, H. S., and Shin, H. (2010). Control of osteogenic differentiation and mineralization of human mesenchymal stem cells on composite nanofibers containing poly[lactic-co-(glycolic acid)] and hydroxyapatite. *Macromol. Biosci.* 10, 173–182. doi:10.1002/mabi.200900169
75. Leven, R. M., Virdi, A. S., and Sumner, D. R. (2004). Patterns of gene expression in rat bone marrow stromal cells cultured on titanium alloy discs of different roughness. *J. Biomed. Mater. Res. A* 70, 391–401. doi:10.1002/jbm.a.30082
76. Liu, D., Xie, Y., Shao, H., and Jiang, X. (2009). Using azobenzene-embedded self-assembled monolayers to photochemically control cell adhesion reversibly. *Angew. Chem. Int. Ed. Engl.* 48, 4406–4408. doi:10.1002/anie.200901130
77. Lutolf, M. P., and Blau, H. M. (2009). Artificial stem cell niches. *Adv. Mater.* 21, 3255–3268. doi:10.1002/adma.200802582
78. Lutolf, M. P., Gilbert, P. M., and Blau, H. M. (2009). Designing materials to direct stem-cell fate. *Nature* 462, 433–441. doi:10.1038/nature08602

79. Macchiarini, P., Walles, T., Biancosino, C., and Mertsching, H. (2004). First human transplantation of a bioengineered airway tissue. *J. Thorac. Cardiovasc. Surg.* 128, 638–641. doi:10.1016/j.jtcvs.2004.02.042

80. Maclaine, S. E., Gadhari, N., Pugin, R., Meek, R. M., Liley, M., and Dalby, M. J. (2012). Optimizing the osteogenicity of nanotopography using block co-polymer phase separation fabrication techniques. *J. Orthop. Res.* 30, 1190–1197. doi:10.1002/jor.22076

81. Matsuoka, F., Takeuchi, I., Agata, H., Kagami, H., Shiono, H., Kiyota, Y., et al. (2013). Morphology-based prediction of osteogenic differentiation potential of human mesenchymal stem cells. *PLoS ONE* 8:e55082. doi:10.1371/journal.pone.0055082

82. McBeath, R., Pirone, D. M., Nelson, C. M., Bhadriraju, K., and Chen, C. S. (2004). Cell shape, cytoskeletal tension, and RhoA regulate stem cell lineage commitment. *Dev. Cell* 6, 483–495. doi:10.1016/S1534-5807(04)00075-9

83. McMurray, R. J., Gadegaard, N., Tsimbouri, P. M., Burgess, K. V., McNamara, L. E., Tare, R., et al. (2011). Nanoscale surfaces for the long-term maintenance of mesenchymal stem cell phenotype and multipotency. *Nat. Mater.* 10, 637–644. doi:10.1038/nmat3058

84. McNamara, L. E., Sjöström, T., Burgess, K. E., Kim, J. J., Liu, E., Gordonov, S., et al. (2011). Skeletal stem cell physiology on functionally distinct titania nanotopographies. *Biomaterials* 32, 7403–7410. doi:10.1016/j.biomaterials.2011.06.063

85. Mei, Y., Saha, K., Bogatyrev, S. R., Yang, J., Hook, A. L., Kalcioglu, Z. I., et al. (2010). Combinatorial development of biomaterials for clonal growth of human pluripotent stem cells. *Nat. Mater.* 9, 768–778. doi:10.1038/nmat2812

86. Mosiewicz, K. A., Kolb, L., van der Vlies, A. J., Martino, M. M., Lienemann, P. S., Hubbell, J. A., et al. (2013). In situ cell manipulation through enzymatic hydrogel photopatterning. *Nat. Mater.* 12, 1072–1078. doi:10.1038/nmat3766

87. Murphy, S. V., and Atala, A. (2013). Organ engineering combining stem cells, biomaterials, and bioreactors to produce bioengineered organs for transplantation. *Bioessays* 35, 163–172. doi:10.1002/bies.201200062

88. Nuttelman, C. R., Tripodi, M. C., and Anseth, K. S. (2006). Dexamethasone-functionalized gels induce osteogenic differentiation of encapsulated hMSCs. *J. Biomed. Mater. Res. A* 76, 183–195. doi:10.1002/jbm.a.30537

89. Ohmuro-Matsuyama, Y., and Tatsu, Y. (2008). Photocontrolled cell adhesion on a surface functionalized with a caged arginine-glycine-aspartate peptide. *Angew. Chem. Int. Ed. Engl.* 47, 7527–7529. doi:10.1002/anie.200802731

90. Oreffo, R. O. C., Cooper, C., Mason, C., and Clements, M. (2005). Mesenchymal stem cells: lineage, plasticity, and skeletal therapeutic potential. *Stem Cell. Rev.* 1, 169–178. doi:10.1385/SCR:1:2:169

91. Ott, H. C., Matthiesen, T. S., Goh, S. K., Black, L. D., Kren, S. M., Netoff, T. I., et al. (2008). Perfusion-decellularized matrix: using nature's platform to engineer

a bioartificial heart. *Nat. Med.* 14, 213–221. doi:10.1038/nm1684

92. Paszek, M. J., Zahir, N., Johnson, K. R., Lakins, J. N., Rozenberg, G. I., Gefen, A., et al. (2005). Tensional homeostasis and the malignant phenotype. *Cancer Cell* 8, 241–254. doi:10.1016/j.ccr.2005.08.010

93. Petersen, S., Alonso, J. M., Specht, A., Duodu, P., Goeldner, M., and del Campo, A. (2008). Phototriggering of cell adhesion by caged cyclic RGD peptides. *Angew. Chem. Int. Ed. Engl.* 47, 3192–3195. doi:10.1002/anie.200704857

94. Pittenger, M. F. (2008). Mesenchymal stem cells from adult bone marrow. *Methods Mol. Biol.* 449, 27–44. doi:10.1007/978-1-60327-169-1_2

95. Pouille, P. A., Ahmadi, P., Brunet, A. C., and Farge, E. (2009). Mechanical signals trigger myosin II redistribution and mesoderm invagination in *Drosophila* embryos. *Sci. Signal.* 2, ra16. doi:10.1126/scisignal.2000098

96. Prusty, D., Park, B.-H., Davis, K. E., and Farmer, S. R. (2002). Activation of MEK/ERK signaling promotes adipogenesis by enhancing peroxisome proliferator-activated receptor gamma (PPARgamma) and C/EBPalpha gene expression during the differentiation of 3T3-L1 preadipocytes. *J. Biol. Chem.* 277, 46226–46232. doi:10.1074/jbc.M207776200

97. Putnam, A. J., Schultz, K., and Mooney, D. J. (2001). Control of microtubule assembly by extracellular matrix and externally applied strain. *Am. J. Physiol. Cell Physiol.* 280, C556–C564.

98. Qin, D., Xia, Y., and Whitesides, G. M. (2010). Soft lithography for micro- and nanoscale patterning. *Nat. Protoc.* 5, 491–502. doi:10.1038/nprot.2009.234

99. Rahman, M. S., Akhtar, N., Jamil, H. M., Banik, R. S., and Asaduzzaman, S. M. (2015). TGF-beta/BMP signaling and other molecular events: regulation of osteoblastogenesis and bone formation. *Bone Res.* 3, 15005. doi:10.1038/boneres.2015.5

100. Rawsterne, R. E., Todd, S. J., Gough, J. E., Farrar, D., Rutten, F. J., Alexander, M. R., et al. (2007). Cell spreading correlates with calculated logP of amino acid-modified surfaces. *Acta Biomater.* 3, 715–721. doi:10.1016/j.actbio.2007.02.006

101. Rim, N. G., Shin, C. S., and Shin, H. (2013). Current approaches to electrospun nanofibers for tissue engineering. *Biomed. Mater.* 8, 014102. doi:10.1088/1748-6041/8/1/014102

102. Riveline, D., Zamir, E., Balaban, N. Q., Schwarz, U. S., Ishizaki, T., Narumiya, S., et al. (2001). Focal contacts as mechanosensors: externally applied local mechanical force induces growth of focal contacts by an mDia1-dependent and ROCK-independent mechanism. *J. Cell Biol.* 153, 1175–1186. doi:10.1083/jcb.153.6.1175

103. Ruoslahti, E., and Pierschbacher, M. D. (1987). New perspectives in cell adhesion: RGD and integrins. *Science* 238, 491–497. doi:10.1126/science.2821619

104. Shemesh, T., Geiger, B., Bershadsky, A. D., and Kozlov, M. M. (2005). Focal adhesions as mechanosensors: a physical mechanism. *Proc. Natl. Acad. Sci. U.S.A.* 102, 12383–12388. doi:10.1073/pnas.0500254102

105. Sjöström, T., Dalby, M. J., Hart, A., Tare, R., Oreffo, R. O., and Su, B. (2009). Fabrication of pillar-like titania nanostructures on titanium and their interactions with human skeletal stem cells. *Acta Biomater.* 5, 1433–1441. doi:10.1016/j.actbio.2009.01.007

106. Sjöström, T., McNamara, L. E., Meek, R. M. D., Dalby, M. J., and Su, B. (2013). 2D and 3D nanopatterning of titanium for enhancing osteoinduction of stem cells at implant surfaces. *Adv. Healthc. Mater.* 2, 1285–1293. doi:10.1002/adhm.201200353

107. Sjöström, T., McNamara, L. E., Yang, L., Dalby, M. J., and Su, B. (2012). Novel anodization technique using a block copolymer template for nanopatterning of titanium implant surfaces. *ACS Appl. Mater. Interfaces* 4, 6354–6361. doi:10.1021/am301987e

108. Teixeira, A. I., McKie, G. A., Foley, J. D., Bertics, P. J., Nealey, P. F., and Murphy, C. J. (2006). The effect of environmental factors on the response of human corneal epithelial cells to nanoscale substrate topography. *Biomaterials* 27, 3945–3954. doi:10.1016/j.biomaterials.2006.01.044

109. Todd, S. J., Farrar, D., Gough, J. E., and Ulijn, R. V. (2007). Enzyme-triggered cell attachment to hydrogel surfaces. *Soft Matter* 3, 547–550. doi:10.1039/b618256a

110. Tourniaire, G., Collins, J., Campbell, S., Mizomoto, H., Ogawa, S., Thaburet, J. F., et al. (2006). Polymer microarrays for cellular adhesion. *Chem. Commun.* 2118–2120. doi:10.1039/b602009g

111. Trappmann, B., Gautrot, J. E., Connelly, J. T., Strange, D. G., Li, Y., Oyen, M. L., et al. (2012). Extracellular-matrix tethering regulates stem-cell fate. *Nat. Mater.* 11, 642–649. doi:10.1038/nmat3339

112. Tsimbouri, P. M., McMurray, R. J., Burgess, K. V., Alakpa, E. V., Reynolds, P. M., Murawski, K., et al. (2012). Using nanotopography and metabolomics to identify biochemical effectors of multipotency. *ACS Nano* 6, 10239–10249. doi:10.1021/nn304046m

113. Tsimbouri, P. M., Murawski, K., Hamilton, G., Herzyk, P., Oreffo, R. O., Gadegaard, N., et al. (2013). A genomics approach in determining nanotopographical effects on MSC phenotype. *Biomaterials* 34, 2177–2184. doi:10.1016/j.biomaterials.2012.12.019

114. Visse, R., and Nagase, H. (2003). Matrix metalloproteinases and tissue inhibitors of metalloproteinases – structure, function, and biochemistry. *Circ. Res.* 92, 827–839. doi:10.1161/01.RES.0000070112.80711.3D

115. Watt, F. M., and Hogan, B. L. M. (2000). Out of Eden: stem cells and their niches. *Science* 287, 1427–1430. doi:10.1126/science.287.5457.1427

116. Weber, L. M., Hayda, K. N., Haskins, K., and Anseth, K. S. (2007). The effects of cell-matrix interactions on encapsulated beta-cell function within hydrogels functionalized with matrix-derived adhesive peptides. *Biomaterials* 28, 3004–3011. doi:10.1016/j.biomaterials.2007.03.005

117. Wei, S. C., Fattet, L., Tsai, J. H., Guo, Y., Pai, V. H., Majeski, H. E., et al. (2015).

Matrix stiffness drives epithelial-mesenchymal transition and tumour metastasis through a TWIST1-G3BP2 mechanotransduction pathway. *Nat. Cell Biol.* 17, 678–688. doi:10.1038/ncb3157

118. Weiss, P., and Garber, B. (1952). Shape and movement of mesenchyme cells as functions of the physical structure of the medium – contributions to a quantitative morphology. *Proc. Natl. Acad. Sci. U.S.A.* 38, 264–280. doi:10.1073/pnas.38.3.264

119. Wen, J. H., Vincent, L. G., Fuhrmann, A., Choi, Y. S., Hribar, K. C., Taylor-Weiner, H., et al. (2014). Interplay of matrix stiffness and protein tethering in stem cell differentiation. *Nat. Mater.* 13, 979–987. doi:10.1038/nmat4051

120. Wilkinson, C. D. (2004). Making structures for cell engineering. *Eur. Cell. Mater.* 8, 21–26.

121. Wirkner, M., Alonso, J. M., Maus, V., Salierno, M., Lee, T. T., García, A. J., et al. (2011a). Triggered cell release from materials using bioadhesive photocleavable linkers. *Adv. Mater. Weinheim* 23, 3907–3910. doi:10.1002/adma.201100925

122. Wirkner, M., Weis, S., San Miguel, V., Álvarez, M., Gropeanu, R. A., Salierno, M., et al. (2011b). Photoactivatable caged cyclic RGD peptide for triggering integrin binding and cell adhesion to surfaces. *Chembiochem* 12, 2623–2629. doi:10.1002/cbic.201100437

123. Xiao, G., Jiang, D., Gopalakrishnan, R., and Franceschi, R. T. (2002). Fibroblast growth factor 2 induction of the osteocalcin gene requires MAPK activity and phosphorylation of the osteoblast transcription factor, Cbfa1/Runx2. *J. Biol. Chem.* 277, 36181–36187. doi:10.1074/jbc.M206057200

124. Yamada, K. M. (1991). Adhesive recognition sequences. *J. Biol. Chem.* 266, 12809–12812.

125. Yamato, M., Konno, C., Utsumi, M., Kikuchi, A., and Okano, T. (2002). Thermally responsive polymer-grafted surfaces facilitate patterned cell seeding and co-culture. *Biomaterials* 23, 561–567. doi:10.1016/S0142-9612(01)00138-7

126. Yang, C., Tibbitt, M. W., Basta, L., and Anseth, K. S. (2014). Mechanical memory and dosing influence stem cell fate. *Nat. Mater.* 13, 645–652. doi:10.1038/nmat3889

127. Yang, X., Harkins, L. K., Zubanova, O., Harrington, A., Kovalenko, D., Nadeau, R. J., et al. (2008). Overexpression of Spry1 in chondrocytes causes attenuated FGFR ubiquitination and sustained ERK activation resulting in chondrodysplasia. *Dev. Biol.* 321, 64–76. doi:10.1016/j.ydbio.2008.05.555

128. Yeo, W. S., Yousaf, M. N., and Mrksich, M. (2003). Dynamic interfaces between cells and surfaces: electroactive substrates that sequentially release and attach cells. *J. Am. Chem. Soc.* 125, 14994–14995. doi:10.1021/ja038265b

129. Yim, E. K. F., Pang, S. W., and Leong, K. W. (2007). Synthetic nanostructures inducing differentiation of human mesenchymal stem cells into neuronal lineage. *Exp. Cell Res.* 313, 1820–1829. doi:10.1016/j.yexcr.2007.02.031

130. Zelzer, M., Scurr, D. J., Alexander, M. R., and Ulijn, R. V. (2012). Development

and validation of a fluorescence method to follow the build-up of short peptide sequences on solid 2D surfaces. *ACS Appl. Mater. Interfaces* 4, 53–58. doi:10.1021/am2015266

131. Zhang, Y., Ouyang, H., Chwee, T. L., Ramakrishna, S., and Huang, Z. M. (2005). Electrospinning of gelatin fibers and gelatin/PCL composite fibrous scaffolds. *J. Biomed. Mater. Res. Part B Appl. Biomater.* 72, 156–165. doi:10.1002/jbm.b.30128

4
CHAPTER

BONE DEFECT REGENERATION BY A COMBINATION OF A β-TRICALCIUM PHOSPHATE SCAFFOLD AND BONE MARROW STROMAL CELLS IN A NON-HUMAN PRIMATE MODEL

Tomokazu Masaoka, Toshitaka Yoshii, Masato Yuasa, Tsuyoshi Yamada, Takashi Taniyama, Ichiro Torigoe, Kenichi Shinomiya, Atsushi Okawa, Sadao Morita, Shinichi Sotome

Keywords: Bone marrow-derived stromal cells, bone regeneration, long bone defect, non-human primate, tissue engineering, β-tricalcium phosphate

INTRODUCTION

Autologous bone grafts, allografts and alternative biomaterials have been used to reconstruct large bone defects. Among them, autologous grafts have the highest osteogenic capability and sufficient mechanical strength, are free from virus transmission, and do not induce immune responses. However, the amount of autologous bone available for grafting is limited and the harvesting of bone grafts is associated with a relatively high risk of donor site morbidity, hematoma, and nerve injury [1-3]. Allografts offer osteoconductivity and mechanical strength at least immediately after surgery, and the use of allograft bone is unaffected by supply limitations. However, the characteristics of the allografts vary depending on the type of allograft and the preparation method. Furthermore, a relatively high complication rate has been reported for massive intercalary grafts in the treatment of osseous neoplasms, and for patients receiving adjuvant therapy, the survival rate of the allograft decreases to 50% within 10 years [4]. Synthetic calcium phosphate bonegraft substitutes composed of

Citation: Tomokazu Masaoka, Toshitaka Yoshii, Masato Yuasa, Tsuyoshi Yamada, Takashi Taniyama, Ichiro Torigoe, Kenichi Shinomiya,Atsushi Okawa, Sadao Morita, Shinichi Sotome, Bone Defect Regeneration by a Combination of a β-Tricalcium Phosphate Scaffold and Bone Marrow Stromal Cells in a Non-Human Primate Model, DOI: 10.2174/1874120701610010002.

hydroxyapatite and/or tricalcium phosphates (TCPs) were developed to address these drawbacks,and the use of these materials is not hindered by the risk of virus transmission or limited availability. The osteogenic capacityof such grafts has been increased through continuous developmentof synthetic bone-graft substitutes; however,the osteogenic capabilityis still not sufficient for treating large bone defects.

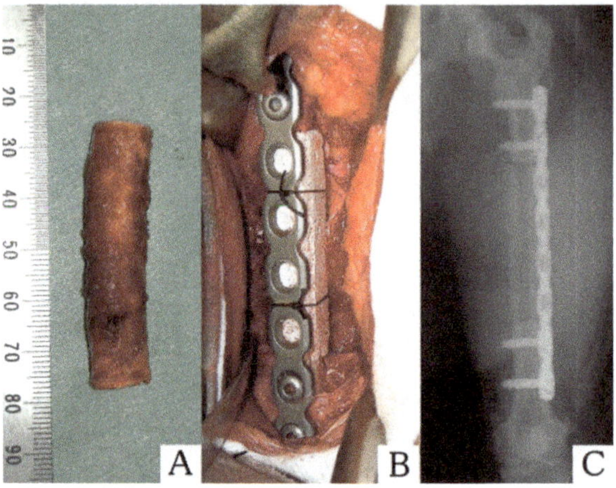

Figure 1: Transplantation of a β-TCP block (control) in a large bone-defect model in macaques. Here, a 5-cm-long diaphysis segment was resected from the left femur (A). A β-TCP block was then transplanted into the bone defect and fixed to a titanium plate with two sutures (B). X-ray image of the transplanted femur (C).

Bone marrow-derived stromal cells (BMSCs) expanded by common culture protocols can differentiate into not only osteogenic cells but also chondrogenic, adipogenic, and other mesenchymal lineages [5]. Following the demonstration of bone formation by BMSCs, tissue engineering approaches using BMSCs have attracted attention for large bone-defect reconstruction [6]. Various studies have been conducted to augment the osteogenic capability of implants prepared using BMSCs to realize large bone-defect regeneration. However, satisfactory results have not been reported to date.

In this study, we present a combination of three modifications to the original concept of BMSC-based bone tissue engineering: culturing of BMSCs with continuous dexamethasone treatment [7] loading of cells into porous scaffolds under low pressure [8] and cell loading using autologous plasma as a cell loading medium [9]. Each of these modifications improved the bone formation capability by several fold compared with the conventional technique. Therefore, the total improvement achieved by the combined effect was greater than 10 fold. The aim of this study was to evaluate the effectiveness of porous β-TCP/BMSC hybrid implants prepared by combining these modifications for regeneration of large bone defects in a non-human primate model and to assess the resulting bone union capacity, which is an essential property for bone tissue and regenerated bone.

MATERIALS AND METHODS

All animal experiments were approved by the animal committee of Tokyo Medical and Dental University and were conducted according to the guidelines provided by the committee.

Study Design

A primary surgery was performed to assess the osteoconductivity of a porous β-TCP block without cells in a 5-cm-long femur bone defect. A secondary surgery was conducted to evaluate the effectiveness of β-TCP combined with BMSCs for regeneration of the large bone defect. To emphasize the effectiveness, the secondary surgery was conducted at the same site as the primary surgery, where the environment was considered to be more disadvantageous for bone regeneration than that of the native bone subjected to the primary surgery. In a third surgery, osteotomy of the femur was performed to evaluate the bone union capability of the regenerated bone.

Primary Surgery: Transplantation of β-TCP

Nine skeletally mature cynomolgus monkeys (male, 5.7 to 7.2 kg) were used in this study and were divided into two groups: a periosteum-preserved group (n=4) and a periosteum-resected group (n=5). Under general anesthesia achieved by intramuscular administration of medetomidine hydrochloride (0.5 mg/kg) and ketamine hydrochloride (25 mg/kg), the animals were intubated, and general anesthesia was maintained with isoflurane. Each monkey was placed in the right lateral position, and the lateral side of the left femur was shaved. Following intramuscular injection of an antibiotic (cefazolin, 40mg/kg), the lateral aspect of the femur was sterilized with povidone iodine and covered with sterilized drapes, except for at the operative site. A 12-cm longitudinal incision was made at the lateral aspect of the femur, and the femur shaft was exposed by an intermuscular approach between the vastuslateralis and the biceps femoris. In the periosteum-preserved group, the periosteum was gently detached using a raspatrium, and a six-hole titanium alloy plate was contoured to the lateral aspect of the diaphysis and fixed with screws at the two proximal holes and two distal holes. A long bone segment (5 cm) was resected from the mid-diaphysis of the femur using a surgical saw. In the periosteum-resected group, when the resection site was approached, the thin layers of muscle surrounding the diaphysis were left attached to the femur to enable complete resection of the periosteum with the diaphysis. After plate fixation, the diaphysis, including the periosteum, was resected. In both groups, the resected segment was filled with hollowed porous β-TCP (Osferion®; Olympus, Tokyo, Japan). The specifications of the implant were as follows: porosity, 75%; dimensions, 1 x 1 x 5 cm; and diameter of the hollow, 3 mm. The implant was fixed to the plate by surgical nylon sutures, and the operative site was closed and sutured (Fig. 1). After surgery, the monkeys were allowed unlimited activity in the breeding cage.

Preparation of BMSCs

Bone marrow was harvested to obtain BMSCs 11 to 12 days prior to the secondary surgery. Under general anesthesia conducted as described above, 2.5-5.0 ml of bone marrow was aspirated from the bilateral iliac crest and the bilateral greater trochanters of the femurs of each macaque using a bone marrow biopsy needle (Cardinal Health, Dublin, OH) and combined with 30 ml of Dulbecco's modified Eagle medium (DMEM; Sigma Chemical, St. Louis, MO) containing 200 IU of sodium heparin. The bone marrow was centrifuged (450 g, 5 min), and the bone marrow cell sediment was suspended in DMEM containing 10% fetal bovine serum, 1% antibiotic-antimycotic (10,000 units/ml penicillin G sodium, 10 mg/ml streptomycin sulfate and 0.025 mg/ml amphotericin B; Life Technologies, Carlsbad, CA, USA) and 100 nM dexamethasone (Sigma-Aldrich, St. Louis, MO). The bone marrow was plated in 225-cm^2 culture flasks (BD Biosciences, Franklin Lakes, NJ) and cultured at 37°C in a humidified atmosphere with 5% CO_2. The culture medium was replaced every 3 to 4 days, and nonadherent cells were removed. After 7 days of culture, attached BMSCs were detached with 0.25% trypsin containing 1 mM EDTA (Life Technologies) and reseeded in 225-cm^2 culture flasks. The cells were detached and used for transplantation 4 to 5 days after subculture.

Preparation of the BMSC-Loaded Implant

To prepare autologous plasma as a carrier for BMSCs, 18 ml of venous blood was collected from the femoral vein into a polypropylene tube containing 2 ml of citrate phosphate dextrose (CPD) solution (2.63% sodium citrate, 0.327% citric acid, 2.32% dextrose, and 0.251% sodium dihydrogenphosphate; TERUMO, Tokyo, Japan). The blood was then centrifuged at 2400 g for 15 min, and the supernatant was transferred to a new tube as autologous plasma and stored at room temperature until the following cell loading procedure. To load the BMSCs into the porous β-TCP scaffold, our original cell loading method was used, based on spontaneous penetration under low-pressure conditions and the use of an original apparatus (Fig. 2). Briefly, the porous scaffold was set in a tube, as shown in Fig. (2). and the air inside the apparatus was removed by suction using a 100 ml syringe until the pressure reached 25 to 50 mmHg.

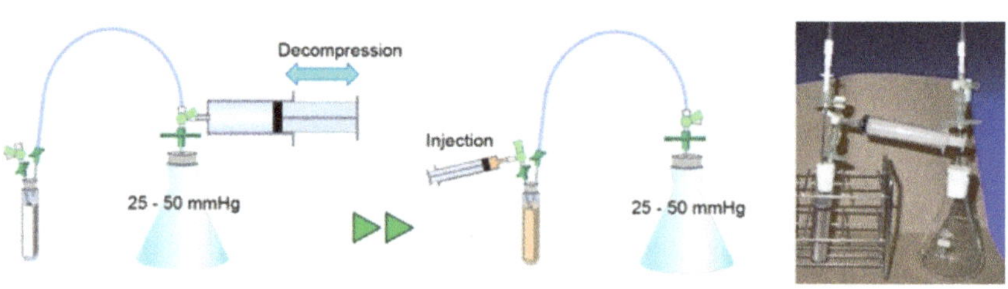

Figure 2: Introduction of a cell suspension into a porous β-TCP block. The inside of the device was decompressed to 25-50 mmHg by a syringe connected to a three-way stopcock. A cell suspension was injected into the evacuated tube in which the β-TCP block was placed, and the pressure was then regained by opening the stopcock.

The detached BMSCs were suspended in 7 ml of autologous plasma and transferred to a 10 ml syringe. Immediately after 1 ml of 2% $CaCl_2$ solution was added to initiate fibrin gel formation, the cell suspension was injected *via* a three-way stopcock into the bottom of the tube containing the scaffold. When the injection was complete, the tube was tapped to remove any bubbles attached to the scaffold, and the three-way stopcock was then released to recover normal pressure inside the apparatus. Within several minutes, gelation of the cell suspension was initiated, and the implant was withdrawn from the tube immediately before transplantation. The final cell concentration in the loaded fibrin gel was 1.3 x 10^6 to 4.1 x 10^6/ml.

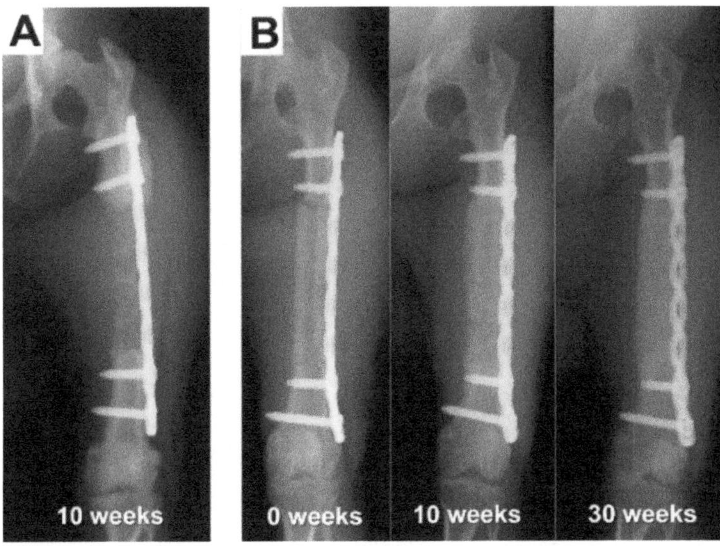

Figure 3: Transplantation of β-TCP blocks without cells. In the periosteum-resected group, bone regeneration was not achieved, and the β-TCP blocks were resorbed (A), except in one case. In this case, vigorous callus formation was observed at 10 weeks after surgery, and the regenerated bone matured (B).

Secondary Surgery: Transplantation of the BMSC-loaded Implant

Seven of the nine macaques that had undergone primary surgery 7 to 12 months before hand under went a secondary surgery in which a β-TCP scaffold combined with BMSCs was transplanted into the same defect site as in the primary surgery (Table 1). The interval between the primary surgery and the secondary surgery depended on how long it had taken to confirm the results of the primary surgery, as the nature of the second surgery performed depended on the results of the first surgery. In cases of bone regeneration failure, the secondary surgery had to be performed before the atrophy of the remnant bone progressed, and in the case of successful bone regeneration, the second surgery was performed after the bone maturation was confirmed radiographically. In the case of successful bone regeneration by the primary surgery, the regenerated bone was resected with the surrounding periosteum-like tissue and replaced with the implant. In the case of bone regeneration failure following the primary surgery, the soft tissue and remnant bone tissue formed at the transplantation site were resected with the fascia of the surrounding muscles facing the transplantation site to remove the periosteum completely, and a bone stump with the normal bone marrow cavity exposed was formed using a steel burr before transplantation.

Third Surgery: Evaluation of the Bone Union Capability of the Regenerated Bone

The bone union capability of the bone regenerated using the β-TCP/BMSC composite was evaluated in a femur osteotomy model. Five macaques whose femurs were successfully regenerated by the second surgery were included in this study 8 to 15 months after the second surgery (Table 1). Here, a 13-mm-long segment of the femur was resected from the center of the regenerated bone. The screws were removed from the two distal screw holes, and the plate was cut using a plate cutter at 13 mm from the distal end of the plate. The distal part of the femur was then fixed again at the two distal screw holes. Consequently, the femur was shortened, and the facing bone stumps were conjugated to the other because the interval between the screw holes was 13 mm. The resected bone segment was fixed in 10% neutral buffered formalin and used for histological evaluation.

Evaluation

For radiographic evaluation: antero-posterior and lateral X-ray images (60kV / 10mA / 0.3 sec) were collected at 2- to 4-week intervals under general anesthesia achieved by intramuscular administration of medetomidine hydrochloride (0.5 mg/kg) and ketamine hydrochloride (25 mg/kg), and bone regeneration and union were evaluated by two orthopaedic surgeons. For histological evaluation, the resected regenerated bone segments from the third surgery were fixed in formalin, decalcified with K-CX solution (Falma, Japan), dehydrated, embedded in paraffin, sectioned at a 5-μm thickness, and stained with hematoxylin and eosin.

Table 1: Schedules of implant surgery, surgical conditions and the results of bone regeneration

ID number	Transplantation of β-TCP (Primary surgery)		Interval (months)	Transplantation of the BMSC-loaded implant (Second surgery)			Interval (months)	Bone union capability (Third surgery)
	Periosteum	Result		Periosteum	Total cell number	Result		Result
1	(+)	Absorption	8	(-)	3.3×10^7	Bone regeneration	15	Union
2	(+)	Absorption	7	(-)	1.7×10^7	Bone regeneration	12	Union
3	(+)	Bone regeneration	10	(-)	1.0×10^7	Bone regeneration	12	Union
4	(+)	Bone regeneration	12	(-)	1.8×10^7	Bone regeneration	8	Non-union
5	(-)	Absorption	8	(-)	1.5×10^7	Bone regeneration	12	Union
6	(-)	Absorption	7	(-)	1.5×10^7	Absorption		
7	(-)	Absorption	12	(-)	3.3×10^7	Absorption		
8	(-)	Absorption						
9	(-)	Bone regeneration						

RESULTS

Transplantation of Porous β–TCP Without BMSCs

All of the animals, including those whose femurs were not regenerated, were able to walk and move freely throughout the experimental period, indicating that the plate fixation provided sufficient strength. In the periosteum-preserved group, two cases showed bone regeneration throughout the defect site, whereas the other two cases showed only partial and intermittent bone formation, and most of the transplanted β-TCP was resorbed within 12 weeks. In the periosteum-resected group, one case unexpectedly showed complete bone regeneration (Fig. 3B, Table 1), whereas four of the five cases failed to achieve bone regeneration, as predicted (Fig. 3A, Table 1). In the bone-regenerated cases, bone formation appeared to occur not only from the osteotomy stumps but also evenly throughout the transplanted site and surrounding area, indicating that bone-forming osteoblasts originated from not only the adjacent bone marrow but also the surrounding periosteum or muscle tissue.

Transplantation of the Porous β–TCP/BMSC Hybrid

Regardless of the results of the primary surgery, all four macaques in the periosteum-preserved group and three macaques in the periosteum-resected group were used for evaluation of the BMSC-loaded implant. Five of the seven cases showed successful bone regeneration (Fig. 4, Table 1), and two cases resulted in failure. A statistical comparison with the control without BMSCs was not performed because the number of animals was small and because the environment at the transplanted sites was different from that at the sites of the first surgery. There was no correlation between the bone regeneration results and the transplanted cell number.

Bone Union Capability of the Regenerated Femurs

Five regenerated femurs were tested for their bone union capability, which is one of the most important characteristics of natural living bone. Four of the five shortened regenerated bones showed bone union that could easily be identified from X-ray images (Fig. 5, Table 1). In the case of bone union failure, the gap between the bone stumps was relatively large (1.5 to 2.0 mm) because of poor surgical technique, and a higher amount of β-TCP remnants was recognized in the resected bone tissue by macroscopic observation compared with the other cases (Fig. 6B).

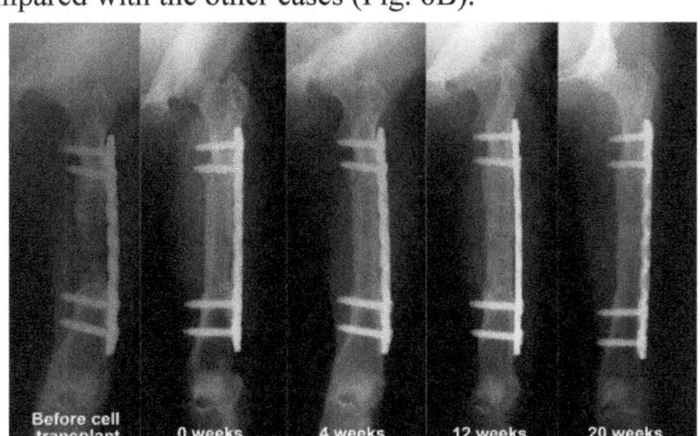

Figure 4: Transplantation of β-TCP with BMSCs. After the bone tissue remnants and the scar

tissue formed at the defect site were removed, a β-TCP block combined with BMSCs was transplanted into the defect. The X-ray images correspond to before cell transplantation; at transplantation; and 4, 12, and 20 weeks after transplantation.

Histology

The center portion of the regenerated bone resected in the third surgery was used for histological evaluation. The bone tissue on the medial side of the regenerated femur was dense and matured nearly equally to normal cortical bone. In contrast, the bone tissue on the titanium plate side was not as dense and mature as that on the medial side because of stress shielding. In contrast to the normal diaphysis, which consists of a hollow cortical bone and fatty marrow that fills the cavity, most of the regenerated bone was cancellous bone-like tissue exhibiting blood vessels and incorporated β-TCP remnants (Fig. 6A). The regenerated bone in the case with union failure included more abundant β-TCP remnants, as also determined by macroscopic observation. However, more osteoclast-like multinucleated cells were attached to the remnants. Therefore, the abundance of remnants would have likely decreased if harvesting had been conducted at a later time point, and bone union may have been achieved.

DISCUSSION

In this study, we succeeded in the regeneration of 5 cm long bone defects using porous β-TCP blocks with or without BMSCs in a non-human primate model. The success rate of the β-TCP/BMSC hybrid was higher than that of β-TCP alone, although a statistical analysis was not performed. The regenerated bone exhibited bone union capability, which is one of the most important characteristics of natural living bone.

The reconstruction of large bone defects caused by bone tumors, trauma, and infection is a major challenge in the orthopedic field. Many studies have attempted the reconstruction of large bone defect, and large animal models have been used in such studies to verify the practicality of the results. Mastrogiacomo *et al.* reported the osteoconductivity of a scaffold composed of hydroxyapatite and silicon-stabilized TCP in a 4.8 cm long tibia defect model [10] and then reported enhanced osteoconductivity when using the same scaffold combined with BMSCs ina 4.5 cm tibia defect model [11]. These findings indicate the insufficiency of scaffold transplantation alone and the efficacy of scaffold-BMSC transplantation for large bone defect reconstruction. Other reports have also demonstrated the effectiveness of BMSCs for reconstruction of large bone defects [12-15].

To augment bone formation by BMSCs using the conventional method developed by Caplan *et al.* [6] various methods, such as gene transfer and perfusion culture, have been attempted. In the present study, we implemented three modifications to the conventional method to facilitate large scale bone regeneration.

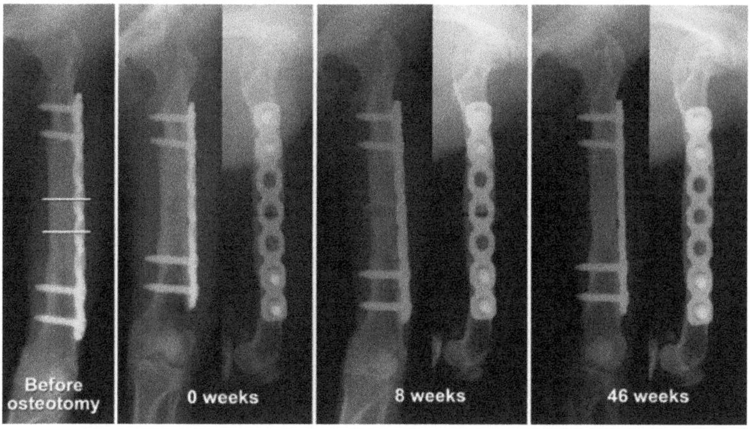

Figure 5: The center portion of the regenerated bone (between the white lines, length of 13 mm) was resected, and the femur was shortened and fixed to a plate. Callus formation at the osteotomy site was observed at 8 weeks after surgery, and bone union was completed by 46 weeks.

The first modification involved optimization of the cell culture method to obtain BMSCs with a higher differentiation capability. A popular osteogenic induction protocol for BMSCs uses dexamethasone only during the induction of differentiation with ascorbic acid phosphate and β-glycerophosphate. In contrast to the standard protocol, the culture protocol used in this study used dexamethasone during the entire BMSC proliferation period. A previous study demonstrated that human BMSCs proliferated in dexamethasone-containing medium presented higher enhanced differentiation not only into the osteogenic lineage but also into the chondrogenic and adipogenic lineages, and furthermore that the bone formation capability of macaque BMSCs that proliferated in the presence of dexamethasone was at least two-fold higher than that in control medium [7].

The second modification that we applied was cell loading under a low pressure system. To efficiently infiltrate liquid into porous materials, it is important to remove the air inside the pores; therefore, low pressure has been generally applied after immersion of the material to remove residual air. However, the complete removal of residual air from the immersed porous material is prevented by the surface tension of the surrounding liquid. In the present study, low pressure was thus applied to the porous scaffolds before immersion in the cell suspension to more efficiently remove the air from the porous materials. Using 5 mm cubic, porous β-TCP blocks and a heterotopic bone formation model with rat BMSCs, previous studies demonstrated that the cell loading efficiency and bone formation of hybrid implants prepared under the low pressure cell loading method were increased by 2 and 2.5 fold, respectively, compared with preparation by removal of air after immersion [8].

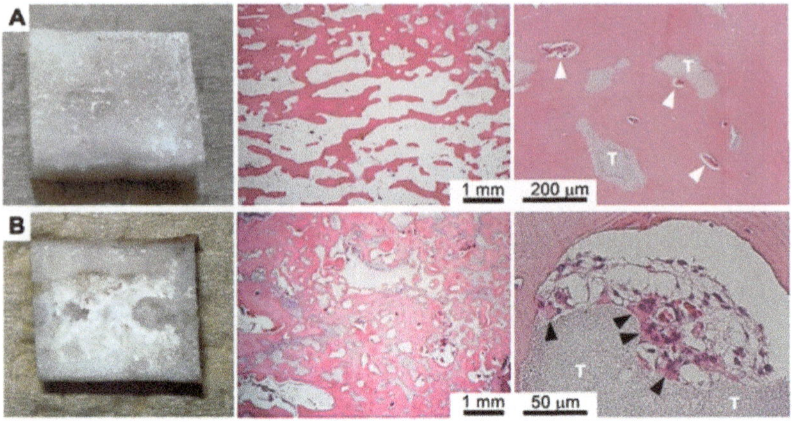

Figure 6: Resected diaphysis at the osteotomy surgery site and histological specimens stained with hematoxylin and eosin. Most of the β-TCP was absorbed and replaced by bone tissue and bone marrow tissue (A). In the case of bone union failure, more β-TCP persisted than in the other cases (B). However, continued β-TCP absorption by osteoclast-like cells was also confirmed. T: remnant of β-TCP. The white arrowheads indicate blood vessels. The black arrowheads indicate osteoclast-like cells.

The third modification that we applied was related to the cell loading medium. When BMSCs were introduced into the porous scaffold, we used autologous blood plasma as a cell suspension medium; in contrast, BMSCs are suspended in the culture medium in conventional methods. Because the introduced plasma formed a fibrin gel within minutes in the pores of the porous scaffolds and the BMSCs were firmly maintained within the gel, the implant could be transplanted without waiting for cell attachment to the scaffold. Thus, this method would be convenient for use in the clinic; furthermore, preparation of BMSCs in this manner has been shown to augment bone formation in heterotopic bone formation models. In particular, for bone formation using a macaque heterotopic bone formation model, it was shown that a hybrid implant of a porous scaffold and BMSCs prepared using autologous plasma required one-tenth of the number of cells needed when culture medium was used as the cell loading medium [9]. Thus, BMSCs suspended in plasma showed a ten-fold increase in bone formation compared to the same number of BMSCs prepared using conventional techniques.

The combination of these modifications should greatly augment bone formation capability relative to the conventional method and contribute to the regeneration of 5 cm long bone defects. However, in the present study, some cases of control implants that did not receive BMSCs also achieved bone regeneration, and in such cases, bone formation did not necessarily occur from the femur stumps. Recently, intramuscular osteoinduction by biomaterials has been reported [16-22] and this osteoinduction was associated with two common factors: the use of a large-animal model, such as baboons, dogs, or sheep [22] and the use of a material with a macroporous or microporous structure to increase the specific surface area [19, 21]. The present study used a macaque large-animal model, and the porous β-TCP had macropores and micropores.The findings reported herein demonstrate that porous β-TCP has strong osteoconductivity and possibly osteoinductivity, and that β-TCP can function as a fourth factor in addition to the three modifications we made to the BMSC preparation protocol to augment bone formation in large bone defects.

This study demonstrated the efficacy of β-TCP/BMSC hybrid transplantation for 5 cm long critical-size bone defects using a non-human primate model and revealed the bone union capability of the regenerated bone. However, two of the seven BMSC transplanted cases failed to show bone regeneration, and the extent of regeneration was not correlated with the transplanted cell number. This finding suggests that the quality of the BMSCs used for transplantation is more important than the number of transplanted BMSCs as reported in the literature [23]. Criteria for appropriate preparation of BMSCs for transplantation should be established for safe and reliable BMSC based clinical bone regeneration.

ACKNOWLEDGEMENTS

This work was supported by a Grant-in-Aid for Scientific Research from the Ministry of Education, Culture, Sports, Science and Technology of Japan. We also acknowledge Olympus Co. for kindly donating the β-TCP ceramic blocks.

REFERENCES

1. N.A. Ebraheim, H. Elgafy, and H.B. Semaan, "Computed tomographic findings in patients with persistent sacroiliac pain after posterior iliac graft harvesting", Spine (Phila Pa 1976), vol. 25, pp. 2047-2051, 2000.
2. D.H. Kim, R. Rhim, L. Li, J. Martha, B.H. Swaim, R.J. Banco, L.G. Jenis, and S.G. Tromanhauser, "Prospective study of iliac crest bone graft harvest site pain and morbidity", Spine J., vol. 9, no. 11, pp. 886-892, 2009.
3. C. Myeroff, and M. Archdeacon, "Autogenous bone graft: donor sites and techniques", J. Bone Joint Surg. Am., vol. 93, no. 23, pp. 2227-2236, 2011.
4. E. Ortiz-Cruz, M.C. Gebhardt, L.C. Jennings, D.S. Springfield, and H.J. Mankin, "The results of transplantation of intercalary allografts after resection of tumors. A long-term follow-up study", J. Bone Joint Surg. Am., vol. 79, no. 1, pp. 97-106, 1997.
5. M.F. Pittenger, A.M. Mackay, S.C. Beck, R.K. Jaiswal, R. Douglas, J.D. Mosca, M.A. Moorman, D.W. Simonetti, S. Craig, and D.R. Marshak, "Multilineage potential of adult human mesenchymal stem cells", Science, vol. 284, no. 5411, pp. 143-147, 1999.
6. J. Goshima, V.M. Goldberg, and A.I. Caplan, "The osteogenic potential of culture-expanded rat marrow mesenchymal cells assayed in vivo in calcium phosphate ceramic blocks", Clin. Orthop. Relat. Res., no. 262, pp. 298-311, 1991.
7. H. Oshina, S. Sotome, T. Yoshii, I. Torigoe, Y. Sugata, H. Maehara, E. Marukawa, K. Omura, and K. Shinomiya, "Effects of continuous dexamethasone treatment on differentiation capabilities of bone marrow-derived mesenchymal cells",

Bone, vol. 41, no. 4, pp. 575-583, 2007.

8. I. Torigoe, S. Sotome, A. Tsuchiya, T. Yoshii, M. Takahashi, S. Kawabata, and K. Shinomiya, “Novel cell seeding system into a porous scaffold using a modified low-pressure method to enhance cell seeding efficiency and bone formation”, Cell Transplant., vol. 16, no. 7, pp. 729-739, 2007.

9. I. Torigoe, S. Sotome, A. Tsuchiya, T. Yoshii, H. Maehara, Y. Sugata, S. Ichinose, K. Shinomiya, and A. Okawa, “Bone regeneration with autologous plasma, bone marrow stromal cells, and porous β-tricalcium phosphate in nonhuman primates”, Tissue Eng. Part A, vol. 15, no. 7, pp. 1489-1499, 2009.

10. M. Mastrogiacomo, A. Corsi, E. Francioso, M. Di Comite, F. Monetti, S. Scaglione, A. Favia, A. Crovace, P. Bianco, and R. Cancedda, “Reconstruction of extensive long bone defects in sheep using resorbable bioceramics based on silicon stabilized tricalcium phosphate”, Tissue Eng., vol. 12, no. 5, pp. 1261-1273, 2006.

11. P. Giannoni, M. Mastrogiacomo, M. Alini, S.G. Pearce, A. Corsi, F. Santolini, A. Muraglia, P. Bianco, and R. Cancedda, “Regeneration of large bone defects in sheep using bone marrow stromal cells”, J. Tissue Eng. Regen. Med., vol. 2, no. 5, pp. 253-262, 2008.

12. G. Liu, L. Zhao, W. Zhang, L. Cui, W. Liu, and Y. Cao, “Repair of goat tibial defects with bone marrow stromal cells and β-tricalcium phosphate”, J. Mater. Sci. Mater. Med., vol. 19, no. 6, pp. 2367-2376, 2008.

13. M.B. Nair, H.K. Varma, K.V. Menon, S.J. Shenoy, and A. John, “Tissue regeneration and repair of goat segmental femur defect with bioactive triphasic ceramic-coated hydroxyapatite scaffold”, J. Biomed. Mater. Res. A, vol. 91, no. 3, pp. 855-865, 2009.

14. X. Liu, X. Li, Y. Fan, G. Zhang, D. Li, W. Dong, Z. Sha, X. Yu, Q. Feng, F. Cui, and F. Watari, “Repairing goat tibia segmental bone defect using scaffold cultured with mesenchymal stem cells”, J. Biomed. Mater. Res. B Appl. Biomater., vol. 94, no. 1, pp. 44-52, 2010.

15. J. Huang, L. Zhang, B. Chu, X. Peng, and S. Tang, “Repair of bone defect in caprine tibia using a laminated scaffold with bone marrow stromal cells loaded poly (L-lactic acid)/β-tricalcium phosphate”, Artif. Organs, vol. 35, no. 1, pp. 49-57, 2011.

16. U. Ripamonti, B. Van den Heever, and J. Van Wyk, “Expression of the osteogenic phenotype in porous hydroxyapatite implanted extraskeletally in baboons”, Matrix, vol. 13, no. 6, pp. 491-502, 1993.

17. U. Ripamonti, “Osteoinduction in porous hydroxyapatite implanted in heterotopic sites of different animal models”, Biomaterials, vol. 17, no. 1, pp. 31-35, 1996.

18. Z. Yang, H. Yuan, W. Tong, P. Zou, W. Chen, and X. Zhang, “Osteogenesis in extraskeletally implanted porous calcium phosphate ceramics: variability among different kinds of animals”, Biomaterials, vol. 17, no. 22, pp. 2131-2137, 1996.

19. S. Fujibayashi, M. Neo, H.M. Kim, T. Kokubo, and T. Nakamura, “Osteoinduction

of porous bioactive titanium metal", Biomaterials, vol. 25, no. 3, pp. 443-450, 2004.

20. D. Le Nihouannen, G. Daculsi, A. Saffarzadeh, O. Gauthier, S. Delplace, P. Pilet, and P. Layrolle, "Ectopic bone formation by microporous calcium phosphate ceramic particles in sheep muscles", Bone, vol. 36, no. 6, pp. 1086-1093, 2005.
21. P. Habibovic, T.M. Sees, M.A. van den Doel, C.A. van Blitterswijk, and K. de Groot, "Osteoinduction by biomaterials-physicochemical and structural influences", J. Biomed. Mater. Res. A, vol. 77, no. 4, pp. 747-762, 2006.
22. N. Akiyama, M. Takemoto, S. Fujibayashi, M. Neo, M. Hirano, and T. Nakamura, "Difference between dogs and rats with regard to osteoclast-like cells in calcium-deficient hydroxyapatite-induced osteoinduction", J. Biomed. Mater. Res. A, vol. 96, no. 2, pp. 402-412, 2011.
23. T. Yamada, M. Yuasa, T. Masaoka, T. Taniyama, H. Maehara, I. Torigoe, T. Yoshii, K. Shinomiya, A. Okawa, and S. Sotome, "After repeated division, bone marrow stromal cells express inhibitory factors with osteogenic capabilities, and EphA5 is a primary candidate", Bone, vol. 57, no. 2, pp. 343-354, 2013.

5
CHAPTER

MESENCHYMAL STEM CELL MORPHOLOGY AND MIGRATION ON MICROTEXTURED TITANIUM

Brittany L. Banik, Thomas R. Riley, Christina J. Platt and Justin L. Brown

Keywords: Cell–material interactions, titanium (alloys), PEEK, spinal implant, regenerative medicine

INTRODUCTION

Spinal fusion surgery combines (or fuses) two or more vertebrae together to reduce discomfort by immobilizing a painful vertebral motion segment and restoring spinal stability (Williams et al., 2005;Nouh, 2012; Obrigkeit et al., 2012). Following surgery, it can take 6–12 months for the fusion process to occur (Obrigkeit et al., 2012). During the fusion process, implant osseointegration is critical (Olivares-Navarrete et al., 2010).

Autografts and allografts are often viewed as the "gold standard" in many biomedical applications; however, bone material donations have complications. Specifically for spinal fusion cages, the issues include an unpredictable nature due to an inconsistency in mechanical strength, machining challenges, and migration issues (Rihn et al., 2009; Obrigkeit et al., 2012). Titanium and polyetheretherketone (PEEK) implants are among the most common alternatives to bone (Abernathie and Pfeiffer, 2011;Cabraja et al., 2012; Obrigkeit et al., 2012).

Citation: Banik BL, Riley TR, Platt CJ and Brown JL (2016) Mesenchymal Stem Cell Morphology and Migration on Microtextured Titanium. Front. Bioeng. Biotechnol. 4:41. doi: 10.3389/fbioe.2016.00041.

Cell–material interactions are of particular interest in biomedical implants because the initial contact between the cells and the biomaterial can define the success of the device. As part of the tissue microenvironment presented to the cells, the surface morphology and chosen material are integral in this interaction and the cellular response – adhesion, spreading, migration, proliferation, and differentiation – ultimately contributing to the fate of the cells and tissue formation (Bächle and Kohal, 2004; Anselme and Bigerelle, 2005; Zhao et al., 2011). The surface features on the fusion host environment have key roles in the fusion process.

Textured surface features are of specific interest because cells interact with the extracellular environment through micro- (e.g., organelles) and nanoscale (e.g., protein complexes, such as focal adhesions). When a surface demonstrates a characteristic dimension on the same order of magnitude as protein complexes up to organelles, the response of the cell can be modulated through a myriad of intracellular signaling and mechanotransduction events, leading to altered gene transcription and potentially regulating the differentiation of stem and progenitor cells (Anselme et al., 2010; Ozdemir et al., 2013; Higgins et al., 2015). We believe that the presentation of textured surfaces to cells is a non-toxic, material-independent option to induce beneficial cellular responses for medical devices and serve as a tool to help design more therapeutically effective biomedical implants.

This research investigates the effects of spinal fusion cage surface morphology on initial cellular responses. Adhesion, spreading, migration, proliferation, and differentiation are important phenotypic considerations. This article directly addresses spreading and migration through morphology, speed of movement, differentiation markers, and directionality data, and indirectly suggests potential differentiation outcomes through circularity and cell spreading (*via* aspect ratio) measurements. Surface characteristics influence numerous fields, including proliferation, gene expression activity, phenotype commitment, cell adherence, protein adsorption, and cell shape (Deligianni et al., 2001; Olivares-Navarrete et al., 2010). These cell–material interactions are significant toward discerning the potential for bacterial growth on the implant and in turn suggest the chance for a biomaterial-associated infection (BAI).

The term "race for the surface" is used to describe competition at the implant surface between microbial adhesion and tissue integration (Gristina, 1987; Subbiahdoss et al., 2009; Caraca-Huber et al., 2012). The goal is to have tissue cells win the race against bacteria to prevent biofilm formation, which obstructs cellular functions and healthy tissue formation (Subbiahdoss et al., 2009). Additional complications caused by implant-associated infections include: BAIs are very difficult to manage and often require removal of the implant (Gorth et al., 2012); treatment costs are overwhelmingly expensive (Kurtz et al., 2008); and BAIs are very painful and debilitating to patients. For these reasons and as the number of implantations continue to rise, gaining a better understanding of how cells interact with biomaterial surfaces is critical. The sizes of the surface-fouling microorganisms are typically 1–2 μm (Graham and Cady, 2014), characteristically have less deformable membranes (compared to eukaryotic cells), and present distinctive structures (Anselme et al., 2010); therefore, using textured biomaterial surfaces may be an advantageous method to disrupt adhesion and mobility mechanisms of bacteria and limit biofilm formation. In this article, increased cell spreading and random migration suggest better surface coverage and movement, which could help reduce the potential of BAIs. The cell aspect ratio and circularity data provide information about projected phenotype lineage commitment based on published literature investigating cell differentiation on surfaces similar to those presented (Matsuoka et al., 2013), and the differentiation data presented support these previous findings. This information will suggest effects of surface features presented to the cell based on common spinal fusion cage materials: textured rough titanium, smooth titanium, and PEEK. We hypothesize that the acid-etched endoskeleton surface will lead to cellular responses indicative of successful spinal implants by demonstrating cellular responses that suggest microtopography may be a possible key parameter in preventing biofilm formation. This research enhances the current understanding of cellular responses to biomaterials, detailed toward spinal fusion research, by giving insight into cellular responses as correlated with surface morphology of common biomaterials for spinal implants. In turn, this research could aid in improving the functional integrity and performance of spinal fusion devices.

MATERIALS AND METHODS

Substrate Preparation

Substrates were 15-mm diameter disks machined from titanium alloy (Ti6Al4V ELI per ASTM F136) and PEEK (ASTM F2026) to create relatively smooth surfaces (Titan Spine, LLC, Mequon, WI, USA). To create the roughened surface texture, titanium disks were treated with the proprietary endoskeleton acid-etch process. Figure 1 presents the surface topographies of PEEK, smooth titanium, and acid-etched titanium (Matteson et al., 2015). All disks were sterilized by immersion in 70% ethanol for 30 min (Kummer et al., 2013; Vidal et al., 2013; Hirano et al., 2014) and rinsed with 1× phosphate-buffered saline (PBS) prior to use.

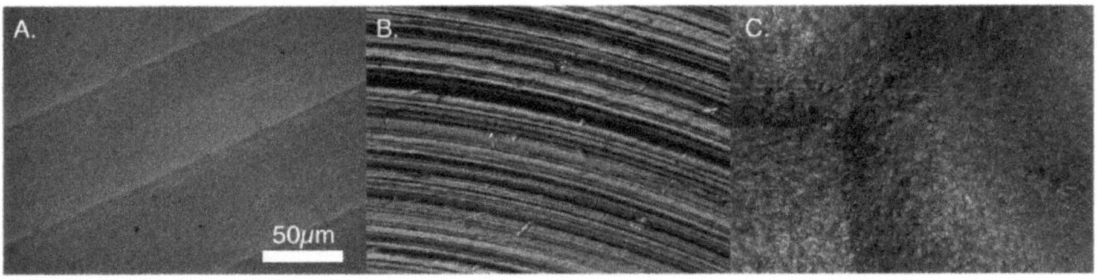

Figure 1: Surface morphology of PEEK and titanium samples. (A) PEEK, (B) smooth titanium, and (C) rough, acid-etched endoskeleton surface.

Cell Culture

Human mesenchymal stem cells (MSCs) were obtained from Lonza and were grown to appropriate numbers in a humidified incubator at 37°C and 5% CO_2, and then seeded onto surfaces at 1000 cells/cm^{2}for early morphology and early migration experiments. A lower seeding value, compared with the typical seeding value of 10000 cells/cm^2, was chosen in order to be able to better characterize the morphology, spreading, and migration events. At the time of seeding, the MSCs were at passage 6. The MSCs were maintained in a basal growth media for all early morphology and early migration experiments. The basal growth media consisted of alpha modified MEM (Life Technologies, Carlsbad, CA, USA) supplemented with 10% fetal bovine serum (FBS, Atlanta Biologics, Atlanta, GA, USA) and 1% penicillin/streptomycin (Life Technologies, Carlsbad, CA, USA). The media was changed every 2 days during the culture period. For the differentiation studies, samples were seeded at 10000 cells/cm^2 with a culture period of 10 days. Alpha-modified MEM basal growth media was switched to osteogenic media 12 h after seeding. Osteogenic media consisted of alpha modified MEM (Life Technologies, Carlsbad, CA, USA) supplemented with 10% fetal bovine serum (FBS, Atlanta Biologics, Atlanta, GA, USA), 1% penicillin/streptomycin (Life Technologies, Carlsbad, CA, USA), 100-nM dexamethasone (Sigma-Aldrich, St. Louis, MO, USA), 50 μg/mL ascorbic acid (Sigma-Aldrich, St. Louis, MO, USA), and 10-mM beta-glycerophosphate (Sigma-Aldrich, St. Louis, MO, USA).

Early Morphology

Mesenchymal stem cells on surfaces used for early morphology were stained with the DiI derivative, DiR (Life Technologies, Carlsbad, CA, USA) to fluorescently label the cell membrane. The staining was carried out by incubating the MSCs in a solution of 0.5% DiR in basal media, from a stock DiR solution concentration of 1 mg/mL in ethanol, for 30 min in a humidified incubator at 37°C. The samples were maintained in the incubator and removed at 2, 6, and 24 h to acquire images. At each time point, a minimum of 31 cells was imaged for analysis for each sample. Due to the depth of the surface, *z*-stacks were acquired and processed using the extended depth of field plugin for ImageJ. The subsequent images were analyzed with MATLAB to create image masks and with CellProfiler to quantify cell morphology. A minimum $n = 30$ was used for each sample.

Early Migration

Mesenchymal stem cells on surfaces used for early migration quantification were stained with a Qtracker 705 Cell Labeling kit (Life Technologies, Carlsbad, CA, USA) prior to being seeded. This allowed long-term evaluation of the cell centroid based on endocytosis of quantum dots. The quantum dot-loaded cells were imaged every 10 min for 12 h. Similar to the cell morphology, *z*-stacks were acquired at each time point and processed with the extended depth of field plugin for ImageJ. CellProfiler was used to quantify the migration velocities and directions. A minimum $n = 6$ was used for each sample.

Differentiation Markers

At 10 days, samples were lysed with 200-μL radioimmunoprecipitation assay buffer.

The lysates were used to quantify alkaline phosphatase (ALP), osterix (OSX) (SP7) transcription factor levels, and double-stranded DNA. General protocols for the immunodetection ALP substrate kit (Bio-Rad, Hercules, CA, USA), Quant-iT™ Picogreen® dsDNA reagent kit (Invitrogen, Molecular Probes), and Human SP7/Osterix ELISA Kit (LifeSpan BioSciences, Inc., Seattle, WA, USA) were followed as written. Sample volumes run in the assays were 5 μL.

Late Nuclear Morphology and Immunostaining

At 24 h and 7 days, samples were removed and fixed for immunostaining in addition to analysis of nuclear morphology. The samples to be stained for imaging at the 24-h time point were quickly washed with cold PBS and then fixed with 3.7% paraformaldehyde for 15 min followed by permeabilization in 0.1% Triton X-100 in 2% bovine serum albumin for 1 h. The cells were incubated with a mouse monoclonal anti-vinculin antibody (Sigma-Aldrich, St. Louis, MO, USA) at 1:400 in the permeabilization buffer for 1 h at room temperature. The samples were washed with PBS three times and then incubated in phalloidin conjugated to Atto 490LS (Sigma-Aldrich, St. Louis, MO, USA) at 1:1000, DAPI at 1:1000, and Dylight 488 anti-mouse secondary antibody (Life Technologies, Carlsbad, CA, USA) at 1:200 for 1 h at room temperature. Finally, the samples were washed three times with PBS and imaged. The samples imaged after 7 days were prepared as above; however, the vinculin primary and 488 secondary were omitted since vinculin was not needed to determine morphology. Nuclear morphology was quantified with CellProfiler.

Statistics

One-way ANOVAs with Tukey *post hoc* tests were used to determine significant differences for morphology features measured, migration velocity and migration directionality, and nuclear area and axial rotation. A ^{2} was used to evaluate the alignment of nuclei in each sample relative to a predicted random distribution.

RESULTS

Early Morphology

Mesenchymal stem cell morphology was examined both quantitatively from 2 to 24 h and qualitatively at 24 h. Figure 2 presents the quantitative cell morphology results on smooth PEEK, smooth Ti, and acid-etched endoskeleton surfaces. Figure 2A presents the areas of MSCs on each surface and shows an increasing trend for MSCs on the acid-etched endoskeleton surface: 6801 ± 533 μm^2 at 2 h, 7016 ± 647 μm^2 at 6 h, and ending with 8795 ± 841 μm^2 at 24 h. Similarly, the spreading area of MSCs on the smooth Ti increased at each time point: 5047 ± 634 μm^2 at 2 h, 5971 ± 562 μm^2 at 6 h, and 6041 ± 396 μm^2 at 24 h. However, the smooth PEEK was the only surface to demonstrate a maximal value followed by a decrease: 5292 ± 442 μm^2 at 2 h, 7008 ± 702 μm^2 at 6 h, and falling back to 5791 ± 565 μm^2 at 24 h. Only the acid-etched endoskeleton surface demonstrated significance with respect to area, demonstrating more spreading area per cell at 24 h when compared to the other surfaces at 24 h in addition to the earlier time points on the acid-etched surface. Next, the circularity of MSCs on the surfaces was analyzed. Circularity was defined as

$$\text{Circularity} = \frac{4\pi A}{P^2}$$

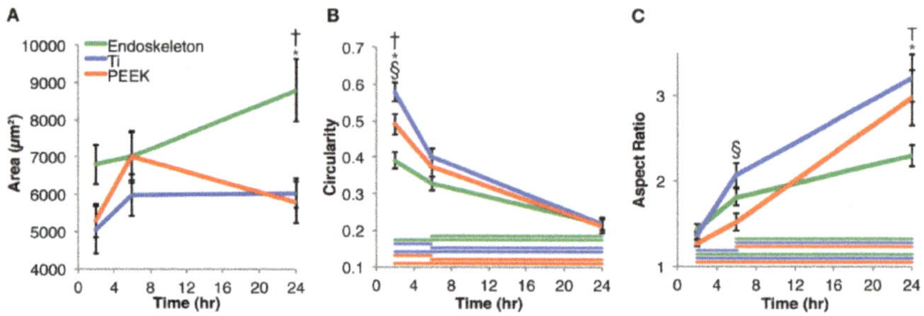

Figure 2: Morphological changes of mesenchymal stem cells analyzed at 2, 6, and 24 h post-seeding. (A) Area, (B) circularity, and (C) aspect ratio measurements were taken. The results indicate that stem cells on the acid-etched endoskeleton surface spread the most over 24 h. The circularity of the three surfaces began dissimilar, but converged at 24 h. The aspect ratio of stem cells initially began close to 1, but over 24 h, the smooth surfaces, Ti and PEEK, increased significantly higher than the rough, acid-etched endoskeleton surface. Taken together, the aspect ratio and circularity indicate that stem cells on smooth surfaces move toward a spindle or fibroblastic morphology, whereas those on the rough, acid-etched endoskeleton surface moved toward a stellate or star-like morphology. Within a single time point, * indicates significance, $p < 0.05$ between acid-etched Ti and PEEK, †indicates significance between acid-etched Ti and Ti, and § indicates significance between PEEK and Ti. Color-coded bars demonstrate significance between time points for a single surface.

Mesenchymal stem cells on all three surfaces demonstrated a significant decrease in the circularity of the cells at each time point. Smooth Ti surfaces demonstrated the highest circularity at 2 h, whereas the acid-etched endoskeleton surfaces demonstrated the lowest circularity at 2 h. The final shape factor analyzed was aspect ratio. All three surfaces demonstrated an increasing aspect ratio at each subsequent time point. The two smooth surfaces reached a final aspect ratio at 24 h of approximately 3, whereas the acid-etched endoskeleton surface reached a final aspect ratio of approximately 2. At 24 h, samples were stained to qualitatively examine morphology. Figure 1 illustrates the surface topography of the samples; reflected DIC was used to obtain the images. Figure 3 depicts the results from the qualitative staining, which are stained for phalloidin (red), the adhesion protein vinculin (green), and nuclear DNA (blue). In each image, a reflected DIC image of the surface is overlaid with the fluorescence channels in gray. In Figures3A,B, it is evident that MSCs on the smooth surfaces demonstrate an elongated spindle-like morphology. In contrast to Figures 3A–C, demonstrates MSCs with cuboidal and stellate (star-shaped) morphologies on the acid-etched endoskeleton surface.

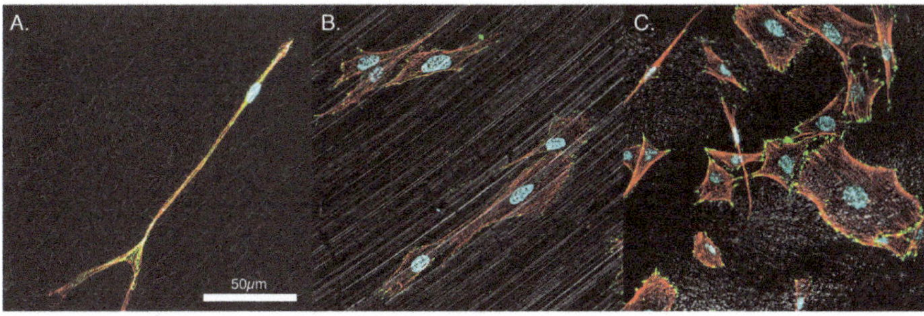

Figure 3: Representative morphologies of MSCs. (A) PEEK, (B) smooth titanium, and (C)rough, acid-etched endoskeleton surface, at 24 h. Immunofluorescence was carried out to examine the focal adhesion protein vinculin (green), the actin cytoskeleton (red), and the cell nuclei (blue). Additionally, a gray scale depiction of the surface was obtained with reflected DIC. The results demonstrated the trends observed in Figure 2 with cells on the smooth surfaces moving toward an elongated spindle-shaped morphology, whereas the cells on the rough surface demonstrated a range of morphologies from spindle-shaped cells to cuboidal and stellate-shaped cells. In particular, the cuboidal and stellate cells in C. are representative of morphologies expected of osteoblastic differentiation. Scale bar indicating 50 μm applies to (A–C).

Early Migration

In addition to the morphology shift on each of the three surfaces, the rate and direction of migration were assayed beginning at 6 h post-seeding and continuing for 12 h. Figure 4 depicts the quantitative migration data. In Figure 4A, rose plots (circular histograms) are provided to demonstrate the direction of travel. The MSCs on both smooth surfaces (e.g., PEEK and Ti) demonstrate migration along predominantly one axis. In contrast, the MSCs on the acid-etched endoskeleton surface demonstrate migration in multiple directions. The velocity on the samples is depicted in Figure 4B. The highest average velocity was found in MSCs on the smooth Ti, 28.24 ± 1.62 μm/h, followed by the acid-etched endoskeleton, 21.39 ± 1.38 μm/h, and the lowest average velocity was observed on smooth PEEK, 16.16 ± 1.46 μm/h. Velocities on each surface were significantly different than all other surfaces. Finally, the directionality of the cells on each surface was measured. Directionality was defined as

$$\text{Directionality} = \frac{\text{end-to-end distance}}{\text{total distance}}$$

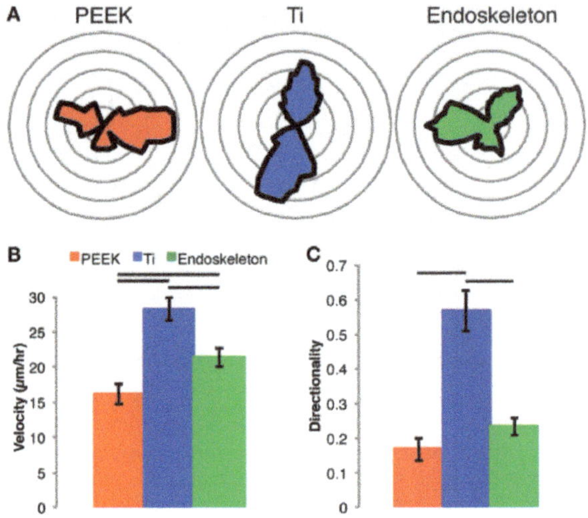

Figure 4: Stem cell migration on each surface was assessed from 6 to 18 h post-seeding. The results demonstrate random migration on the PEEK and acid-etched endoskeleton surfaces indicated by the rose plots in (A), a histogram of the angle of migration for each cell monitored in (B), and the graph of directionality in (C), which demonstrates significance between PEEK and acid-etched endoskeleton surfaces when compared to the smooth titanium surface. Furthermore, the non-random migration on smooth titanium followed the grooves created by milling the surface, and this non-random migration resulted in an expected velocity increase, which was significantly higher than both the PEEK and acid-etched endoskeleton surfaces. Between the two surfaces demonstrating random migration, the MSCs on the acid-etched endoskeleton surface demonstrated a significantly higher velocity than those on PEEK. Significance, $p < 0.05$, is demonstrated by bars between groups in (B,C).

The directionality was again highest on the smooth Ti, 0.57 ± 0.06, followed by the acid-etched endoskeleton, 0.23 ± 0.03, and the lowest directionality was observed on smooth PEEK, 0.17 ± 0.03. The smooth Ti was significantly higher as compared to both the smooth PEEK and the acid-etched endoskeleton surface.

Differentiation Markers

The early osteogenic differentiation marker ALP and mid-differentiation marker OSX were investigated after 10 days on the three surfaces. dsDNA was quantified to normalize the ALP and OSX values. Figure5A demonstrates that early maker, ALP, increased on the smooth Ti surface relative to PEEK, while the mid-marker OSX increased on the acid-etched endoskeleton surface. There was a significant difference between the ALP values for smooth Ti, 12.16 ± 1.37 U/μg, compared to PEEK, 8.19 ± 0.28 U/μg. The OSX value for the acid-etched endoskeleton surface was significantly higher than PEEK, 12.28 ± 1.59 and 7.31 ± 1.79 ng/μg, respectively. PEEK had decreased values for both ALP and OSX. Figure 5B shows a general increase of dsDNA from smooth Ti to PEEK to the acid-etched endoskeleton surface, 310.28 ± 131.90 to 342.41 ± 21.14 to

441.63 ± 60.45 ng/mL, with the acid-etched endoskeleton surface exhibiting the highest dsDNA value.

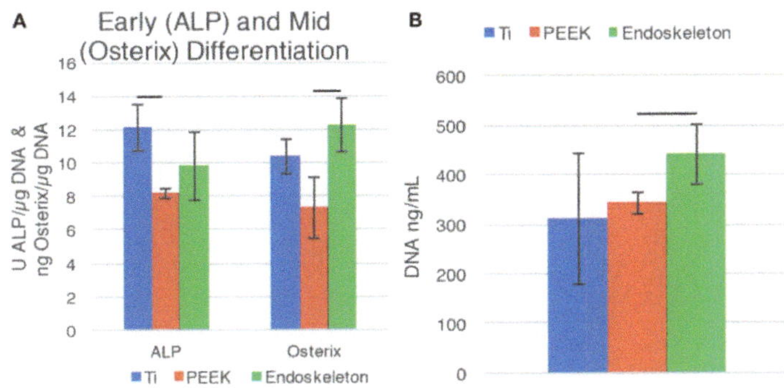

Figure 5: Early differentiation marker alkaline phosphatase (ALP) and osterix (OSX), a transcription factor significant for osteoblast differentiation, were normalized to dsDNA. (A) Early differentiation marker, ALP, is increased on the smooth Ti surface, while the mid-differentiation marker OSX increased on the acid-etched endoskeleton surface. The PEEK surface fell short for both ALP and OSX. This suggests that hMSC differentiation is moving toward bone formation for the Ti surfaces. (B) Seeding densities for all samples were equal. The dsDNA value for the acid-etched endoskeleton surface is the highest amongst the surfaces, which suggests that there is improved cell attachment and/or proliferation for the acid-etched endoskeleton surface compared to the smooth Ti and PEEK substrates.

Late Nuclear Morphology

After 7 days, the nuclei morphologies were analyzed as a predictor of cell morphology. The cell morphology could not be assessed directly at 7 days due to the cells being confluent; however, nuclear morphology has previously demonstrated a correlation over the general cell morphology (Maniotis et al., 1997; Li et al., 2014; Ramdas and Shivashankar, 2015). First, we examined the axial ratio and nuclear area on all three surfaces, shown in Figure 6A. The axial ratios were similar on the PEEK and smooth Ti, 1.88 ± 0.03 and 1.89 ± 0.03, respectively. The axial ratio for nuclei on the acid-etched endoskeleton surface, 1.60 ± 0.02, was significantly lower than both of the smooth surfaces. The acid-etched endoskeleton surface also demonstrated the lowest nuclear area, 340.5 ± 9.3 µm^2, as compared to the PEEK and smooth Ti surfaces, 1406.4 ± 31.4 and 2037.6 ± 70.8 µm^2. All nuclear areas were significantly different from all others, illustrated in Figure 6B. Finally, the alignment of the nuclei was quantified by examining the angle of the long axis of each nucleus. This data is presented in a histogram in Figure 6C. Additionally, the inset of Figure 6C provides a cumulative distribution plot of the histogram data with a dotted line corresponding to a random distribution. A X^2 (chi-squared) test demonstrated that both the PEEK and smooth Ti had nuclei aligned in a single direction, which was significantly different than an expected random distribution. In contrast, the nuclei on the acid-etched endoskeleton surface were not significantly different from an expected random distribution.

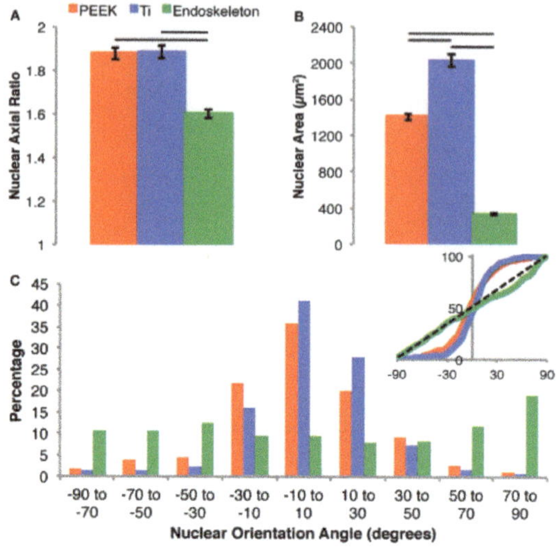

Figure 6: Nuclear morphology was examined to assess the general cell morphology after 7 days when the populations were confluent and cell borders were difficult to identify. The nuclear morphology on PEEK and Ti surfaces were very similar in regards to axial ratio (A), whereas the nuclei on the rough acid-etched endoskeleton surface had a significantly lower axial ratio than either the PEEK or smooth Ti surface indicating more circular nuclei on the acid-etched endoskeleton surface. The nuclear area (B) followed a similar trend to axial ratio with the smooth surfaces demonstrating significantly more nuclear area than the rough acid-etched endoskeleton surface. Finally, the orientation of nuclei (C) was assessed establishing 0° as the average orientation direction. The inset provides a plot of the cumulative distribution and clearly demonstrates that PEEK and smooth Ti surfaces were different than the rough, acid-etched endoskeleton surface. Nuclei on PEEK and smooth Ti were grouped very close to 0° indicating that most cells presented an elongated nucleus in the same direction; however, on the acid-etched endoskeleton surface, the nuclei were randomly oriented with only one range, 70–90°, demonstrating a slight increase. The black dotted line in the inset of (C) provides the expected cumulative distribution for random orientation; *p*values were calculated for each of the three samples with a ^{2} test and yielded *p* values of 10^{-10}, 10^{-19}, and 1.0 for PEEK, Ti, and acid-etched endoskeleton, respectively. Taken together, these results indicated that the aligned spindle morphology observed early on the PEEK and smooth Ti surfaces persists when the stem cells are confluent, and likewise, the random cuboidal/stellate morphology on the acid-etched endoskeleton surface also persists to the confluent cell layer observed after 7 days.

The quantitative data above are represented by the immunofluorescence images presented in Figures 7A–C. Figures 7A,B show confluent layers of MSCs on the PEEK and smooth Ti surfaces. In each, it is clear that the nuclei are elongated and are primarily organized along a single axis. In contrast, the acid-etched endoskeleton surface presents a more random distribution of MSC morphologies.

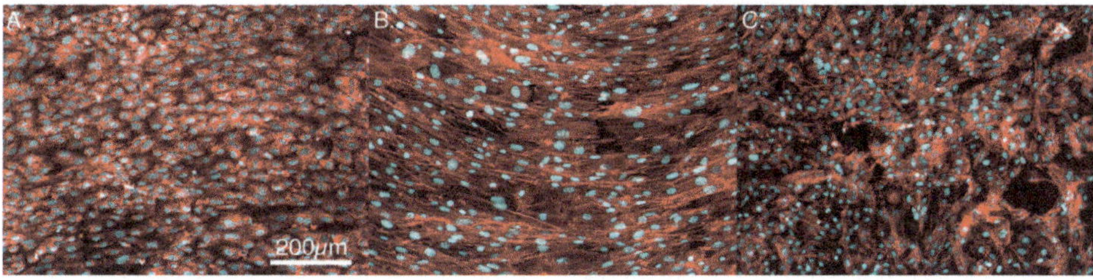

Figure 7: Representative images of confluent cells stained for actin (red) and the cell nuclei (blue). (A) PEEK, (B) smooth titanium, and (C) rough, acid-etched endoskeleton surface, after 7-day culture. The cells on PEEK and smooth titanium demonstrate an elongated morphology in a uniform direction, whereas cells on the acid-etched endoskeleton surface demonstrate a branched random morphology. Scale bar indicating 200 μm applies to (A–C).

DISCUSSION

The advantages of the acid-etched endoskeleton surface in promoting osteoblast differentiation are well established in the literature (Gittens et al., 2012; Olivares-Navarrete et al., 2012, 2013). The goals of the present study were to examine the early responses of MSCs to each of the surfaces, and identify if the early response was predictive of the known long-term osteoblastic differentiation and establishment of MSC migration and morphology. The project objective was to demonstrate data characterizing the events preceding phenotype development on rough titanium since material and surface characterization and cell differentiation data with respect to rough versus smooth surfaces have been well studied. A key feature of successful implants is winning the "race for the surface" (Gristina et al., 1989). This can be defined by examining key features: rate of initial cell adhesion and spreading and the rate of random cell migration. Random cell migration is significant in generating the uniform population distribution that will lead to uniform coverage of the surface by the MSCs (Gail and Boone, 1970). Examination of the data from the cell area measurements clearly reveals that MSCs on the acid-etched endoskeleton surface spread at a higher rate than on either of the smooth surfaces. This was demonstrated by a 40% increase in spreading area per cell by 2 h for MSCs on the acid-etched endoskeleton surface, which increased to nearly 50% more spreading area per cell by 24 h. A 50% increase in the cell spreading area dramatically reduces the time required for the surface to be covered by MSCs. Furthermore, the shape of these spreading cells revealed interesting trends. Initially, all MSCs were circular, or nearly circular, as demonstrated by high circularity values and low aspect ratios. As time progressed, MSCs on the smooth surfaces moved toward spindle-shaped morphologies. These elongated and aligned spindle-shaped cells are typical morphology of fibroblastic tissue (Dalby et al., 2007). This is evident from the combination of a high aspect ratio, 3:1 at 24 h, coupled with low circularity. Together, these two characteristics suggest long slender cells that are further supported by the immunostaining images at 24 h presented in Figure 3. In contrast, MSCs on the acid-etched endoskeleton surface demonstrated more stellate or cuboidal morphologies at 24 h, indicated by lower aspect ratios and similar circularities. The similar circularity indicates that MSCs on the acid-etched endoskeleton surface have a high perimeter:area ratio, but the lower circularity indicates that the long axis and short axis of the cell are not dramatically different. Together, these two properties lead to the conclusion that MSCs on the acid-etched endoskeleton surface have multiple processes and are stellate in morphology. Figure 3 demonstrates MSCs on the acid-etched endoskeleton surface showing varied morphologies from stellate to spindle-shaped. The cuboidal and stellate morphologies observed on the acid-etched endoskeleton surface are expected for cells undergoing osteogenic differentiation (Dalby et al., 2007; Hong et al., 2010). Furthermore, the differentiation data illustrated in Figure 5A support that the cells were indeed moving toward the osteogenic lineage as indicated by increased levels of ALP and OSX compared to PEEK (Pinzone et al., 2016). The increased ALP on smooth Ti and increased OSX on acid-etched endoskeleton surface together suggest that osteogenic differentiation was dramatically enhanced on the acid-etched endoskeleton surface, with smooth Ti being moderately enhanced relative to PEEK. The dsDNA data in Figure 5B also suggest improved cell attachment and/or proliferation for the acid-etched endoskeleton surface based on the increased dsDNA value for that surface and the fact that initial seeding densities across the samples were equal.

The examination of migration further supported the acid-etched endoskeleton surface. MSCs on both of the titanium surfaces were faster than those on PEEK. The MSCs on the acid-etched endoskeleton surface did not present the highest velocity; however, they did present both a moderately high velocity coupled with a low directionality. The low directionality and histogram of migration vectors indicate the MSCs on the acid-etched endoskeleton surface were moving in a random way. In contrast, MSCs on the smooth titanium exploited contact guidance generated by machining the titanium. This contact guidance resulted in high directionality with migration occurring primarily on one axis. The MSCs on PEEK presented random migration; however, the MSCs velocities were significantly lower than either of the two titanium surfaces.

Together, the morphology and migration data support the acid-etched endoskeleton surface as the best option for randomly and uniformly distributing the cell population in addition to covering the available area when compared to either of the smooth surfaces. Furthermore, the acid-etched endoskeleton surface promoted bone differentiation markers after 10 days and stellate and cuboidal cell morphologies as early as 24 h, which are the expected morphologies of MSCs undergoing osteogenic differentiation. Finally, the long-term examination of nuclear morphology at 7 days indicates that the morphologies observed at 24 h persisted on the surfaces. Both of the smooth surfaces presented spindle-shaped cells, and at 7 days, the nuclei were elongated along a uniform axis. Therefore, it may be concluded that the cells are still spindle-shaped when confluent. In contrast, MSCs on the acid-etched endoskeleton surface did not demonstrate preferential nuclei alignment, which indicates that MSCs on the acid-etched endoskeleton surface maintained a cuboidal or stellate morphology at 7 days. In closing, the unique rough surface presented by the acid-etched endoskeleton surfaces promotes morphology and migration behavior consistent with successful implants.

AUTHOR CONTRIBUTIONS

BB contributed to the acquisition of data, drafting of manuscript, and critical revision. TR and CP contributed to the acquisition and analysis of the data. JB contributed through study design, analysis and interpretation of data, and drafting of the manuscript. All authors critically reviewed the work, approved the final version to be published, and agree to be accountable for the work.

CONFLICT OF INTEREST STATEMENT

The authors declare that the research was partially funded by Titan Spine, LLC.

FUNDING

We thank Titan Spine, LLC for supplying the samples for analysis and funding support.

REFERENCES

1. Abernathie, D. L., and Pfeiffer, F. M. (2011). *Spinal Fusion Cage, Method of Design, and Method of Use*. US 8,057,548 B2.
2. Anselme, K., and Bigerelle, M. (2005). Topography effects of pure titanium substrates on human osteoblast long-term adhesion. *Acta Biomater.* 1, 211–222. doi: 10.1016/j.actbio.2004.11.009
3. Anselme, K., Davidson, P., Popa, A. M., Giazzon, M., Liley, M., and Ploux, L. (2010). The interaction of cells and bacteria with surfaces structured at the nanometre scale. *Acta Biomater.* 6, 3824–3846. doi:10.1016/j.actbio.2010.04.001
4. Bächle, M., and Kohal, R. J. (2004). A systematic review of the influence of different titanium surfaces on proliferation, differentiation and protein synthesis of osteoblast-like MG63 cells. *Clin. Oral Implants Res.* 15, 683–692. doi:10.1111/j.1600-0501.2004.01054.x
5. Cabraja, M., Oezdemir, S., Koeppen, D., and Kroppenstedt, S. (2012). Anterior cervical discectomy and fusion: comparison of titanium and polyetheretherketone cages. *BMC Musculoskelet. Disord.* 13:172. doi:10.1186/1471-2474-13-172
6. Caraca-Huber, D. C., Fille, M., Hausdorfer, J., Pfaller, K., and Nogler, M. (2012). Evaluation of MBEC™-HTP biofilm model for studies of implant associated infections. *J. Orthop. Res.* 30, 1176–1180. doi:10.1002/jor.22065
7. Dalby, M. J., Gadegaard, N., Tare, R., Andar, A., Riehle, M. O., Herzyk, P., et al. (2007). The control of human mesenchymal cell differentiation using nanoscale symmetry and disorder. *Nat. Mater.* 6, 997–1003. doi:10.1038/nmat2013
8. Deligianni, D. D., Katsala, N., Ladas, S., Sotiropoulou, D., Amedee, J., and Missirlis, Y. F. (2001). Effect of surface roughness of the titanium allow Ti-6Al-4V on human bone marrow cell response and on protein adsorption. *Biomaterials* 22, 1241–1251. doi:10.1016/S0142-9612(00)00274-X
9. Gail, M. H., and Boone, C. W. (1970). The locomotion of mouse fibroblasts in tissue culture. *Biophys. J.* 10, 980–993. doi:10.1016/S0006-3495(70)86347-0

10. Gittens, R. A., Olivares-Navarrete, R., McLachlan, T., Cai, Y., Hyzy, S. L., Schneider, J. M., et al. (2012). Differential responses of osteoblast lineage cells to nanotopographically-modified, microroughened titanium-aluminum-vanadium alloy surfaces. *Biomaterials*33, 8986–8994. doi:10.1016/j.biomaterials.2012.08.059

11. Gorth, D. J., Puckett, S., Ercan, B., Webster, T. J., Rahaman, M., and Bal, B. S. (2012). Decreased bacteria activity on Si3N4 surfaces compared with PEEK or titanium. *Int. J. Nanomed.* 7, 4829–4840. doi:10.2147/IJN.S35190

12. Graham, M. V., and Cady, N. C. (2014). Nano and microscale topographies for the prevention of bacterial surface fouling. *Coatings* 4, 37–59. doi:10.3390/coatings4010037

13. Gristina, A. (1987). Biomaterial-centered infection: microbial adhesion versus tissue integration. *Science* 237, 1588–1595. doi:10.1126/science.3629258

14. Gristina, A., Naylor, P., and Myrvik, Q. (1989). Infections from biomaterials and implants: a race for the surface. *Med. Prog. Technol.* 14, 205–224.

15. Higgins, A. M., Banik, B. L., and Brown, J. L. (2015). Geometry sensing through POR1 regulates Rac1 activity controlling early osteoblast differentiation in response to nanofiber diameter. *Integr. Biol.* 7, 229–236. doi:10.1039/c4ib00225c

16. Hirano, M., Kozuka, T., Asano, Y., Kakuchi, Y., Arai, H., and Ohtsu, N. (2014). Effect of sterilization and water rinsing on cell adhesion to titanium surfaces. *Appl. Surf. Sci.* 311, 498–502. doi:10.1016/j.apsusc.2014.05.096

17. Hong, D., Chen, H.-X., Yu, H.-Q., Liang, Y., Wang, C., Lian, Q.-Q., et al. (2010). Morphological and proteomic analysis of early stage of osteoblast differentiation in osteoblastic progenitor cells. *Exp. Cell Res.* 316, 2291–2300. doi:10.1016/j.yexcr.2010.05.011

18. Kummer, K. M., Taylor, E. N., Durmas, N. G., Tarquinio, K. M., Ercan, B., and Webster, T. J. (2013). Effects of different sterilization techniques and varying anodized TiO_2 nanotube dimensions on bacteria growth. *J. Biomed. Mater. Res. B Appl. Biomater.* 101, 677–688. doi:10.1002/jbm.b.32870

19. Kurtz, S. M., Lau, E., Schmier, J., Ong, K. L., Zhao, K., and Parvizi, J. (2008). Infection burden for hip and knee arthroplasty in the United States. *J. Arthroplasty* 23, 984–991. doi:10.1016/j.arth.2007.10.017

20. Li, Q., Kumar, A., Makhija, E., and Shivashankar, G. V. (2014). The regulation of dynamic mechanical coupling between actin cytoskeleton and nucleus by matrix geometry. *Biomaterials* 35, 961–969. doi:10.1016/j.biomaterials.2013.10.037

21. Maniotis, A. J., Chen, C. S., and Ingber, D. E. (1997). Demonstration of mechanical connections between integrins, cytoskeletal filaments, and nucleoplasm that stabilize nuclear structure. *Proc. Natl. Acad. Sci. U.S.A.* 94, 849–854. doi:10.1073/pnas.94.3.849

22. Matsuoka, F., Takeuchi, I., Agata, H., Kagami, H., Shiono, H., Kiyota, Y., et al. (2013). Morphology-based prediction of osteogenic differentiation potential of human mesenchymal stem cells. *PLoS ONE* 8:e55082. doi:10.1371/journal.

pone.0055082

23. Matteson, J. L., Greenspan, D. C., Tighe, T. B., Gilfoy, N., and Stapleton, J. J. (2015). Assessing the hierarchical structure of titanium implant surfaces. *J. Biomed. Mater. Res. Part B*. doi:10.1002/jbm.b.33462

24. Nouh, M. R. (2012). Spinal fusion-hardware construct: basic concepts and imaging review. *World J. Radiol.* 4, 193–207. doi:10.4329/wjr.v4.i5.193

25. Obrigkeit, D. D., Koenen, J., Schumann, D. O. A., and Smit, L. (2012). *Spinal Fusion Cage*. US 2012/0046750 A1.

26. Olivares-Navarrete, R., Gittens, R. A., Schneider, J. M., Hyzy, S. L., Haithcock, D. A., Ullrich, P. F., et al. (2012). Osteoblasts exhibit a more differentiated phenotype and increased bone morphogenetic protein production on titanium alloy substrates than on poly-ether-ether ketone. *Spine J.* 12, 265–272. doi:10.1016/j.spinee.2012.02.002

27. Olivares-Navarrete, R., Hyzy, S., Hutton, D., Erdman, C., Wieland, M., Boyan, B. D., et al. (2010). Direct and indirect effects of microstructured titanium substrates on the induction of mesenchymal stem cell differentiation towards the osteoblast lineage.*Biomaterials* 31, 1–15. doi:10.1016/j.biomaterials.2009.12.029

28. Olivares-Navarrete, R., Hyzy, S. L., Gittens, R. A. I, Schneider, J. M., Haithcock, D. A., Ullrich, P. F., et al. (2013). Rough titanium alloys regulate osteoblast production of angiogenic factors. *Spine J.* 13, 1563–1570. doi:10.1016/j.spinee.2013.03.047

29. Ozdemir, T., Xu, L.-C., Siedlecki, C., and Brown, J. L. (2013). Substrate curvature sensing through Myosin IIa upregulates early osteogenesis. *Integr. Biol.* 5, 1407–1416. doi:10.1039/c3ib40068a

30. Pinzone, J. J., Hall, B. M., Thudi, N. K., Vonau, M., Qiang, Y., Rosol, T. J., et al. (2016). The role of Dickkopf-1 in bone development, homeostasis, and disease. *Blood* 113, 517–526. doi:10.1182/blood-2008-03-145169

31. Ramdas, N. M., and Shivashankar, G. V. (2015). Cytoskeletal control of nuclear morphology and chromatin organization. *J. Mol. Biol.*427, 695–706. doi:10.1016/j.jmb.2014.09.008

32. Rihn, J. A., Patel, R., Makda, J., Hong, J., Anderson, D. G., Vaccaro, A. R., et al. (2009). Complications associated with single-level transforaminal lumbar interbody fusion. *Spine J.* 9, 623–629. doi:10.1016/j.spinee.2009.04.004

33. Subbiahdoss, G., Kuijer, R., Grijpma, D. W., van der Mei, H. C., and Busscher, H. J. (2009). Microbial biofilm growth versus tissue integration: "the race for the surface" experimentally studied. *Acta Biomater.* 5, 1399–1404. doi:10.1016/j.actbio.2008.12.011

34. Vidal, G., Blanchi, T., Mieszawska, A. J., Calabrese, R., Rossi, C., Vigneron, P., et al. (2013). Enhanced cellular adhesion on titanium by silk functionalized with titanium binding and RGD peptides. *Acta Biomater.* 9, 4935–4943. doi:10.1016/j.actbio.2012.09.003

35. Williams, A. L., Gornet, M. F., and Burkus, J. K. (2005). CT evaluation of lumbar

interbody fusion: current concepts. *Am. J. Neuroradiol.*26, 2057–2066.

36. Zhao, C., Cao, P., Ji, W., Han, P., Zhang, J., Zhang, F., et al. (2011). Hierarchical titanium surface textures affect osteoblastic functions. *J. Biomed. Mater. Res. A* 99, 666–675. doi:10.1002/jbm.a.33239

6
CHAPTER

MODELING OF DRUG DELIVERY BY A PUMP DRIVEN MICRO-NEEDLE ARRAY SYSTEM

Kai Chen, Min Pan, Zhi-Gang Feng

Keywords: Drug delivery system, fluid infusion, micro-needle, infusion flow

INTRODUCTION

Although patch-based transdermal drug delivery has been used for clinical application over decades, it faces the challenge of overcoming stratum corneum as a natural barrier to large molecular drugs. Other physical or chemical enhancing methods are inconvenient and rarely used in practice. Ordinary sized needles are associated with problems such as pain, trauma, bleeding, etc. Micro-needle array, a technology having both the non invasive feature of a drug patch and the effectiveness of a hypodermic needle, has been reported to increase the drug permeability in skin by several orders of magnitude [1, 2]. Solid micro-needles were first fabricated from microelectronic industry in 1980s, and are often coated with drugs for rapid bolus administration. Hollow micro-needles were fabricated using a silicon nitride shell on top of a silicon substrate subsequently. They are often combined with a micro pump or a syringe to create a controlled drug delivery system [1, 2]. The micro-needle system can also be integrated with other techniques such as optical trapping, to trap, store and deliver drug molecules/ cells to specific targets [3]. Through decades of research, different techniques have been developed and improved for the fabrication of micro-needle array that originates from microelectronics industry [4-7]. A dissolvable polymer material was proposed for the fabrication of a micro-needle patch. The new micro-needles can be dissolved into

Citation: Kai Chen, Min Pan, Zhi-Gang Feng, Modeling of Drug Delivery by A Pump Driven Micro-Needle Array System, DOI: 10.2174/18741207016100010019.

bodily fluid after being pierced into the skin [8, 9]. Lots of investigation has been done to understand physical mechanism involved in the injection of micro-needle delivery, in order to optimize the system variables and improve the performance of the micro-needle transdermal delivery. Sanders et al. [10] developed constitutive models that describe skin response to stretching force. Kong and Wu [11] studied the penetration of a sharp tip into human skin. Gomaa et al. [12] studied the effects of micro-needle length, density, insertion time on enhancing drug flux through measurements of trans epidermal water loss. The propagation of drug after its initial infusion has been studied by Lv et al. [13] and Zhang et al. [14]. Recent research found that achieving larger flow rates has been difficult, apparently due to the low flow conductivity in the skin, and the compression of dense dermal tissue during micro-needle insertion, which increases the resistance to flow [15, 16]. However, micro jets interaction with the skin and the jet behavior under the skin have not been fully understood. Theoretical models so far mostly focus on the piecing process for solid micro-needles [17]. Shergold & Fleck [18] developed a micromechanical model for the needle penetration of a soft solid. The authors have developed an analytic model based on liquid expansion in a soft solid to calculate the initial infusion of a micro-needle array driven by a micro-pump [19].

Ideally, hollow micro-needles shall have more clinical applications than solid micro-needles for its feature of continuous and controlled drug release. However, it has generally received less attention and has been less used due to its practical problems. Most studies on hollow micro-needles were of in vitro experimental performance. There are currently few theoretical models developed that can describe the flow behavior of the micro jets inside the skin. Our previous study has presented an analytic model based on the liquid expansion in a soft solid for the initial infusion of the drug through a micro-needle system [19]. The model assumes that the soft solid is an incompressible, hyperelastic, isotropic material, and the amount of energy delivered by the micro-pump is equal to the energy used for the expansion of soft skin due to micro-needle drug infusion. However, the human skin, especially dermis structure underneath the epidermis is a non homogeneous porous material. The process of liquid diffusion will be dominant after the initial expansion process during the injection of micro-needle system. The presented model consists of two parts: an expansion part and a diffusion part. The diffusion part is based on the mass conservation, and the soft tissue is treated as uniform porous medium with uniform properties. The analytic model can be described by a set of ordinary differential equations. Numerical solutions to these coupled equations are obtained. For a typical commercial piezoelectric micro pump, the flow expansion stops instantly and the flow rate quickly drops to zero, unless the pressure from the micro-pump is increased. If the jet flow rate remains constant, the diameter of the diffusion boundary first increases and then tapes off as a constant, indicating the diffusion process keeps going. Preliminary experiments of micro-needle injection on silicon rubber and polyacrylamide gel were carried out, revealing some qualitative results that match with the results from the modeling work. The present study may shed light on the optimization of the micro-needle system.

DESCRIPTION OF MATHEMATICAL MODEL

General Conservation of Mass and Energy

As shown in Fig. (1), a typical hollow micro-needle drug delivery system consists of a drug reservoir, a micro-pump, and a micro-needle array. The micro-needles just pierce across epidermis to produce micro sized channels for further infusion of the drug. The energy used to cause drug infusion and expansion in skin should be equal to the energy delivered by the micro-needles. However, part of the energy provided by the micro-pump is lost due to the minor and major losses in the flow system.

The following expression is obtained after the conservation of energy is applied for the flow system [20].

$$Q\left(\frac{P_{in}}{\rho g}+\frac{V_{in}^{2}}{2g}+Z_{in}\right)+Q\frac{P_{pump}}{\rho g}=Q_{out}\left[\frac{P_{out}}{\rho g}+\frac{V_{out}^{2}}{2g}+Z_{out}\right]+\text{total major loss}+\text{total minor loss}, \tag{1}$$

where ρ is the liquid density, V is the liquid velocity, Q is the liquid flow rate from the output of the micro pump, and g is the gravitational constant, Z is the vertical position, P_{pump} is the pressure that the micro-pump could raise. The subscripts in and out denote the inlet (drug reservoir) and outlet (micro-needles), respectively. The above expression assumes each micro-needle has the same output parameters. The total major loss due to friction in the tube is:

$$\textit{total major loss} = Q\lambda\frac{L}{D_1}\frac{V_D^{2}}{2g}, \tag{2}$$

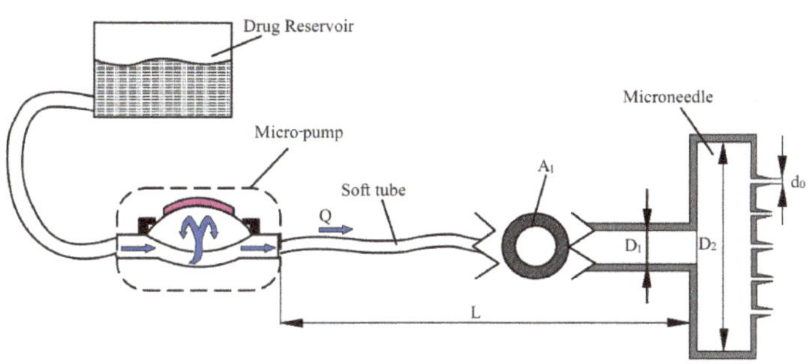

Figure 1: A pump driven micro-needle drug delivery system.

where V_D is the flow velocity in the soft tube, D_1 is the inner diameter of the soft tube, L is the length of the soft tube, and λ is the friction factor. The total minor loss due to sudden expansion or contractions is:

$$\textit{total minor loss} = Q\left[\sum K_1\frac{V_D^{2}}{2g}+\sum K_2\frac{V_{out}^{2}}{2g}\right], \tag{3}$$

where $\sum K_1$ is the total minor loss coefficient that liquid sustains before it flows into the micro-needles, and $\sum K_2$ is the total minor loss coefficient of flow in the micro-needle section. Obviously, $V_D = \frac{Q}{\pi D_1^2/4}$, and $V_{out} = \frac{Q/N}{\pi d_o^2/4}$, where d_0 is the diameter of a single micro-needle on the array, and N is the total number of micro-needles on the array. By changing the notation of P_{out} to P_o, the actual energy that micro-needle can deliver is:

$$P_o = P_{pump} - \left(\lambda \frac{L}{D_1} + \sum K_1\right)\frac{\rho}{2}\left(\frac{Q}{\pi D_1^2/4}\right)^2 - \left(1+\sum K_2\right)\frac{\rho}{2}\left(\frac{Q/N}{\pi d_o^2/4}\right)^2 \quad (4)$$

Friction factor λ depends upon the viscosity, the state of the flow and the wall smoothness of micro-needles.

$\sum K_1$ and $\sum K_2$ can be estimated by the following formula [20]:

$$\sum K_1 = \left(1 - \frac{A_1}{A_2}\right)^2 = \left(1 - \frac{D_1^2}{D_2^2}\right), \quad (5)$$

And

$$\sum K_2 = 0.42\left(1 - \frac{A}{A_2}\right)^2 = \left(1 - \frac{Nd_0^2}{D_2^2}\right)^2, \quad (6)$$

where A_1, A_2 and A are the cross sectional area of soft tube, intracavity of micro-needle array, and micro-needles, respectively. D_2 is the diameter of micro-needle intracavity as shown in Fig. (1).

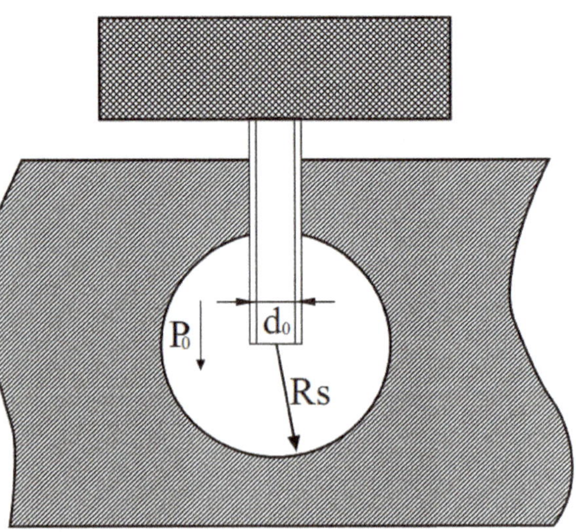

Figure 2: Liquid expansion of single micro-needle in a soft solid.

The Model of Spherical Expansion

Due to the relatively higher pressure, the liquid coming out of the micro-needle will push the soft skin aside to form an expansion, as shown in Fig. (2). It is assumed in the current model that the initial liquid infusion through a micro-needle follows a spherical pattern of expansion. The mass and energy should be conserved in the liquid infusion process.

For incompressible liquid, the conservation of mass yields:

$$V = \frac{4}{3}\pi R_S^3 = \int_0^T \frac{Q(t)}{N}dt\,, \tag{7}$$

where V is the volume of total drug delivered from the beginning of infusion through time T for a single micro-needle; Q(t)/N is the volume flow rate of a single micro-needle; R_s is the expansion radius through time T.

From the expansion model given by Shergold & Fleck [18], the work done by the injected liquid through a single micro-needle is equivalent to the stored strain energy in the infinite medium of soft material:

$$\int_0^{R_s} 4\pi r^2 P_o dr = \frac{4}{3}\pi R_s{}^3 \int_1^\infty \frac{2\mu}{\alpha^2} h\left(\eta', \frac{d_o}{2R_s}\right) d\eta'\,, \tag{8}$$

where P_o is the liquid pressure coming out of a micro-needle, as described in Equation (4), and r is the radius of the sphere during expansion.α is a strain hardening exponent, μ is the shear modulus under infinitesimal straining of the soft material. η', a dimensionless number, and the function h(), are explained in [19]. If the integration part of the R.H.S is noted as

$$G = \int_1^\infty \frac{2\mu}{\alpha^2} h\left(\eta', \frac{d_o}{2R_s}\right) d\eta'\,, \tag{9}$$

The following equation can be derived

$$\frac{dR_s}{dt} = \frac{P_o - \left(G + \frac{1}{3} R_s \frac{dG}{dR_s}\right)}{4\pi NAR_s{}^2}\,. \tag{10}$$

The unknown variables P_o, R_s can be calculated through Equation (4) and (10), if the micro-pump variables (P_{max} and Q), the variables of micro-needle system (N and D_1, D_2, d_o) and mechanical properties of soft material (α and μ) are provided.

The Model of Spherical Diffusion

In addition to expansion, the drug solution diffuses into the skin due to its concentration gradient and natural flow between soft tissues, as shown in Fig. (3). The drug absorption along its flow path gradually decreases. For simplicity, the surrounding tissues are divided into "Saturated Tissues" and "Unsaturated Tissues" by an imaginary diffusion boundary. Within the spherical space inside the moving interface of diffusion boundary, the solution is saturated anywhere at anytime, whereas outside the diffusion boundary the concentration of the drug solution is unsaturated [13].

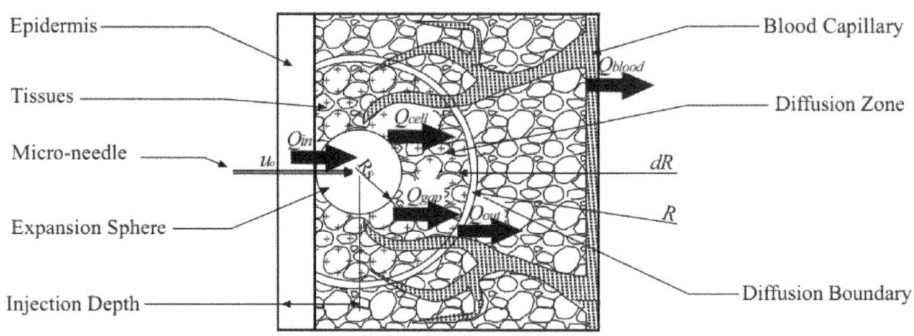

Figure 3: The diffusion model of single micro-needle in the skin after expansion.

Similar to the model proposed by Lv, et al., the following four parts contribute to the diffusion of drug solution into the skin: The first part is absorption of the tissue cells (represented by Q_{cell} in flow volume), with an absorption rate defined as γ. The second part is taken away by blood vessels (represented by Q_{blood} in flow volume), which is proportional to the total volume by a proportion coefficient expressed as β. The third part is the solution that fills the spaces between the tissues (represented by Q_{gap} in flow volume), which is also proportional to the total volume by a volumetric porosity ε. The fourth part is the drug diffusion through concentration gradient through the diffusion boundary (represented by $Q_{diffusion}$ in flow volume).

The flow volume of drug solution into the skin during a time period of dt can be expressed as:

$$Q_{in} = \frac{Q}{N} dt \quad (11)$$

The four parts of the diffusion of the drug solution can be expressed as:

$$Q_{blood} = \beta(2\pi R^2 dR + 2\pi R^3 / 3 - 2\pi R_s^{\ 3} / 3)dt \, , \quad (12)$$

$$Q_{gap} = 2\varepsilon\pi R^2 dR \, , \quad (13)$$

$$Q_{cell} = 2\gamma(1-\varepsilon)\pi R^2 dR \, , \quad (14)$$

$$Q_{diffusion} = 2\pi R^2 D \frac{\partial C}{\partial R} M / \rho \,, \tag{15}$$

Where R is the radius of diffusion boundary, D is the diffusion coefficient of the drug solution in the skin, C is the concentration of the drug solution, $\rho(kg/m^3)$ is the density of the drug solution, and M (g/mol) is the molar mass of drug solution. The following equation can be obtained from the conservation of mass flow:

$$\frac{Q}{N} dt = \beta(2\pi R^2 dR + 2\pi R^3/3 - 2\pi R_s^{\ 3}/3)dt + 2\varepsilon\pi R^2 dR + 2\gamma(1-\varepsilon)\pi R^2 dR + 2\pi R^2 D \frac{\partial C}{\partial R} M / \rho \tag{16}$$

The concentration gradient $\partial C/\partial R$ is very small close to the boundary, and the diffusion coefficient D is also very small. dR·dt is a much smaller term than dt or dR. The above equation can be simplified as:

$$\left[\frac{Q(t)}{N} - \frac{2}{3}\pi\beta(R^3 - R_s^{\ 3})\right] dt = 2\pi R^2(\varepsilon + \gamma - \gamma\varepsilon) dR \tag{17}$$

Again, the diffusion boundary R can be calculated if the micro-pump performance (Q), the variables of micro-needle system (N) and mechanical properties of the skin material (β, ε, and γ) are provided.

CALCULATION RESULTS

The coupled equations (Equation (4), and (10)) for the expansion model of the micro-needle drug delivery system derived in the previous section are numerically solved by a Runge-Kutta integration method.

The human skin is generally a highly organized, stratified structure mainly consisting of four layers: the stratum corneum (SC), epidermis, dermis and hypodermis. Ideally, the micro-needles penetrate the SC and reach the viable epidermis or hypodermis for painless injection. Gerling and Thomas [21] presented the mechanical properties of skin as a Young's Modulus of 1.36×10^5 Pa for the epidermis, 8.0×10^4 Pa for the dermis, 3.4×10^4 Pa for the subcutaneous fat with a Poisson's Ratio of 0.48 for each layer. The shear modulus (μ) can be thus calculated according to the relationship:

$$\mu = \frac{E}{2(1+\nu)}, \tag{18}$$

where E is Young's modulus, ν is poisson's ratio.

For a typical micro-pump of piezoelectric diaphragm type, Q and P_{pump} follow the reverse linear relationship, that is:

$$P_{pump} = P_{max}\left(1 - \frac{Q}{Q_{max}}\right), \tag{19}$$

where P_{max} and Q_{max} are pump characteristics provided by the manufacturer. A piezoelectric micro pump provided by Bartels Mikrotechnik was chosen for the calculation. For its MP6 pump, P_{max} = 550 mbar, Q_{max} = 6 ml/min, and the inner diameter and the length of soft tube are set at 1.3 mm and 500 mm respectively, and thus, A_1 = 1.33 mm^2. It is also assumed that the diameter of micro-needle chamber is constant (D_2 = 11 mm), and thus A_2 = 95 mm^2. A= d_o^2/ 4 is dependent upon the inner diameter of micro-needle (d_o). For the selected pump, the friction factor λ is estimated in the range of 0.6~1.0. For further simplification of calculation, a fixed number of λ = 0.8 was used in calculation.

In order to evaluate the effects of soft material properties and micro-needle system parameters on injection flow characteristics, four groups of calculation were carried out: 1): different strain hardening exponent (α); 2): different shear modulus (μ); 3): different total number of micro-needle array (N); and 4): different diameter of micro-needle (d_o). The values of α and μ were chosen around the aforementioned values given by [22]. In each calculation, one input variable was changed while others were kept constants. The chosen input variables for the four runs are listed in Table 1.

Table 1: The system parameters used in the expansion model calculation

Diameter d_o (mm)	Number (N)	Shear modulus μ (Pa x10^4)	Strain hardening exponent α	Maximal pressure P_{max} (Pa x10^4)	Maximal flow rate Q_{max} (ml/min)
120	43	1.1	6	5.5	6

The results of D_s ($2R_s$, expansion diameter), Q (flow rate) and P_o (expansion pressure) varying with time for three different α values were presented in Fig. (4). The increase of strain hardening exponent will reduce the expansion diameter as well as the jet flow rate.

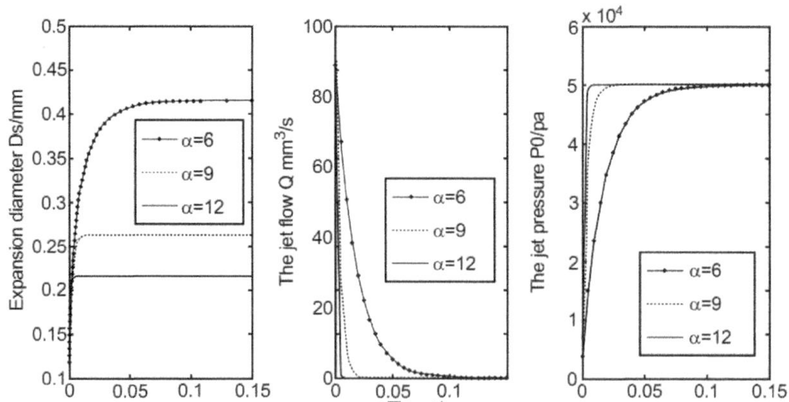

Figure 4: Calculated D_s, Q and P_o (α = 6, 9, 12).

Fig. (5) shows calculated D_s, Q and P_o vs. time for three different shear modulus (μ) values. A bigger shear modulus makes the expansion diameter smaller, and it takes less time for the flow rate to approach to zero.

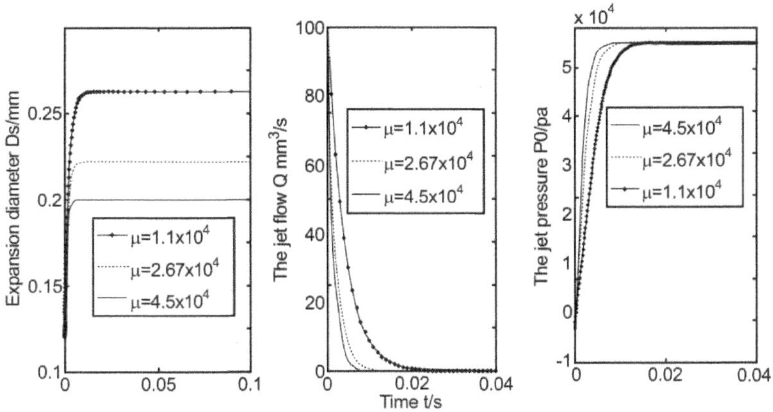

Figure 5: Calculated D_s, Q and P_o ($\mu = 1.1 \times 10^4$, 2.7×10^4, 4.5×10^4).

If the micro-needle array has a denser arrangement, that is, the total number of micro-needles increases, it takes longer time for P_o to reach a constant value and for Q to drop to zero, as shown in Fig. (6). However, the change of micro-needle number does not alter the expansion diameter that the injection can achieve. In other words, the arrangement of the micro-needle array has little influence on the initial infusion effects.

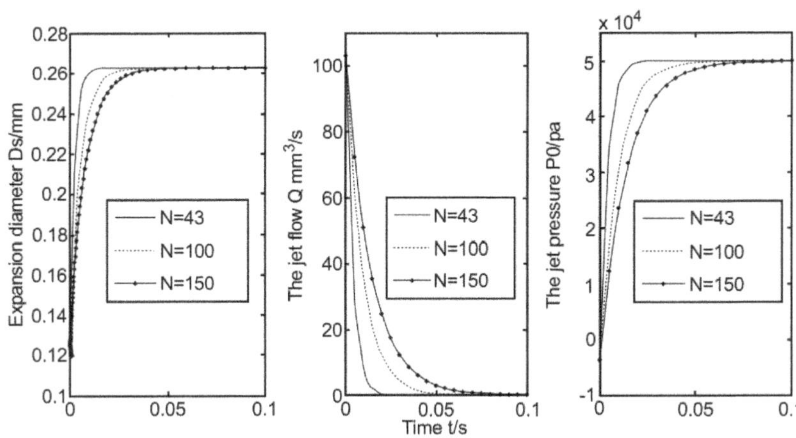

Figure 6: Calculated D_s, Q and P_o (N = 43, 100, 150).

Fig. (7) shows the results of D_s, Q and P_o for the three different values of micro-needle diameter d_o, whereas other variables were kept unchanged. A larger d_o makes the expansion easier. As a result, the expansion diameter increases, and it takes longer time for the flow rate drops to zero. It is also found that the expansion diameter is about 2-3 times of the micro-needle diameter no matter what the micro-needle diameter is.

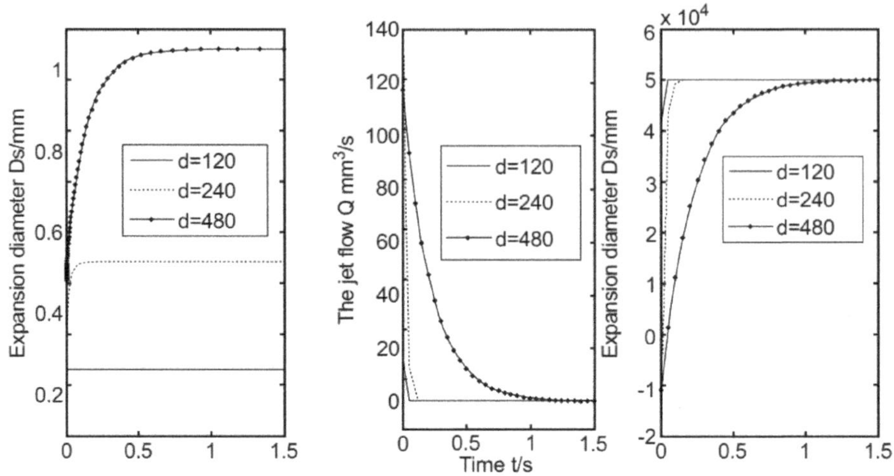

Figure 7: Calculated D_s, Q and P_o (d_o = 120, 240, 480).

The calculation results of expansion model show that the expansion radius levels out instantaneously. The initial infusion of the micro-needle jet is largely restricted by the spherical expansion of the jet.

In calculation of the diffusion boundary, it is assumed that the diffusion is an independent process. The jet flow rate Q(t) from the above expansion calculation thus can be substituted into Equation (17) to obtain the diameter of the diffusion boundary D_f (=2R). The physical properties of the human skin model used for the calculation of the diffusion boundary are listed in Table 2.

Table 2: The physical properties used in the diffusion model calculation

Liquid absorption rate of blood vessel β (s^{-1})	Porosity ε	Liquid absorption rate of cells γ
120	43	0.001

Fig. (8) shows both the diameter of diffusion boundary (D_f) and the expansion diameter (D_s) varying with time from the beginning of the injection, using the flow rate Q(t) from the above expansion calculation with the system parameters listed in Table 1 and Table 2. As shown in Fig. (8), the diffusion boundary increases rapidly from the initial injection, and reaches a peak value in 0.09 to 0.1 seconds and tapers after that. The variation tendency of the diameter of the diffusion boundary is dependent on the jet flow rate, the liquid uptake rate of the cells, the blood vessels, and the space between tissues. At the beginning of the injection, Q(t) starts from a maximum value and then decreases rapidly. The diffusion boundary thus picks up rapidly from the beginning of the injection, reaching a maximum value soon before it decreases to close to the expansion boundary when Q(t) decreases to close to zero.

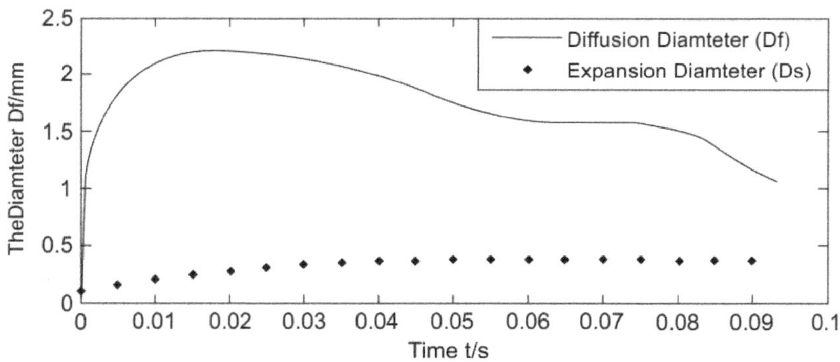

Figure 8: Calculated D_f, D_s vs. injection time.

Since the resistance quickly accumulates during the expansion of the jets, and the flow rate quickly drops to zero for a typical piezoelectric micro-pump, the diffusion also stops quickly. Normally, the diffusion of the micro-needle jets is a relatively slow process. It is thus reasonable to assume that the diffusion process starts after the expansion process nearly stops and it will reach an equilibrium state while Q(t) /N is stable. The following calculation assumes that Q(t) /N remains constant from the point of expansion diameter reaching 0.4mm (injection time=0.9s), while other parameters of the properties in Table 2 varying.

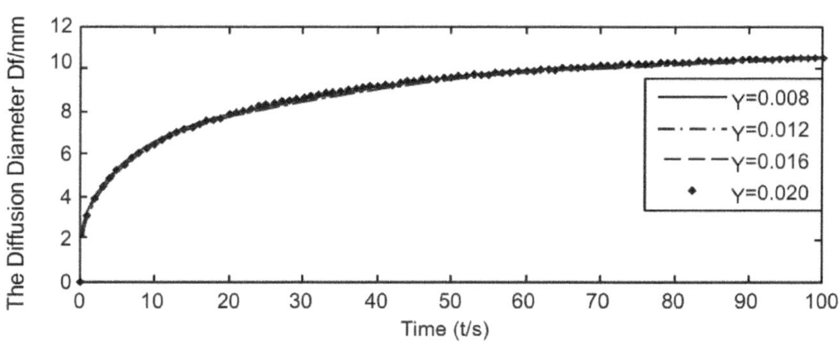

Figure 9: Calculated D_f for different γ ($Q(t)/N = 1.667 \times 10^{-9} m^3/s$).

Fig. (9) shows the results of diffusion boundary diameter D_f, for the three different values of liquid absorption rate of cells γ, whereas other variables were kept unchanged. Figs. (10, 11) show the calculation results of varying absorption rate of the blood vessel β, and the skin porosity ε, whereas other variables were kept constant as shown in Table 2, respectively.

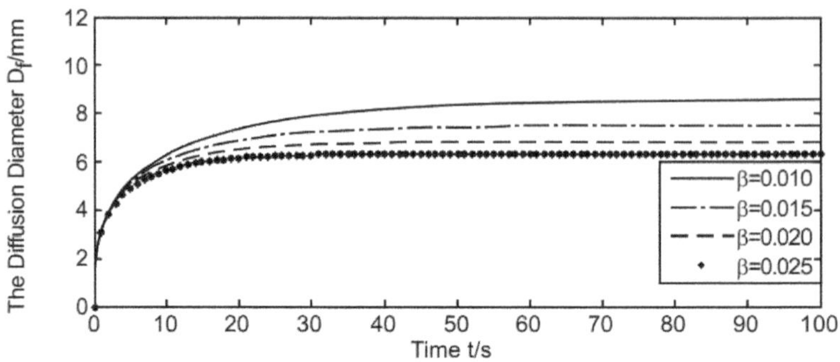

Figure 10: Calculated D_f for different β (Q(t)/N =1.667 × 10^{-9}m³/s).

It is seen from Figs. (9-11). that the diffusion boundary largely depends on the absorption rate of the blood vessel β and the skin porosity ε, and is relatively insensitive to the absorption rate of cells γ. Since γ is normally a magnitude smaller than, and both of them exist in the denominator of the exponential power in Equation (17), it is obvious that γ has little influence on the diffusion boundary. The absorption rate of blood vessel β has a reverse effect on size of the diffusion boundary. The increase of β will limit the permeability of the liquid, thus containing the diffusion boundary. On the contrary, the increase of skin porosity ε will increase the size of the diffusion boundary, thus increasing the permeability of the liquid.

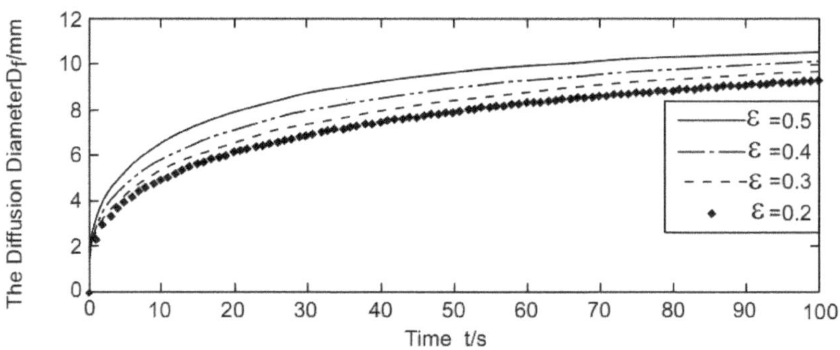

Figure 11: Calculated D_f for different ε (Q(t)/N =1.667 × 10^{-9}m³/s).

If $Q_{max}(t)$ in Table 1 is fixed as a constant, the jet flow rate of Q(t)/N varies as the number of micro-needle varies, and its impact on the diffusion boundary is shown in Fig. (12). (Q(t) /N = $Q_{max}(t)$/N, Other parameters are listed in Table 1 and Table 2). The increase of jet flow rate of Q(t) /N will obviously increase the size of the diffusion boundary.

QUALITATIVE EXPERIMENTS

Since the infusion process of a micro-needle system is difficult to visualize, a single needle driven by a syringe pump was used for experimental study. The needle has inner diameter of 0.14mm and outer diameter of 0.32mm. The infusion syringe pump (Harvard Pump 11 Elite, Provided by InsTech Laboratories, PA, USA, infusion velocity from 1.28 pl/min. to 88.28 ml/min without load) has a microprocessor for actuation and is synchronized with a high speed digital imaging system (provided by Beijing Daheng Imavision, China, Transmission speed: 400Mbit/s, frame rate of 32 frames per second, exposure time 43 ~67s range, automatic shutter).

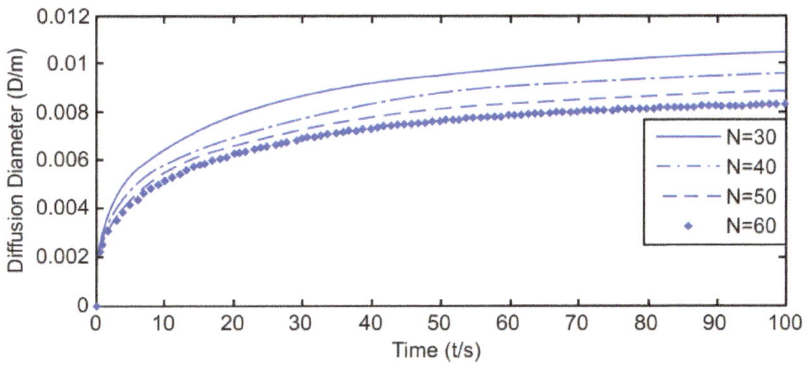

Figure 12: Calculated D_f for different N.

Silicon rubber and polyacrylamide gel were chosen as model soft material for their skin like characteristics. Silicon Rubber is an incompressible, hyperelastic, isotropic, soft solid that is often used to replace human skin. It satisfies the Odgen model of strain energy that the current expansion model is based upon [18]. Polyacrylamide gel has the property of inelastic, absorptive, transparent, and is ideal for visualization. Overall, silicon rubber has the property close to SC and epidermis, and polyacrylamide gel is close to dermis and hypodermis.

In the experiments, liquid silicone rubber which contains A, B two materials (R-705A, R-705B, provided by Chengdu Zhonglan Chemical Engineering Research Institute, China), was mixed with ratio of 10:1, after centrifuged, then put into a drying oven for a period of time. The self made silicon rubber has Shore hardness of 10 HA. Polyacrylamide gel was created by adding initiators to acrylamide solution. 30% Acr/0.8% BisAcrylamide (SDS-PAGE, Provided by Nanjing KeyGen Biotech, China) was mixed with DI water to create acrylamide solutions. Gels were polymerized by the addition of 10% APS (45ml) and TEMED (12ml) to 6ml acrylamide solution, resulting 30% gel. The self-made polyacrylamide gel has Shore hardness of 8 HA.

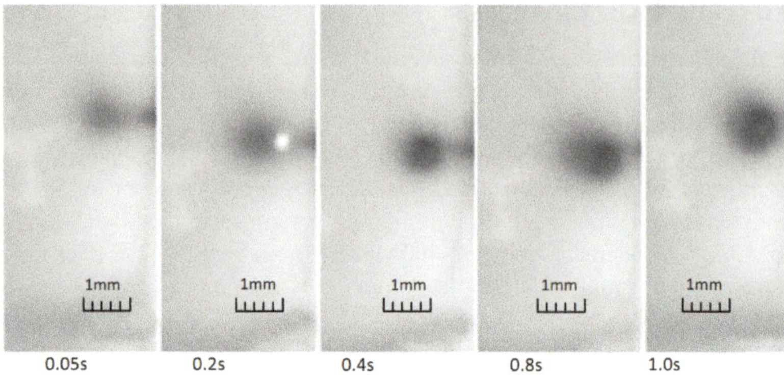

Figure 13: Jet expansion in a silicon rubber through a single needle.

Fig. (13) shows the initial injection of the liquid in the prepared silicon rubber through the needle that was put approximately 2mm underneath the surface. The infusion velocity at the pump is set to be 50ml/min. The silicon rubber was placed under the aforementioned digital imaging system with the exposure time set to 50ms. It can be seen from the figure that the jet expansion quickly stops (within 1s of initial infusion) due to high resistance of surrounding material. The results agree with the analytic results from the expansion model.

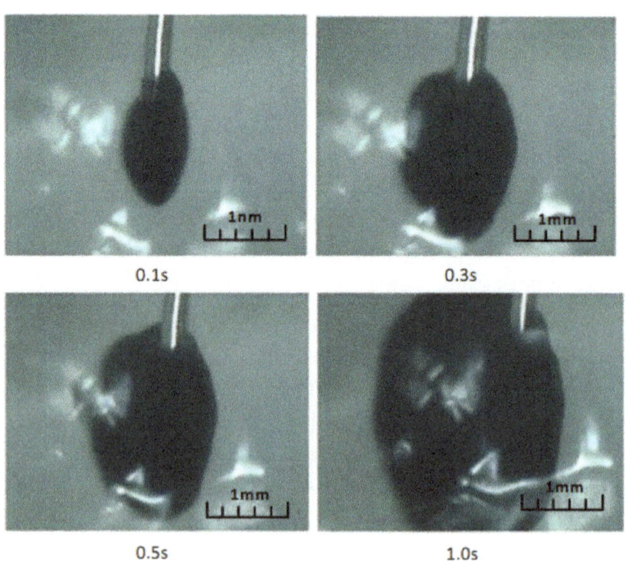

Figure 14: Jet dispersion in a polyacrylamide gel through a single needle.

Fig. (14) illustrates the initial injection of the liquid in the prepared polyacrylamide gel through the same needle and the same velocity setting of the pump. The figure is clearer due to more transparent feature of the polyacrylamide gel. The jet expansion is much bigger than that in silicon rubber, and keeps expanding after 1s. Polyacrylamide gel has the property of good absorption. Therefore, the expansion can be partly viewed as diffusion, and the results qualitatively agree with the analytic results from the dispersion model. In fact, the jet expansion becomes irregular in shape and disperses to particular areas after keeping injection for several seconds.

DISCUSSION

Human skin is a composite material that consists of cells, tissues, nerves, blood vessels, and water. In general, the properties of stratum corneum and epidermis are closer to those of silicon rubber, and the properties of dermis and hypodermis are closer to those of polyacrylamide and water. The current model of micro-needle infusion may have guiding significances on practical micro-needle drug delivery depending on the location of transdermal injection.

Although micro-needle length will usually be greater than the thickness of the stratum corneum (SC) of the skin, the process of micro-needle puncture of the skin will cause deformation and tension of the stratum, result in changes of strain energy and hardness surrounding the micro-needle, and the actual depths of micro-needle insertion are below than expected [17], as shown in Fig. (15). The increase of strain hardening exponent and shear modulus from stratum and epidermis will make the liquid infusion more difficult, as indicated in Fig. (4). and Fig. (5). Many experimental studies show that the infusion through hollow micro-needles into the skin is limited by the resistance to flow caused by compressed dense dermal tissue [15, 16]. It also explains the reason that the commercialization of the micro-needle system driven by a micro-pump is difficult. If the micro-needles are just long enough to pierce through the layer of SC and epidermis without touching the nerves, the diffusion process may dominate and the infusion flow will be improved.

In reality, the dermis structure underneath the epidermis is a non homogeneous porous material that is difficult to be described by a few mechanical properties. The current model also assumes that the infusion expansion by each micro-needle in the array is an independent process. However, when the expansion grows to a certain level such that the expansion diameter or diffusion boundary is comparable to the distance of two neighboring micro-needles, the flow behavior will be affected, which makes the current assumption invalid. The current model describes the initial flow characteristics of the micro-needles infusion when the pump flow pressure is much higher than the capillary resistance pressure. In addition, since most of the liquid drug has low viscosity, it is reasonable to neglect the capillary resistance even the inner radius of the needles is very small.

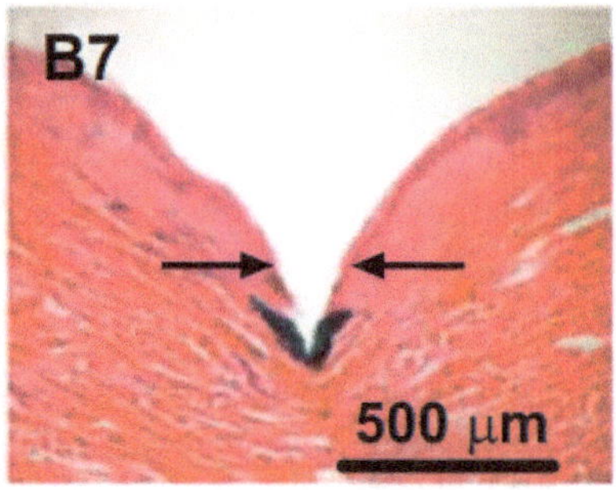

Figure 15: Deformation and tension of skin during insertion of micro-needles (the arrow indicating the site of needle penetration, photo courtesy of [17]).

CONCLUSION

An analytical model is presented to calculate the flow characteristics of the infusion of a micro-needle drug delivery system. It is assumed that the initial liquid infusion through micro-needles forms a spherical expansion and a spherical diffusion. During the expansion process, the skin is treated as a non porous, incompressible, hyper elastic, and isotropic solid. The calculations based on the current model lead to some interesting results: for a typical commercial piezoelectric micro pump, the flow expansion stops instantly and the flow rate quickly drops to zero, unless the pressure from the micro-pump is increased. It is assumed that the diffusion of the micro-needle jet is driven by the jet flow coming out of the micro-needle. The diffusion process is influenced by the absorption of the tissue cells, liquid carrying by blood vessels, and the solution filling the spaces between the tissues, while the diffusion through concentration gradient is neglected. The rapid drop of the jet flow rate resulted from the jet expansion process causes the diameter of the diffusion boundary increasing quickly at the beginning, then tapered off immediately after reaching a maximum value. If the jet flow rate remains constant, the diameter of the diffusion boundary increases with the increasing skin porosity, but decreases with the increasing absorption rate of the blood vessel, and is insensitive to the absorption rate of cells. The experimental results from the jet flow through a single needle in silicon rubber that fits into the assumption of the expansion model also show that the jet expansion as well as jet flow quickly stops after initial infusion. However, the phenomena of the jet flow in polyacrylamide gel show that the jet expansion is much larger and the jet flow will keep going as long as the pump pressure is enough. The polyacrylamide gel has good absorption property, and the results qualitatively agree with the analytic results from the diffusion model.

ACKNOWLEDGEMENTS

The current project is under support of China's National Science Foundation (No. 51275142).

DISCLOSURE

Part of this article has been previously published in Biomedical Engineering and Informatics (BMEI), 4th International Conference 2011, (Volume:2), Pages: 913 - 917; DOI: 10.1109/BMEI.2011.6098420.

REFERENCES

1. M.R. Prausnitz, S. Mitragotri, and R. Langer, "Current status and future potential of transdermal drug delivery", Nat. Rev. Drug Discov., vol. 3, no. 2, pp. 115-124, 2004.
2. M.R. Prausnitz, "Microneedles for transdermal drug delivery", Adv. Drug Deliv. Rev., vol. 56, no. 5, pp. 581-587, 2004.
3. M.A. Jalil, N. Suwanpayak, K. Kulsirirat, S. Suttirak, J. Ali, and P.P. Yupapin, "Embedded nanomicro syringe on chip for molecular therapy", Int. J. Nanomedicine, vol. 6, pp. 2925-2932, 2011.
4. S. Hashmi, P. Ling, G. Hashmi, M. Reed, R. Gaugler, and W. Trimmer, "Genetic transformation of nematodes using arrays of micromechanical piercing structures", Biotechniques, vol. 19, no. 5, pp. 766-770, 1995.
5. T.H. Shikida, and K. Sato, "Fabrication of a hollow needle structure by dicing, wet etching and metal deposition", J. Micromech. Microeng., vol. 16, pp. 2230-2239, 2006.
6. N. Wilke, and A. Morrissey, "Silicon microneedle formation using modified mask designs based on convex corner undercut", J. Micromech. Microeng., vol. 17, pp. 238-244, 2007.
7. H. Huang, and C. Fu, "Different fabrication methods of out-of plane polymer hollow needle arrays and their variations", J. Micromech. Microeng., vol. 17, pp. 393-402, 2007.
8. J.W. Lee, J.H. Park, and M.R. Prausnitz, "Dissolving microneedles for transdermal drug delivery", Biomaterials, vol. 29, no. 13, pp. 2113-2124, 2008.
9. L.Y. Chu, S.O. Choi, and M.R. Prausnitz, "Fabrication of dissolving polymer microneedles for controlled drug encapsulation and delivery: Bubble and pedestal microneedle designs", J. Pharm. Sci., vol. 99, no. 10, pp. 4228-4238, 2010.
10. J.E. Sanders, B.S. Goldstein, and D.F. Leotta, "Skin response to mechanical stress: adaptation rather than breakdown-a review of the literature", J. Rehabil. Res. Dev., vol. 32, no. 3, pp. 214-226, 1995.
11. X.Q. Kong, and C.W. Wu, "Measurement and prediction of insertion force for the mosquito fascicle penetrating into human skin", J. Bionics Eng., vol. 6, pp. 143-152, 2009.
12. Y.A. Gomaa, D.I. Morrow, M.J. Garland, R.F. Donnelly, L.K. El-Khordagui, and V.M. Meidan, "Effects of microneedle length, density, insertion time and multiple applications on human skin barrier function: Assessments by transepidermal water loss", In: Toxicol. In Vitro, vol. 24. 2010, pp. 1971-1978.

13. Y.G. Lv, J. Liu, Y.H. Gao, and B. Xu, "Modeling of transdermal drug delivery with a microneedle array", J. Micromech. Microeng., vol. 16, pp. 2492-2501, 2006.

14. R. Zhang, P. Zhang, C. Dalton, and G.A. Jullien, "Modeling of drug delivery into tissues with a microneedle array using mixture theory", Biomech. Model. Mechanobiol., vol. 9, no. 1, pp. 77-86, 2010.

15. W. Martanto, J.S. Moore, T. Couse, and M.R. Prausnitz, "Mechanism of fluid infusion during microneedle insertion and retraction", J. Control. Release, vol. 112, no. 3, pp. 357-361, 2006.

16. W. Martanto, J.S. Moore, O. Kashlan, R. Kamath, P.M. Wang, J.M. O'Neal, and M.R. Prausnitz, "Microinfusion using hollow microneedles", Pharm. Res., vol. 23, no. 1, pp. 104-113, 2006.

17. S.P. Davis, B.J. Landis, Z.H. Adams, M.G. Allen, and M.R. Prausnitz, "Insertion of microneedles into skin: measurement and prediction of insertion force and needle fracture force", J. Biomech., vol. 37, no. 8, pp. 1155-1163, 2004.

18. O.A. Shergold, and N.A. Fleck, "Mechanisms of deep penetration of soft solids, with application to the injection and wounding of skin", Proc. R. Soc. Lond. A, vol. 460, pp. 3037-3058, 2004.

19. F. Yang, K. Chen, and Z.G. Feng, "Analytical model of initial fluid infusion by a microneedle drug delivery system", Proceeding of The 4th International Conference on BioMedical Engineering and Informatics, BMEI 2011, 2011 Shanghai, China

20. F.M. White, Fluid Mechanics. McGraw-Hill: New York, 2003.

21. G.J. Gerling, and G.W. Thomas, "The effect of fingertip microstructures on tactile edge perception", In: Proceeding of the 1st Joint Eurohaptics Conf. and Symp. on Haptic Interfaces for Virtual Environment and Teleoperator Systems. 2005. Pisa, Italy

22. R.W. Ogden, "Large deformation isotropic elasticity: On the correlation of theory and experiment for incompressible rubberlike solids", Proc. R. Soc. Lond. A Math. Phys. Sci., vol. 326, pp. 565-584, 1972

7

CHAPTER

RECENT PATENTS AND DESIGNS ON HIP REPLACEMENT PROSTHESES

H Derar, M Shahinpoor

Keywords: Total Hip Replacement/Arthroplasty (THR/THA), Revision Surgery, Stemless Prosthesis, Femoral Head Prosthesis, Acetabular Cup Prosthesis

INTRODUCTION

Total Hip Replacement (THR) surgery or Total Hip Arosthroplasty (THA), is a surgery in which the hip joint is replaced with a prosthetic implant. Hip replacement surgery was first performed in 1840 in New York, by Dr. Carnochan who was the first surgeon to insert a wooden piece between the diseased hip joint [1]. In recent years the THR surgery is being considered by most in the field to be a successful elective major procedure especially in restoring mobility to patients. Worldwide, there are approximately one million implants performed annually [2, 3]. The surgery has become a routine with a minimum rate of early complications, offering patients great relief of pain when medications fail. It further offers tremendous improvement in function and consequently quality of life. Therefore, it is one of the most satisfying operations to both patients as well as surgeons. THR is performed as a solution to several degenerative and traumatic processes which affect the hip joint; it is a reconstructive surgical procedure.

In the past five decades, advances that have been made in technology; innovations in materials, surgical techniques, and methods of fixation and sterilization of prostheses, facilitated hip joint implants go through multiple design evolutions seeking better results and longer survivorship for implants. This resulted in the breakthrough of hip surgery;

Citation: H Derar, M Shahinpoor, Recent Patents and Designs on Hip Replacement Prostheses, DOI: 10.2174/1874120701509010092.

nevertheless, not all implants were able to withstand the test of longevity. Although the risks of the surgery are low, there are long term complications that contribute to the failure of the prosthesis; the most problematic is the limited life spanof the prosthesis. Ten percent of the implanted prostheses have a revision surgery within ten years [4]; the average life-span of the prosthesis is fifteen years [2, 4, 5], which is a crucial problem to the growing number of young patients under forty years of age. These young patients usually are more active and therefore they will require multiple revision surgeries throughout their life-time. Revision surgery is substantially more difficult than primary THR surgery due to the involvement of removal of existing implant and fixations, complexity of the procedure, and longer anaesthesia and operative time [6]. Preparation of the operating site has to be performed prior to insertion of the new prosthesis with the use of any necessary fixation methods or reinforcement. Revision surgery has a higher rate of intraoperative fractures than primary THR [7]. Postoperatively, patients are prone to have more complications and rehabilitation takes longer. Therefore, it is more risky [5, 7], costly and inconvenient to the patient than primary surgery.

It was reported by the Swedish National Hip Arthroplasty Register annual report [7] that between the year 1979 and 2004, 73% of revision surgery was due to aseptic loosening of the implants. "Osteolysis, is defined as the process of progressive destruction of periprosthetic bony tissue" [6], which if not treated could lead to aseptic loosening and failure of the implant. As the femoral head articulates against the acetabular cup, particles of a clinically relative size (0.1 – 10 μm) [4] are released from the implant activating macrophages, consequently, causing osteolysis and resulting in aseptic loosening of the implant leading to the failure of the THA and a necessary revision surgery. The high rates of revision surgery are considered to be affected by prosthetic hip design, materials and fixation methods, as well as the patient's age and activity [8]. To decrease the number of revision surgeries, new technical innovations for the prosthesis have been created. This paper presents several patents of various innovations for different components of the prostheses designed to lessen the number of revision surgeries with the intention of increasing the longevity of implants.

The prosthesis typically consists of a femoral stem, a femoral head (ball) that attaches to the stem, an acetabular cup and a fixation agent to secure the stem into the femur and the acetabular cup into the acetabulum in the pelvis, Fig. (1).

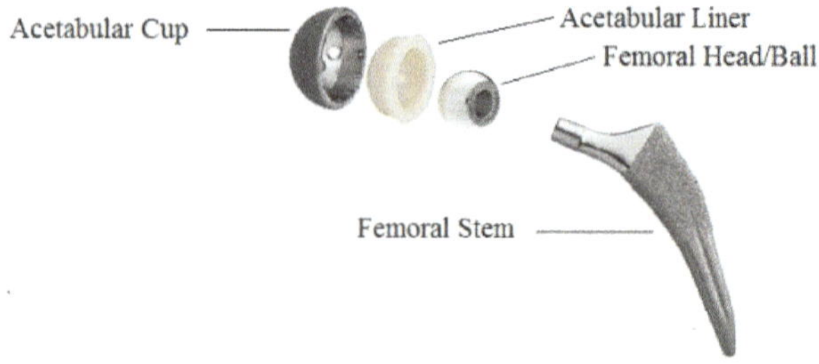

Figure 1: Hip Joint Prosthesis.

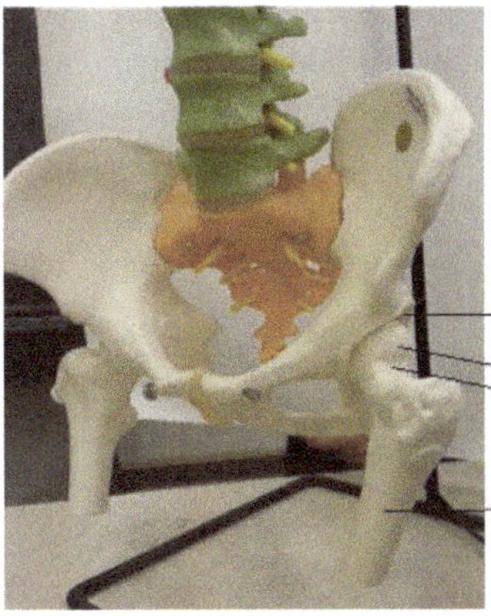

Figure 2: The hip joint, (picture taken by author from a skeleton in our Biomedical Engineering Lab., in UMaine).

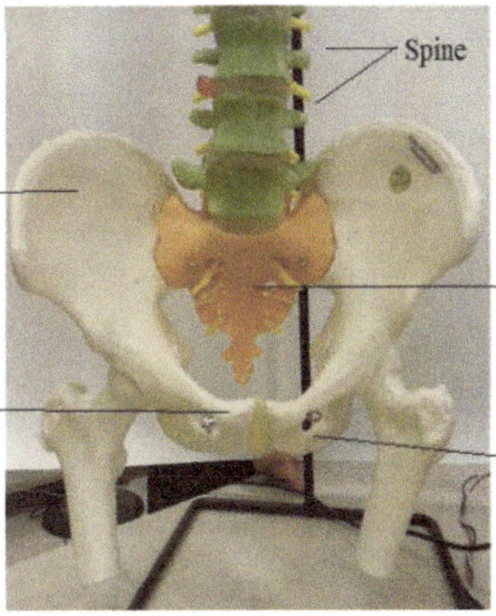

Figure 3: Bones of the pelvis (picture taken by author from a skeleton in our Biomedical Engineering Lab., UMaine).

The hip joint is one of the largest joints in the body, similar to a typical ball and socket joint, see Fig. (2), and it is the most weight-bearing. It is located where the femur, the thigh bone, meets the three bones that make up the pelvis; the ilium is at the rear, the ischium at the lower front and the pubis above it [9], as depicted in Fig. (3). These bones congregate to shape the acetabulum (deep socket) at the outer side of the pelvis. At the top of the femur is the femoral head, a ball-like shape, 2/3 of a sphere, it is attached to the femur by the femoral neck which is a short section of bone. The acetabulum forms approximately half a sphere (concaved). A smooth cushion of shiny white articular cartilage, about one quarter of an inch thick, with rubbery consistency, covers the femoral head and the acetabulum. The articular cartilage is made of tough flexible tissues that are kept slippery by the lubricant fluid made in the synovial membrane (joint lining). The synovial fluid is a viscous and sticky lubricant and combined with the articular cartilage they are very slippery, allowing the joint surfaces to move against each other easily without causing damage.

The femoral head and acetabulum are secured in place and prevented from dislocating by large ligaments, tendons and muscles that surround the hip joint (joint capsule).

BACKGROUND ART

Hip replacement surgery is an old procedure, and one of the most challenging procedures as it plays an important role in helping patients suffering from joint failure due to diseases that include osteoarthritis, avascular necrosis, rheumatoid arthritis, Paget's disease and bone tumors, to name a few [10]. There are three types of hip replacement surgery:

1. total hip replacement THR or total hip arthroplasty THA, in which the whole hip joint, ball and socket, is replaced with femoral stem and prosthetic implant
2. partial hip replacement in which only the femoral head is replaced
3. a hip resurfacing procedure in which the socket or acetabulum is replaced and the femoral head is trimmed, reshaped and then covered with a smooth cap.

Some of the complications may be shared by all three types. Thus, not only several surgical approaches have been introduced to find the ideal hip implant, but many aspects have been studied ranging from the novel designs of the various parts of the prosthesis to the different materials employed and their biocompatibility.

The following section reviews a number of recent patents on hip replacement prosthesis.

U.S. Patent No. 6,248,132 B1, by inventor Charles C. Harris titled "Hip Replacement Prosthesis" [11] and issued June 2001 discusses "Abstract: A hip joint prosthesis including a stem assembly having an outer casing received within the hip socket. The cup assembly outer casing includes threadedly attached upper and lower portions to encapsulate the lining and the lining includes an upper portion having a recess receiving the head and a split lower portion seating the head. The cup assembly also includes an interior spring assembly providing shock absorption between the head and the casing. The stem assembly includes an elongate stem and a cooperating shield attached to the stem, the stem being independently movable following insertion of the stem and shield into the femur."

According to the inventor, an ideal implant should be able to re-produce the mechanism and structure of the original member replaced. It is essential for the femoral head of the implant to be tightly fixed to the stem and that the head is received within the acetabulum. Also, the resulting joint should provide some flexibility or "cushioning".

The inventor [11], presents an improved hip joint replacement over previous arts which surpasses past problems and offers advantages for this invention [11].

The inventor provides a hip prosthesis that delivers a substantial universal joint movement between the stem assembly and the cup assembly. The stem is secured into the femur and the cup assembly receives the femoral head which is received by the prepared hip socket. The socket is being affixed with a tight socket shell. The structural arrangements for the parts provide: rotational movement of the cup assembly about the radial center of the socket and also pivotal movement of the stem about the center of the femoral head while circular movement of the head about the femoral neck axis.

One of the invention aspects is to have the cup assembly consisting of means providing shock absorption between the head and casing.

An additional feature of the invention is that the stem assembly has an extended stem and a shield with means between them allowing the stem to move independently relatively to the shield, after both being inserted into the femur.

According to the inventor [11], the novelty of this invention is to have an implant with the femoral head firmly fixed to the femur and the head "received" within the acetabulum. This invention introduces a less expensive replacement as well as ease of manufacturing and installment. It is considered efficient in providing natural joint movement.

U.S. Patent No. 6,336,941 B1, by inventors; G. V. Subba Rao, Anil K. Goli, titled "Modular Hip Implant With Shock Absorption System" [12] and issued Jan. 2002 introduces "Abstract: A modular hip implant that can be custom fit to an individual patient, including a shock absorption system that absorbs compressive stresses that are imparted to the implant. The size of the femoral ball member, size of the femoral stem, femoral neck length, and tension in the shock absorption system are all individually adjustable parameters, depending on the particular patient. A unique coupling member houses a modular spring mechanism that serves as the shock absorber. The coupling member is received into the ball member to an adjustable depth, the adjustment of which varies the length of the femoral neck. The length of the femoral neck can be adjusted during surgery without requiring additional parts."

The invention [12] presents a device that can absorb compressive stresses conveyed to the implant through the shock absorption system. Additionally, the device may be custom fitted, where the ball and femoral components are selected from a range of ball and femoral members, the selection of the ball depends on the size of the acetabulum socket. This invention [12] also comprises a spring system running through the ball and the neck in order to furnish cushioning between the ball and the femoral stem. The spring is to be chosen from a plurality of springs with different constants and stiffness. The device consisted of two shock absorbers, one attached to the ball and a second attached to the upper part of the femur with a spring between them to cushion the compressive force. This device [12] could be of advantages to the patients as the spring mechanism of contracting and expanding while performing daily activities reduces load bearing, shock and compressive stresses on the implant. This will mean less movement of the implant and hence no loosening resulting in a longer implant life-span. Other advantages of the invention [12] are decreases in complications such as acetabular damage and erosion, and dislocation. Additionally, the spring being custom fitted provides the option of choosing a spring with the right parameters (stiffness). Moreover, the length of the femoral neck can be chosen as required without additional parts since a single coupling member may be installed in the ball to the depth that corresponds to the acquired neck length, this can be adjusted during surgery.

U.S. Patent No. 6,379,390 B1, by inventors, Suresh G. Advani, Michael H. Santare, Freeman Miller, Makarand Joshi, and issued April 2002, introduces "Stemless Hip Prosthesis," [13], in which "Abstract: A stemless hip prosthesis uses one or more cables which wrap around the prosthesis and the femur to mount the prosthesis in place thereby avoiding the need to provide the prosthesis with a stem located in the medullary canal."

According to the inventors; one of the main reasons of THR failure is bone resorption which might be due to stress shielding of bone as a result of a stiff prosthesis being used, plus extra shear stresses where both prosthesis and bone contact. In the classical surgery, the current designs of prostheses use a stem that is inserted in the femur. Therefore, the inventors are introducing a stemless hip implant. To divert the load from being transferred through the stem of the prosthesis the load is applied at the proximal end of the femur. To apply the bending moment through the cross section of the femur with the greater trochanter included would acquire a new fixation technique that decreases the interface shear stresses, relative torsion and stress shielding. Since cables support axial loads, they do not increase the bending stiffness of the bone. The short flexible stem bolt arrangement in the medial calcar area reaches into the femur offering torsional support and fixation, while increasing local interface shear stresses. The cables contacting the tendons increase slightly the local stresses, permitting a "natural" stress spreading through the proximal femur cross section. Hence, stress shielding is at a minimum because the effective bending of the femur is not increased. The notion of this design is to eliminate the "interface shear stresses" by the use of familiar surgical high strength steel cables for fixation, wrapping them around a portion of the femur and prosthesis. The cables uphold axial loads and therefore do not raise the bending stiffness of the bone. Moreover, the inventors [13] believe that this design will simplify revision surgery if needed as it would necessitate the cables being tighter, which is an important feature. The cables and fixture screws are to affix the prosthesis tighter without the use of a stem inserted into the femur.

U.S. Patent No. 6,425,922 B1, by inventors; Bill J. Pope, Jeffrey K. Taylor, Richard H. Dixon, Clayton F. Gardinier, Louis M. Pope, Dean C. Blackburn, Michael A. Vail, Kenneth M. Jensen, and issued July 2002, titled " Prosthetic Hip Joint Having At Least One Sintered Polycrystalline Diamond Compact Articulation Surface," [14] describes "Abstract: Prosthetic joints, components for prosthetic joints, super hard bearing and articulation surfaces, diamond bearing and articulation surfaces, substrate surface topographical features, materials for making joints, bearing and articulation surfaces, and methods for manufacturing and finishing the same, and related information are disclosed, including a prosthetic hip joint having polycrystalline diamond articulation surfaces and at least one sintered polycrystalline diamond articulation surface."This invention is targeting a minimum wear and no debris and therefore longer life-span of prosthesis with expectancy of life-long patient use. Diamonds of various types and super-hard materials are used in this invention in the bearing surfaces because of their low coefficient of friction and resistance to wear, and if particles due to wear are created they will be of no significance. Polycrystalline diamond compacts or super-hard materials are to form one of the articulating surfaces of the implant. This will reduce the incidence of osteolysis which is a major advantage.

US Patent No. 7,641,699 B2 by inventor Anthony S. Unger, titled "Femoral Head Calcar Loading Prosthesis," [15] and issued January 2010 describes "Abstract: Provided is a novel hip replacement implant system that includes a ball assembly having a ball trunnion, the ball assembly being configured as a replacement for the head of the femur and capable of being secured by the ball assembly trunnion to a calcar implant element that can be securely seated in the calcar bone of the femoral neck, thus maintaining the load transfer function of the calcar bone of the femoral neck. A method of using the device is also provided."

Most of the conventional hip replacements include a design of a stem inserted in the femur canal replacing a proximal portion of the femur. This places unnatural stresses on the femur and consequently pain and limitation to the patient's activities. Moreover, the technique used in removing the neck of the femur may cause destruction of the calcar bone and eventually exposes the patient to bone weakness and fractures that could lead to revision surgeries.

This invention presents a solution to the problems of typical hip implants, and provides techniques to replace the conventional one by reproducing the hip joint articulation aspects and also utilizing the natural load transferring femur calcar bone to prevent prosthesis failure and revision surgery. Thus, the inventors [15] present a novel hip implant system comprised of a ball assembly having a ball trunnion or trunnion to facilitate the capability of the ball being affixed to a calcar implant element which can be securely positioned in the calcar bone of the femoral neck and articulating with the ball assembly. Also, included is an acetabular component that is formed and inserted in the hip and articulated with the ball assembly. The ball assembly is of metal as well as the acetabular components; the metal ball is to replace the femoral head and the acetabular component is measured and designed to be inserted in the hip pelvic cavity and articulating with the metal ball component. Additionally, the invention provides a procedure of embedding the hip replacement prosthesis implementing minimally invasive surgery to implant the prosthesis.

U.S. Patent No. 7,833,277 B2, by inventors; Joseph Saladino, Mark E. Nadzadi, Brian Burkinshaw, titled "Femoral Head Assembly With Variable Offset," [16] and issued Nov. 2010, presents "Abstract: A proximal femoral ball assembly having a variable offset that is selectively adjustable to conform to various anatomical conditions encountered during a femoral surgical procedure. The femoral ball assembly generally includes a head, a neck, and an adjustment mechanism. The head has a smooth spherical outer surface that is adapted to engage an acetabular component or native acetabulum. The neck extends outward from the head and removeably connects to the head using a threaded attachment." This invention relates to orthopedic implant prostheses for THA and more specifically to a proximal femoral head assembly of variable offset and selectively adjustable to adapt to any anatomical conditions during surgery. A hip joint implant typically may consist of a femoral stem, a socket or acetabulum, and a femoral head or ball. During surgery, the femur is prepared to receive the implant femoral stem which is then inserted into the intramedullary canal of the femur to the proper depth and orientation, while the appropriate ball is fixed to the proximal end of the stem. The ball is fit into the socket or acetabulum where it facilitates an articulation surface between the femoral prosthesis and acetabulum. Between the femoral head and stem there is a neck or trunnion connected to the stem at one end and in some designs connected to the head, and it is usually of cylindrical shape.

To ensure proper functioning of the prosthesis of this invention [16] after implanting, several crucial features are to be considered. One of these features is the femoral head "offset".

According to the inventors, "femoral head offset is the horizontal distance from the center of rotation of the femoral head to a line bisecting the long axis of the femur from a standing A-P x-ray." The offset of the proximal femoral component is similarly the horizontal distance between the center of rotation of the ball and the stem's long axis. The amount of offset between the ball and the stem implemented by the surgeon during surgery significantly affects the performance and success of the prosthesis. If the patient's natural anatomical needs are not met by the offset, then the prosthesis can be positioned either too far laterally or medially.

Additionally, a decrease in femoral offset medially results in shifts or moves of the femur closer to the pelvis and it can cause in some patients impingement of the prosthesis as well as loosening or laxity of local tissue resulting in implant instability, subluxation and dislocation. A further disadvantage of the offset decrease is that as the abductor muscles balance the pelvis they employ larger force generating discrepancy that might cause a patient's limp, and there is greater polyethylene wear between the ball and the acetabular components.

An increase in the offset laterally on the other hand causes the femur to move or shift further than the pelvis. An increase in offset is sometimes desirable for various reasons such as;

1. may lessen the impingement risk
2. may improve the tension of soft tissues and hence the implant will have more stability
3. the abductor muscles can be appropriately balanced and the patient gait improves, which also results in lesser wear and loosening over time.

Due to the aforementioned disadvantages, hip prostheses are marketed with different offsets. Hence a typical system may have a number of different offsets for each femoral head and therefore the manufacturer will need to have an inventory ranging between 18-30 different femoral heads, which is costly for maintaining and distributing.

Therefore, for the above mentioned disadvantages and others, the inventors [16] present a proximal femoral ball assembly comprised of a head, a neck, and an adjustment mechanism. The ball is of a smooth spherical outer surface to interact smoothly with the acetabular component or the original acetabulum. Further, the neck is extended outwards from the ball and detachably connects with the head by threaded connection.

An additional advantage of the invention is that it furnishes a plurality of small increments of femoral offsets as small as 1 mm increments, and these offsets can range between -10 mm to +10 mm while the inventors think of the possibility of a range up to +30 mm. This enables appropriate matching of the patient's anatomical needs.

In another embodiment of [16], a femoral ball system with different sized heads and spacers are provided that can be employed with a single neck offering several femoral offsets with plurality of various sized spherical balls.

In another embodiment of the above invention [16], two parallel axes that form an acute angle with longitudinal axis of the stem, extend through the femoral ball assembly. The first axis or central axis is concentric with the spherical head body while the second axis or eccentric axis is concentric with the threaded head bore and also concentric with the adjustment mechanism and neck of the femoral head assembly.

Another advantage of the invention is the eccentric neck (or the offset from the femoral head) presents an increased array of movement when attached to the stem, thus the increase replicates the hip motion and stabilizes the prosthesis. Additionally, the eccentric neck presents a femoral prosthesis which will not be prone to impingement, subluxation or dislocation.

U.S. Patent No. 7,931,691 B2; by inventors; Xue Li, Ping Xie, Kerry Y. Xie, titled "External Proximal Femoral Prosthesis For Total Hip Arthroplasty," [17] and issued April 2011 presents "Abstract: A external femoral component for mechanically housing onto exterior remnant of natural femur and coupling with articulation elements in order to use in total hip arthroplasty defines as a hollow shell comprised of asymmetrically bell shaped cup, at least one rigid elongated stem downwardly extended from the lower rim of the cup and a plurality of an cylindrical object upwardly protruded from top of the cup for pairing with articulation elements and coupling with anchoring means and the tension anchoring means fixes the hollow shell on the bone surface through an interlocking mechanisms."

The invention introduces a femoral prosthesis and in particular relating to external proximal femoral element seated in the outside area of the rest of the proximal femur, affixed securely with installation by tension means.

According to the inventors [17] there are disadvantages to the conventional prostheses that have been used in total hip replacement and which comprise stem designs. These disadvantages include:

- The applied bending moment through the stem causes stress concentration at the proximal, medial and the distal lateral ends of the prosthesis, respectively, i.e. in a comparatively small area to the large force applied to the area of the original femoral head.
- High shear stresses result from the transfer of axial loads and torsional moments to the bone through the bone-prosthesis interface.
- Reduced bending displacements because of the prosthesis high stiffness

results in stress shielding between the bone and prosthesis. The discrepancy in stiffness adds to the interface shear stresses.

- Bone features are reduced as a result of insufficient blood circulation at the implant site.

Accordingly, the prostheses with stems may not exist long in the body due to the above reasons, and therefore these prostheses are best for patients over 60 years of age.

Additionally, implanted prostheses generally may cause proximal femoral resorption due to the following:

- Stress shielding under the implant,
- No biocompatibility initially between bone and prostheses causing increased resorption,
- Insufficient femoral head vascularity that leads to osteonecrosis.

The aim of these inventors [17] is to present a femoral component without the need of removing all the femoral neck, and without the insert of the prosthetic stem into the medullar bone of the femur. Using the proposed technique of installing, the prosthesis will spare damages to the intra-medullar femoral canal and bone marrow of proximal femur. Hence, bone growth will not seize.

The inventors [17] also aim to introduce a locking technique for the femoral prosthesis. The advantage of this invention [17] is that it offers the patient a quick recovery and considerable mobility after surgery due to the following reasons:

- The simplicity of the surgical procedure allows it to be performed in short time with the least bone damage.
- The multiple mechanical and biological fastenings used in the prosthesis provide an improved interface between prosthesis and the rest of the femur.

Moreover, the inventors [17] claim that this type of femoral prosthesis is easy to repair, remove or replace by a new one of the same type or a stem one if failure occurs later on. Also, its longevity will extend and therefore will be more promising to younger patients.

U.S. Patent No.7, 947,084 B2, by inventor; Helmut D. Link, titled "Hip Joint Prosthesis With A Shaft To Be Inserted Into The Femur," [18] and issued May, 2011, presents "Abstract: A hip-joint prosthesis includes a shaft which is configured to be inserted into the femur and whose surface has an osteoinductive finish. This finish is provided exclusively in the metaphyseal portion of the shaft and laterally from the line delineating the maximum antero-posterior dimension of the shaft cross section. This ensures a better involvement of the metaphyseal spongiosa in the flow of forces, without compromising the ability to perform follow-up surgery on the prosthesis."

The goal of the inventor [18] here is an improved fixation method of the femoral prosthesis in the bone without a compromise in the ability of performing a follow up surgery. The hip prosthesis in this invention is comprised of a head and a neck that has a shaft to be inserted in the femur. Osteoinductive coating for hip prosthesis with a shaft is performed exclusively on the metaphysical portion where the shaft is placed laterally from the line of maximum antero-posterior (AP) dimension.

The surface area to be finished with osteoinductive substance is defined according to this invention in a different manner than previous arts. The osteoinductive finish is applied at the part of the metaphysical portion where many surface areas have directional normal with lateral components. According to previous experience these surface areas are not expected to have any connection to the bone permitting transmission of tensile forces, while this connection facilitates it to the most part. The earlier application (PCT/EP03/05292 not belonging to the published prior art) proposes arranging the coating on surface areas pointing in the medial direction, the opposite of this invention [18]. It is an advantage that the material can be coated with any type of coating and can be porous.

Immediately after the surgery the effect is that the bone cells quickly develop close and in contact with the prosthetic surface, consequently neither a gap nor a layer of intermediate connective tissue is formed due to the relative movement between the bone and the bone surface, thus intimate connection is more difficult or impossible. The invention [18] provides more rapid accumulation of bone on the trochanteric surface of the prosthesis as well as fast incorporation of bone into the pores resulting in quick permanent fixation of the trochanteric area of the bone to the prosthesis and is thus involved in transmission of forces. In opposition, the connection to the bone on the other surface areas is attained only to the prior anticipated extent. The area outside the trochanteric is ready to access and is non-problematic in a follow up surgery if required. Although the bone might be tightly bound, therefore the physician finds the exact conditions he/she is familiar with when performing follow up surgery. According to the invention, the surface area where the osteoinductive substance consists of pores or undercuts relative to the lateral direction, and the bone substance due to the osteoinduction can both cohere to the surface and anchor firmly onto it.

Portions of the osteoinductively finished surface areas of the prosthesis, which point in the ventral and dorsal directions, are preferably placed at a certain distance closer to the cortex and farther from the mid-plane of the trochanteric bone where it is sometimes less dense than near the cortex. Hence, these surface areas in the AP direction should be not too thin. It is favorable for the thickness and thus distance between dorsal and ventral surface areas to be over 6 mm but more beneficially between 9 and 15 mm according to [18]. Press-fitting of the surface areas can promote growth of new bone cells onto the prosthesis surface and it is beneficial if these areas and their mating surfaces are made of wedge shape in the direction of insertion into the bone. Also, the rasp used to prepare the receiving site for the prosthesis shaft insertion, is of a smaller cross-sectional dimensions. Thus, when the shaft is inserted in the femur these surface areas dislocate bone substance.

U.S. Patent No.8, 133,284 B2, by inventors; K. Scott Ely, Ashok C. Khandkar, Ramaswamy Lakshminarayanan, Aaron A. Hofmann, titled "Hip Prosthesis With Monoblock Ceramic Acetabular Cup," [19] and issued March 2012, introduces "Abstract: An improved hip prosthesis includes an acetabular cup bearing component constructed from a relatively hard and high strength ceramic material for articulation with a ball-shaped femoral head component which may be constructed from a compatible ceramic or metal material. In one form, the acetabular cup further includes a ceramic porous bone ingrowth surface adhered thereto for secure ingrowth attachment to natural patient bone."

Generally hip prostheses are comprised of femoral head or ball-like component, a hip stem component and an acetabular component. The acetabular cup is to receive the femoral head, and the femoral head articulates relatively to the acetabular cup component. Between the acetabular cup and the femoral head, a polymer based bearing insert usually of high density or high molecular weight polyethylene (PE) or similar material is affixed in between the cup and the femoral head for smooth articulation securing low-wear articulation. Studies have illustrated that these polymeric bearing inserts produce substantial wear debris in the long term and may also be partially a contributor to osteolysis [2, 6] and bone resorption and thus prostheses failure. The inventors [19] have introduced an improved hip prosthesis that includes improved implantable and biocompatible materials to achieve ultra-low wear using ceramic-on-ceramic or a ceramic-on-metal articulatory interface. Thus, they propose to eliminate the use of the customary polymer-based bearing insert and the wear debris problems resulting in longer longevity for the prosthesis. Moreover, obtaining a cup with all-round thinner diameter that facilitates the use of a larger head for patients with small bones. Another aspect of the invention [19] is a unipolar prosthesis that consists of a ceramic acetabular cup of a shell shape or cup shape geometry outlining to some extent a low porous substrate combined with a surface of a higher porous bone ingrowth. This higher porous surface extends over the acetabular cup upper surface to be tightly fixed in the prepared acetabulum by bone ingrowth. The low porous substrate defines a partial spherical cavity to seat and articulate with the femoral head. The pores size range between 100 and 500 microns. The head is made of compatible and extremely strong and tough ceramic material or metal material for instance, a biocompatible cobalt chrome alloy or similar.

The ceramic material favoured for the acetabular cup consists of both high flexural strength and high "fracture toughness" material as doped silicon nitride (Si_3N_4), with flexural strength ranging between 700 MPa and 1000 MPa and relatively high fracture toughness ranging between 7 and 10.5 Mega-Pascal [19] for ultra-low wear and a reduced risk of brittle fracture. The unipolar prosthesis is comprised of acetabular cup with a relatively low porosity substrate combined with a higher porosity bone ingrowth surface. The pores size range between 100 and 500 microns.

U.S. Patent No. 8,323,346 B2, by inventor, Slobodan Tepic, titled "Wear-Reducing Geometry of Articulations in Total Joint Replacements," [20] and issued Dec. 2012 discusses "Abstract: The invention reduces wear in total joint articulations by modifications of the shape of either component of the kinematic pair, so as to result in an annular surface contact between the two components. Fluid trapped between the two components within the inner contour of the annular contact area is pressurized under load due to elastic deformation of the components and exuded out through inter-articular gap over the surface of contact, aiding in lubrication and reducing the wear. Reduced to practice for a total hip joint with UHMWPE-metal pair, the wear rate tested in a hip joint simulator up to five million cycles was reduced by factor seven to fifteen compared to conventionally shaped components."

The invention [20] addresses a solution to the most contributing factor to aseptic loosening: wear of Ultra High Molecular Weight Polyethylene (UHMWPE) which leads to shorter lifespan of artificial joints. The notion is to reduce the wear primarily and hence increase the "overall robustness of the joint and possibly relaxing the need for the exacting production technologies."

Through changes in the geometry of the articulating surfaces, a decrease of the contact stresses as well as an improvement in the lubrication of the area of contact will result, and therefore the wear characteristics of the implant is improved. According to this invention [20] the presented changes in the geometry are a combination of either a spherical head with an aspherical cup or an aspherical head in a spherical cup. Note that both assemblies should have a theoretical surface contact over a band that is centered approximately 45 degrees with respect to the revolutionary axis.

U.S. Patent No. 8,372,155 B2, by inventors; Michael Antony Tuke, Andrew Clive Taylor, titled "Acetabular Cup Prosthesis And Method Of Forming The Prosthesis," [21] and issued Feb. 2013, introduces "Abstract: An acetabular cup prosthesis comprising an acetabular cup having a rim and comprising a metal band applied around the outer circumference of the acetabular cup prosthesis and adjacent to said rim."

This invention [21] presents an acetabular cup having a rim and a D-shaped metal band applied around the cup outer circumference and adjacent to the rim. The metal band provides additional strength to the prosthesis plus the hoop compression level required. The acetabular cup may be made of ceramic or of a material with similar ceramic properties such as strength, stiffness and rigidity. An advantage to this invention [21] is that it improves resistance to fracture. Further, the metal band helps to pre-stress the ceramic, where there is a ceramic cup or ceramic liner, since non-stressed ceramic liners while in use are liable to fracture as in previous arts.

The band in this invention [21] is made of any suitable metal, favourably Titanium as well as Cobalt/Chromium. On the outer surface of the band there are ribs extending from the cup, these ribs when in use will facilitate the required torsional stability while interacting with the pelvis. In one arrangement, around the circumference of the band, favourably three ribs may be placed at a plurality of points, or located at three equally spaced positions. The ribs configuration may be the same or differ wherever there is more than one.

The band in this invention [21] can be set on its outer surface to stimulate bone integration, or another aspect is to coat the outer surface with a substance that stimulates bone growth such as hydroxyapatite. The same concept can be performed for the shell. If a Titanium shell is used, the thickness of the Titanium should range between 1 mm to 3 mm.

According to this invention [21] the ceramic cup and liner can be made of any material that is biocompatible, hard and wear resistant with thickness ranging from 2 to 5 mm. The ceramic materials to be used may be silicon nitride or doped silicon nitride, to name a few.

The band thickness will usually be of a few millimeters, and its surface that connects with the cup is usually flat and its outer surface may be curved so the cross-section may be of a D-shape. The thickness at the thickest point may be of 1 to 3mm thick.

There are various techniques to apply the band to the acetabular cup [21]. One of these is to press-fit it, but this might be difficult since the band is a tight fit on the cup. Therefore, one method is to heat the band to fit appropriately. The heating may be by induction which is advantageous as it only affects the metal band and the ceramic cup stays unheated. Depending on the temperature that heats up the band a load may be required for press-fitting. Heating may range from 500 to 700 degrees C while the press-fitting load may be around 5kN [21].

An additional advantage of this invention [21] is that the acetabular cup can withstand any forces while inserting a prosthesis into the acetabulum without damaging or distorting or separating the band. The local compression at the rim of the liner causes a decrease in the diameter. Nonetheless, the spherical shape of the prosthesis is considerably the same.

U.S. Patent No. 8,470,049 B2. By inventors; Bradley Walter, Declan Brazil, Timothy McTighe, titled "Neck Sparing Total Hip Implant System," [22] and issued, Jun. 2013, discusses "Abstract: A femoral prosthesis. The femoral prosthesis includes an implant body having a proximal end a distal end a shoulder at the proximal end, the shoulder being structured and dimensioned for a tight press fit into the neck of a femur. The implant body includes a trunk at the distal end, the trunk having a wedge formed by a tapered portion extending in the direction of the distal end of the implant body. The implant body also includes a medial column extending from the shoulder toward the distal end. The wedge, the medial column, and the lateral column are to provide multi-planar stability for the implant body and surface area for fixation of the implant body."

The disclosure [22] is relating to femoral prosthesis in particular and femoral neck sparing implant. To accomplish implant stability and longevity, a lot of bone loss is involved a problem that was attended to through the years by research and studies and hence tissue sparing plus bone sparing surgical techniques were developed. Bone loss is due mainly to osteolysis and stress shielding. Through improvement of wear properties of modern bearing surfaces loss of bone due to osteolysis was largely decreased. Bone loss due to stress shielding was addressed by "loading the proximal femur with tapered stem geometries or surface replacement devices." These devices have their limitations such as: the procedure requirement of larger exposure, in other words no tissue sparing. Also, there is the possibility of early or late collapse due to the poor foundation of the femoral head, and the likelihood of fracture of femoral neck. Thus, the inventors [22] are minimizing these problems by their invention.

U.S. Patent No. 8,506,644 B1, by inventors; Marie-Christine Ho Ba Tho, Francois Roux, Maximilien Vanleene, titled "Acetabular Prosthesis To Be Fixed Without Cement," [23] and issued Aug. 2013, introduces "Abstract: The invention relates to an acetabular prosthesis comprising an, in general, hemispherically shaped insert (1) having a crown (5) and an apex (4), this insert being provided, on its outer surface (2), With at least one fin. The invention is characterized in that the fin (6) has a face (9) starting from the crown (5) of the insert (1) and extending toward the apex (4) of the insert while forming a crest (10). This crest (10) has an, in particular, curved shape." The invention [23] relates to fixing the acetabular prostheses without cement. The total hip prostheses comprises a femoral prosthesis which includes a stem provided with a femoral head, the stem is to be inserted in the femur, and an acetabular prosthesis to be fixed in the acetabular cavity which receives the femoral head. There are various methods of fixing the acetabular prostheses to the bone such as cemented or uncemented. Note that both methods could be efficient but each has its advantages and disadvantages. The cemented technique which is usually based on PolyMethylMethAcrylate (PMMA) is good in the long-term. However, aseptic loosening frequently results [23]. Another means of fixing without cement is by mechanical means, thus the acetabular prosthesis few months post implantation would be able to have effective mechanical strength of the prosthesis in the bone to stimulate osteointegration or integration of the prosthesis to the bone tissues. Cementless prostheses may consist of a metal cup and a PolyEthylene (PE) insert positioned in the metal cup which is fixed in the bone by pads, screws, fins or pins, also the acetabular implant may be fixed in the bone cavity by what is known as press fit or forced insertion [23]. The invention [23] is proposing to fix the acetabular prosthesis without cement, (as mentioned in the abstract). Introducing the facet may be advantageous as it may distribute the exerted stresses by the insert over the cortical bone, and also the crest of the fin being of a curved shape so the prosthesis is placed in the cancellous bone to avoid damage to the bone tissue. The fins fix the insert in place as the femoral head move and they also provide "mechanical strength of the prosthesis in the bone until osteointegration is sufficient to take over."

In the invention [23] the prosthesis external convex surface has a roughness of 3μm, and is covered with a layer of hydroxyapatite coating, hence facilitating colonization by bone cells and consequently stimulating osteointegration of prosthesis.

Also, the internal surface of the insert, which will be in contact with the femoral head, is coated with Diamond-Like –Carbon (DLC) which consists of large amount of "sp^3 hybrids" that gives it similar properties to diamonds. Using this coating increases the wear resistance properties. Further, the DLC coating has very good biocompatibility.

U.S. Patent No. 8,603,182 B2, by inventors; Richard Lambert, Terry McLean, David Kelman, titled "Hip Prostheses," [24] and issued Dec. 2013 and presents "Abstract: Bipolar prostheses which include various structures and other techniques for optimizing material wear and mechanical strength properties. Such prostheses feature, for example, improved resistance to polyethylene wear while also reducing potential for dislocation of the femoral stem from the prosthesis. Such techniques and structures include varying wear resistance and mechanical strength treatment in various components of the prostheses or portions of those components as desired to improve, accentuate or optimize wear performance and dislocation reduction, locking ring structural features, structures for retaining locking rings in the bipolar prosthesis shell, and structures for limiting or reducing movement or rotation of locking rings and liners in bipolar prosthesis shells."

Bipolar prostheses usually offer two bearing surfaces that are between the femoral head and the acetabulum. The first bearing surface; the shell where its outer surface is usually smooth and made of various materials such as metal, ceramic or other materials. The inner bearing surface is the liner which is mostly made of polyethylene material such as Ultra High Molecular Weight Polyethylene or UHMWP. The liner is to fit securely into the shell where it receives the femoral head and provides smooth articulating movement between the acetabulum and the outer surface of the shell and the relative movement between the femoral head and acetabulum. The two bearing surfaces will absorb the articulation movement and therefore lessen protrusion and erosion of the acetabulum. Thus, in [24] the shear forces are distributed between the inner and outer bearings. The inner bearing also absorbs some of the movement between the acetabular and the femoral head; hence the acetabular wear is subsided. Bipolar or dual bearing surface facilitates more array of motion than unipolar designs or conventional THA.

According to the inventors [24], although there are advantages to the bipolar prostheses but there are disadvantages such as; the possibility for dislocation of femoral head relative to the shell and liner. Further, the polyethylene wear is an additional problem. These issues are also a concern for acetabular components as well as prostheses for other joints. Dislocation is a serious problem since usually it requires revision surgery. Various hip prostheses and bipolar designs were invented to solve this issue. Some designs involved retaining or locking rings. Overemphasis of prevention of dislocation can result in reduction of motion between the femoral stem and the shell/liner. Moreover, other designs addressed this problem by introducing a split in the annulus formed by the locking ring. Nevertheless, these split rings still have problems such as contracting and expanding of the diameter after installation which may lead to polyethylene wear according to [24].

Polyethylene wear is known as one of the major problems to hip prostheses. Several methods have been undertaken to reduce polyethylene wear such as specialized treating of polyethylene, metal and other surfaces. Further processes were enhancements of polyethylene wear performance for instance irradiation, plus procedures that will increase the cross-linking or features of other materials in polyethylene. Although this is of benefit, it has an effect on the polyethylene mechanical and physical characteristics, e.g., yield strength, tensile, elongation and impact strength as it reduces these characteristics. Polyethylene liners and locking rings are also affected in the manner that they are unable to hold the femoral stem head and avoid dislocation.

To resolve the aforementioned issues the inventors in [24] present several techniques and structures to reduce polyethylene wear while neither compromising nor lessening the ability of the shell/liner in preventing dislocation of the femoral stem head. They also introduce a change in the material properties of parts of the shell/liner, shell and locking ring which are at pre-set locations, by treating the material at these sites to "emphasize wear performance." On the other hand, other sites can be also changed or unchanged or not treated to highlight features as yield strength, tensile strength, elongation and impact strength among others.

The said invention [24] exploits optimum performance properties of various types of irradiated polyethylene materials to exhibit improved wear performance when placed in articulating and non-articulating relationships with metal and other surfaces, certain structures and processes to optimize cross linking of various regions of the liner which are in a position to accept increased load from the femoral stem head.

U.S. Patent No. 8,679,188 B2, by inventors; Jeffrey J. Shea, Vincent W. Shotton, David C. Kelman, titled "Universal Liner," [25] and issued March 2014, introduces "Abstract: The present invention relates to universal liner assemblies for use during hip joint replacement surgeries. The universal liners allow the surgeon a greater degree of selection of liners and shells, without being tied to typical liner/shell connections based on material connection constraints."

According to [25], when the surgeon is making her/his choice of implant she/he takes under consideration several factors such as age, weight, gender, level of activity and approach of surgery, among others. Then there are factors concerning the implant itself such as design, materials used, and methods of fixation. There is also the choice of the liner and shell combined as they both are material and design specific. For instance they could be ceramic liner and metal shell or metal on metal, or Polyethylene liner and metal shell. The ceramic liner metal shell uses for connection what is known as Morse taper connection [25] where the tapered outer surface of the liner and the taper on the inner surface of the shell join. The tapers secure the connection and so the liner locks in the shell. On the other hand, when the liner is made of polyethylene and the shell is made of metal, this may not happen because the polyethylene has a low push-out force resistance and so the liner tends to "push" outwards of the shell as polyethylene warms up due to the body temperature and therefore the liner tends to pop out. Thus, there are other types of locking connections for polyethylene-metal components such as axial locking and rotational locking features. Sometimes, the surgeon chooses to use a shell and a liner independent of each other that might be of benefit to the patient. Hence to secure their connection some surgeons used cement, nonetheless there is no available system to furnish this flexibility.

Hip implants have a limited longevity mostly due to the wear debris caused by the articulation movement between the various parts of the implant. Therefore, it would be advantageous to have a universal liner that "can cooperate with a currently-implanted shell" to reduce shell removal trauma on the patient [25].

This invention [25] embraces several embodiments of the universal liner assemblies. The invention also includes different kits of a variety of universal liners in addition to techniques of manufacturing and implanting.

Universal liners would provide the surgeon with the choice of various liner-shell connections prior to surgery. Another advantage is that the components of implants can be exchanged, e.g. liners of several materials used with different kinds of shells. Thus, it is advantageous to the surgeon in a revision surgery to have the variety of materials that can be used with an existing shell. Additional advantage of the invention [25], the band assembly and the liner component are assembled as one piece to form a universal liner.

U.S. Patent No. 8,700,198 B2, by inventors; Justin Steve Conway, Ryan L. Landon, Jeffrey Joel Shea, and titled "Implant Components and Methods," [26] and issued April 2014, presents "Abstract: Systems, devices, and methods are provided for orthopedic implants. The implants may include a base member, such as an acetabular shell or an augment that is configured to couple with; an augment, flange cup, mounting member, or any other suitable orthopedic attachment. Any of the implantable components may include one or more porous surfaces. The porous surface may be textured by protrusions that connect to and extend from the surface. The sizes and concentration of the protrusions may be varied for specific applications to accommodate different implants and patient anatomies. A porous implant may also include one or more internal or external solid portions that strengthen the implant."

According to the inventors [26] when a hip joint is affected by degenerative disease or other reasons and requires replacement, often the prostheses replacing the original joint comprise two bearing surfaces between the femoral head and the acetabulum. The first is a prosthesis shell or acetabular cup where the second is a liner. The two bearings vary in their materials according to inventors. The liner is usually fitted securely within the shell offering inner bearing surface to receive the prosthetic femoral head, and allow a smooth articulating movement between the femur and the acetabulum.

According to the inventors [26], there are problems and shortcomings with previous arts and to overcome these issues they present systems, devices and methods for modular implants, besides improved features such as bone screws, coatings, and various augment removal and insertion options for a modular implant. The implants may consist of a base member as an acetabular shell or a configured augment to connect with an augment, flange cup, mounting member or any appropriate connection. Furthermore, the connections may be capable of adjusting about the base member. Several techniques of affixation are used between the components of the implant. In other arrangements there are surface characteristics which will facilitate friction permitting ingrowth of bone between the implants and the patient's bone regardless of the bone quality.

- An example of the invention: an implant device consists of a surface that connects to the joint of the patient. The implant may have at its surface spread pores. The protrusions at the surface may be of any form and of any density, also may expand to any appropriate height ranging between about 50 μm and about 2000 μm. The optimum surface will be with protrusions that are adequately large to produce the appropriate friction between the bone and implant, but at the same time not too small to permit a high degree of bone ingrowth through the porous surface.

- Another example: a porous implant may comprise internal or external "strengthening ribs" to support adjacent porous structures.

- The systems, methods, and devices described in the invention [26], having both a profiled macrostructure and a porous microstructure, are beneficial to an orthopedic surgeon as they can allow utilizing customizable, "patient-specific" implant.

CONCLUSION

There have been numerous fairly recent inventions addressing hip prostheses. Nevertheless, there are still problems that affect prostheses functions and longevity. In this paper a few selected patents that have addressed various problems associated with the design of different parts of the hip prostheses are presented. These patents also introduce a number of design novelties that are discussed in this paper. The patents chosen for this paper were of special interest as each discussed a different significant issue whether in design, materials or fixation methodologies and presented a set of diverse solutions. For instance:

- Introducing solutions to femoral stem implants and their consequent complications due to insertion of a stem into the excavated femur. Thus to overcome the disadvantages, stemless implants were presented and with different methods of fixation. Although, these designs may be beneficial but they may still encounter installation and stability issues in early stages. Further studies need to be performed.
- Introducing shock absorption systems with adjustable parameters such as size of femoral ball, stem and neck length, where each could be individually adjusted.
- To reduce the problem of wear debris generation, various approaches were addressed such as: wear-reducing geometry of articulation. Also, using different materials for coating since coating increases the wear resistance features, such as in DLC coating which has very good compatibility. The materials can also be porous.
- Use strong material such as diamonds, which are known for their low coefficient of friction and resistance to wear, to minimize wear debris during motion and hence extend the implant survivorship. The material is to form one of the articulating surfaces.
- Implants that spared the removal of the femoral neck and without insertion of stem in the medullar bone with locking techniques for femoral prosthesis. These implants will lead to quick recovery and considerable mobility after surgery.
- Introducing a design that spares the calcar bone and the method of using the device.
- Femoral head assembly with variable offset that is selectively adjusted.

Each patent focuses on a different problem area of the hip prostheses, making a simple comparison of the patents unhelpful. However, even though the patents differ in the approach with which each addresses the problem of hip failure all have the same objective to obtain the optimum implant with the extended life-span for the patient and possibly no revision surgery.

REFERENCES

1. J.V. Bono, J.C. McCarthy, T.S. Thornhill, B.E. Bierbaum, and R.H. Turner, Eds, Revision Total Hip Arthroplasty, Springer-Verlag: New York, 1999.
2. J. Gallo, P. Kaminek, V. Ticha, P. Rihakova, and R. Ditmar; "Theory of periprosthetic osteolysis: a review", Biomedical Papers, vol. 146, no. 2, pp. 21-28, 2002.
3. L.A. Reynolds and E.M. Tansey, Eds, Early development of total hip replacement, Wellcome Witnesses to Twentieth Century Medicine, vol. 29. Wellcome Trust Centre for the History of Medicine at UCL: London 2007.

4. Sargeant, and T. Goswami, Hip implants: Paper V. Physiological effects, Elsevier Materials and Design, vol. 27, pp. 287-307, 2006.

5. S. Srimongkol, "A review of mathematical modelling in total hip replacement", International Mathematical Forum, vol. 7, no. 52, pp. 2561-2569, 2012.

6. K.J. Saleh, I. Thongtrangan, and E.M. Schwarz, "Osteolysis: medical and surgical approaches", Clinical Orthopaedics and Related Research, no. 427, pp. 138-147, October 2004.

7. D. Snyder, R. Chapell, W. Bruening, K. Schoelles, J. Kaczmarek, E. Kuserk, and E. Erinoff, "Horizon Scan on Hip Replacement Surgery", ECRI Evidence-Based Practice Center, Rockville, MD, Rep. 290-02-0019, December 22, 2006.

8. S. Sivarasu, P. Beulah, and L. Mathew. "Optimization of skeletal hip implant cross-sections", In: National Conference on Computational Instrumentation-NCCI, April 19-20, 2010, pp. 37-43.

9. C. Schmidler. Hip anatomy, function and common problems Online.. Available: http://www.healthpages.org/anatomyfunction/hip-structure-function-common-problems/ , (2010, July 28).

10. S. Pramanik1, A. K. Agarwal, and K. N. Rai, "Chronology of total hip joint replacement and materials development", Trends in Biomaterial and Artificial Organs, vol 19, no 1, pp.15-26, 2005.

11. C.C. Harris, "Hip replacement prosthesis", U.S. Patent 6,248,132 B1, June 19, 2001.

12. G.V. Subba Rao, and A.K. Goli, "Modular hip implant with shock absorption system", U.S. Patent 6,336,941 B1, January 8, 2002.

13. S.G. Advani, M.H. Santare, F. Miller, and M. Joshi, "Stemless hip prosthesis", U.S. Patent 6,379,390 B1, April 30, 2002.

14. B.J. Pope, J.K. Taylor, R.H. Dixon, C.F. Gardinier, L.M. Pope, D.C. Blackburn, M.A. Vail, and K.M. Jensen, "Prosthetic hip joint having at least one sintered polycrystalline diamond compact articulation surface", U.S. Patent 6,425,922 B1, July 30, 2002.

15. S. Unger, "Femoral head calcar loading prosthesis", U.S. Patent 7, 641, 699 B2, January 5, 2010.

16. J. Saladino, M.E. Nadzadi, and B. Burkinshaw, "Femoral head assembly with variable offset", U.S. Patent 7,833,277 B2, November 16, 2010.

17. X. Li, P. Xie, and K.Y. Xie, "External proximal femoral prosthesis for total hip arthroplasty", U.S. Patent 7,931,691 B2, April 26, 2011

18. H.D. Link, "Hip joint prosthesis with a shaft to be inserted into the femur", U.S. Patent 7,947,084 B2, May 24, 2011.

19. K.S. Ely, A.C. Khandkar, R. Lakshminarayanan, and A.A. Hofmann, "Hip prosthesis with monoblock ceramic acetabular cup". U.S. Patent 8,133,284 B2, March 13, 2012.

20. S. Tepic, "Wear-reducing geometry of articulations in total joint replacements",

U.S. Patent 8,323,346 B2, December 4, 2012.

21. M.A. Tuke, and A.C. Taylor, "Acetabular cup prosthesis and method of forming the prosthesis". U.S. Patent 8,372,155 B2, February 12, 2013.
22. B. Walter, D. Brazil, and T. McTighe, "Neck sparing total hip implant system", U.S. Patent 8,470,049 B2, June 25, 2013.
23. M-C. Ho Ba Tho, F. Roux, and M. Vanleene, "Acetabular prosthesis to be fixed without cement", U.S. Patent 8,506,644 B1, Aug13, 2013.
24. R. Lambert, T. McLean, and D. Kelman, "Hip prostheses", U.S. Patent 8, 603, 182 B2, December 10, 2013.
25. J.J. Shea, V.W. Shotton, and D.C. Kelman, "Universal liner", U.S. Patent 8, 679, 188 B2, March 25, 2014.
26. J.S. Conway, R.L. Landon, and J.J. Shea, "Implant components and methods", U.S. Patent 8,700,198 B2, April 15, 2014.

8
CHAPTER

IMPROVED ESTIMATION OF THE CARDIAC GLOBAL FUNCTION USING COMBINED LONG AND SHORT AXIS MRI IMAGES OF THE HEART

Hossam ElRewaidy and Ahmed S. Fahmy

Keywords: Cardiac function, Volume estimation, Geometric models, MRI

BACKGROUND

Accurate calculation of the volumes enclosed by the left ventricular (LV) surfaces is required to assess the global functional parameters of the heart [1, 2, 3, 4]. Cine Magnetic Resonance Imaging (MRI) has become the reference standard for the assessment of the LV volume and global function [5, 6]. Current clinical protocols include the acquisition of a stack of parallel 2D short-axis (SAX) s, or slices, of the heart from base to apex using standard MRI pulse sequences. Nine to twelve consecutive SAX slices are usually acquired and used to calculate the LV volume. The process begins with delineating the LV endocardium and epicardium contours in all slices [7]. Then, a geometric model that uses these contours to approximate the shape of the heart is used to calculate the LV volumes. This process is repeated for the end-diastole and end-systole phases of the cardiac cycle to calculate differential parameters such as the ejection fraction. It is worth noting that the acquisition of each slice requires the patient not to move and hold his/her breath for few seconds until a cross-section is imaged. Patient motion during the scan and/or failure to properly perform the breath-hold, can lead to severe distortion of the acquired images. This means that, in some cases, it is inevitable to estimate the volume from small number of slices. As will be shown below, this leads to reducing the accuracy of estimating the LV volume. The most widely used-method for calculating the

Citation: Hossam El-Rewaidy and Ahmed S. Fahmy, Improved estimation of the cardiac global function using combined long and short axis MRI images of the heart, DOI: 10.1186/s12938-016-0156-3.

myocardium volume from number of parallel SAX contours is the modified Simpson's (mSimp) method [8, 9, 10, 11]. In mSimp method, the LV volume is approximated by a number of parallel discs. The number of discs is equal to the number of the acquired SAX slices, N. The volume, v_i, of the ith disc in the stack is estimated as follows,

$$v_i = A_i \cdot (t + l), \tag{1}$$

where, i=1,2,…,N;A_i is the area enclosed by the myocardium contour in the ith slice; t is the slice thickness; and l is the inter-slice gap. The total volume is then calculated by taking the summation over all discs. When the number of slices, N, is sufficiently large, the mSimp method provides accurate and reliable results even at LV shape anomalies [11]. Nevertheless, the performance of the mSimp method is significantly impacted when the number of the SAX slices decreases due to the inaccurate approximation of large LV segments using simple discs. To avoid these inaccuracies, several models have been proposed to calculate the LV volume from a few planar s of the heart [12, 13, 14]. The models assume simplified geometric LV shapes such as ellipsoids and concatenated cylinders and hemispheres. While these models were originally proposed for analyzing echocardiography images, attempts of applying these models to MRI data have been reported by Thiele et al. [14]. However, the accuracy of these models is very limited due to the over-simplification of the cardiac shape that is not valid especially in patients with cardiac anomalies [14, 15].

In this work, we propose a simple geometric model that can be used to estimate the LV volume from a few number of slices; i.e. image acquisitions. The model incorporates information from SAX and long axial (LAX) s to better estimate the shape of the LV at the inter-slice gaps. In the next section, a derivation of the model equations is presented and it will be shown that the volume can be calculated from a simple equation that includes calculating simple geometric parameters such as the areas enclosed by the SAX and LAX contours and the angle between the LAX and SAX planes. The proposed model is validated using 3D cardiac surface generated from Computed Tomography (CT) acquisitions from five human subjects. In addition, real cardiac MRI datasets from twenty five patients have been used to evaluate the accuracy of the proposed method relative to other existing methods.

METHODS

In the methods described below, it is assumed that the volume of the heart is to be estimated from N SAX slices and one LAX slice. Our default LAX orientation is the four-chamber of the heart; i.e. horizontal LAX. Nevertheless, the effect of changing this orientation will be studied as discussed in "Results and discussion" section. The proposed methodology is identical for calculating the volume enclosed by the epicardium and the volume enclosed by the endocardium at any timeframe. Therefore, for simplicity, we will use the general terms of myocardium contours and cardiac volume when discussing calculating the volume enclosed by a set of contours (epicardium or endocardium) at a specific timeframe.

Problem formulation

Given a number, NN, of SAX slices and one LAX slice, the myocardium boundaries are delineated to obtain a set of N SAX and one LAX contour respectively. Ignoring delineation errors and misregistration due to different levels of breath-holds, these contours can be thought of as a coarse grid representing the intersection between the different image planes and the myocardium surface. It is therefore required to calculate the cardiac volume enclosed by the myocardium surface represented by these contours. As can be seen in Fig. 1, a number of N parallel SAX planes can virtually divide the heart into N chunks (ignoring the part above the most-basal plane). The plane of the LAX contour intersects with the contour of the upper and lower surfaces of the ith chunk and results in a line segments of length $d_i(h,0)$ and $d^i(0, 0)$, respectively, where h is the height of the chunk from the lower surface to the upper.

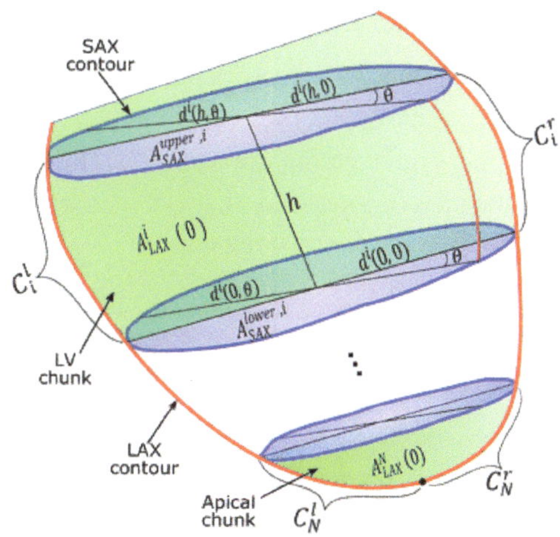

Figure 1: 3D schematic plot for the LV showing the SAX contours (blue) and the LAX contour (red). A number of N SAX image planes (purple areas) can divide the LV into N chunks. Green areas annotate the LAX cross-sectional area of the different chunks.

In general, within the ith chunk, the diameter of the upper and lower surfaces at any given angle, θ, are denoted by $d^i(h, \theta)$ and $d^i(0, \theta)$, respectively, where θ is measured from the plane containing the LAX contour. To account for the unsymmetrical shape of the LAX contour, the right and left parts of the LAX contour within the ith chunk are denoted by, C_i^r and C_i^l, respectively. We further define $A_{LAX}^i(0)$ as the area enclosed by the curves $d^i(0, 0)$, C_i^r, $d^i(h, 0)$, and C_i^l. As can be shown in Fig. 1, the area below the most apical slice, $A_{LAX}^N(0)$, is enclosed by two curves only: $d^N(0,0)$, C_N^r, and C_N^l. 1. For all the myocardium chunks, $A_{LAX}^i(0)$ is numerically calculated by computing the area of a polygon formed by the points on the surrounding curves.

Having defined the basic quantities that are used in the proposed method, the following section describes a simple geometric model that can be used to estimate the cardiac volume of the ith chunk from the contour areas, $A_{LAX}^i(0)$, and diameters, $d^i(h, 0)$

and $d^i(0, 0)$. Adding the volumes of all chunks yields the required total cardiac volume.

Cross-sectional modeling using equivalent trapezoids

To simplify the volume calculations, a simple trapezoid is used to approximate the shape of any given long-axial cross-section of an LV chunk. For a given chunk, i, all modeling trapezoids are assumed to have the same height, h_i, but different lengths of the upper and lower sides depending on the orientation of the LAX plane. For a LAX plane making angle θ, with the acquired LAX image plane, upper, $d^i(h, \theta)$ and lower, $d_i(0,\theta)$, sides of its modeling trapezoid is calculated from the line segments representing the intersection between this LAX plane and the upper and lower SAX contours. The trapezoid height, h_i, can be calculated by setting the trapezoid area equal to the cross-sectional area $A^i_{LAX}(0)$ described above. That is,

$$h_i = \frac{2A^i_{LAX}(0)}{d^i(h,0) + d^i(0,0)} \tag{2}$$

For any virtual LAX plane intersecting the ith chunk and making an angle, θ, with the acquired LAX plane, the area of intersection, $A^i_{LAX}(0)$, may also be represented by a trapezoid of height, h_i, and thus can be estimated by,

$$A^i_{LAX}(\theta) = \frac{d^i(h,\theta) + d^i(0,\theta)}{2} h_i \tag{3}$$

Substituting from Eqs. (2) and (3), the area of the equivalent trapezoid at any angle θ can be written in terms of$A_{LAX}(0, i)$ as follows,

$$A^i_{LAX}(\theta) = \frac{d^i(h,\theta) + d^i(0,\theta)}{d^i(h,0) + d^i(0,0)} A^i_{LAX}(0) \tag{4}$$

If the equivalent trapezoid is rotated with infinitesimal angle, dθ, a wedge-like structure is obtained (as shown in Fig. 2) with volume given by,

$$V_{wedge}(\theta, i) = \frac{A^i_{LAX}(\theta)}{2} \times \frac{(d^i(h,\theta) + d^i(0,\theta))/2}{2} d\theta \tag{5}$$

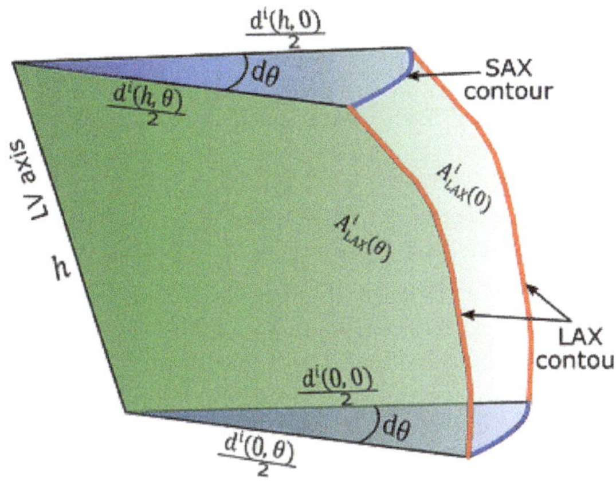

Figure 2: Rotation of a half LAX slice area around the axis of the LV chunk, h, with infinitesimal angle, dθ, results into a wedge-like shape. Its volume can be determined knowing the rotated area, the distance from the axis to the LAX contour segment, and the rotation angle.

That is, the volume of the ith chunk, V_i, can be obtained by integrating Eq. (5) from θ equal zero to 2π. Substituting from Eq. (4) into (5), it can be shown that,

$$V_i = \frac{0.5A^i_{LAX}(0)}{d^i(h,0)+d^i(0,0)} \int_0^{\pi} \left(\frac{d^i(h,\theta)+d^i(0,\theta)}{2}\right)^2 d\theta \tag{6}$$

Since the SAX contours are available, the diameters $d^i(h, \theta)$ and $d_i(0,\theta)$ can be readily calculated and the integration in Eq. (6) can be numerically solved. Observing that the integration in Eq. (6) is done over the square of the mean diameter at angle, θ, i.e., $d^i_{mean}(\theta) \equiv \frac{d^i(h,\theta)+d^i(0,\theta)}{2}$, then it can be approximated by double the area of a virtual SAX contour with diameter $d^i_{mean}(\theta)$. The area of this virtual contour can be further approximated by the average area of the upper and lower SAX contours; that is,

$$V_i \cong \frac{A^i_{LAX}(0)}{d^i(h,0)+d^i(0,0)} \left(A^{upper,i}_{SAX} + A^{lower,i}_{SAX}\right) \tag{7}$$

It is worth noting that, in the most apical chunk (at i = N), the lower base of the chunk is a single point representing the cardiac apex. That is, the LAX cross-section is approximated by a triangle where the values of $d^N(0,0)$ and $A^{lower,N}_{SAX}$, N are set to zero. That is, the volume of the most-apical chunk is calculated using the following equation,

$$V_N = \frac{A^N_{LAX}(0) \cdot A^{upper,N}_{SAX}}{2d^N(h,0)} \tag{8}$$

Equation (7) can also be used to calculate the LV volume represented by the LAX contour segments that extend above the most-basal SAX slice (as shown in Fig. 1). First, these free LAX contour segments are used to define a virtual chunk above the most basal SAX plane with volume, V_0. Then, the volume of this virtual chunk is calculated by respectively setting the area $A_{SAX}^{upper,0}$ and the diameter $d^0(h, 0)$ equal to $A_{SAX}^{lower,0}$ and $d^0(0, 0)$. It can be shown that this approximation results in a volume of a virtual chunk with identical upper and lower surfaces and height equal to the average heights of the two LAX segments extending above the most basal plane. It is worth noting that this volume is excluded from the calculations because there is no reported standard method, and thus a ground truth, for calculating it. It is worth noting that the misregistration between SAX and LAX slices can be corrected by various intensity and contour based methods (as proposed by [16, 17]). Nevertheless, due to imperfect segmentation of the myocardium boundaries in both LAX and SAX images, slight misalignment of the contours causes the LAX contour not to be intersecting with each SAX contour in exactly two points. This gives two possible values for the LV diameter, $d^i(h, 0)$ and $d_i(0,0)$. In this work, the diameters $d^i(h, 0)$ and $d^i(0, 0)$ are calculated from the LAX contours. This is because the LAX slices are less prone to the boundary blurring caused by the partial volume effects and thus the LAX contours are usually more accurate in delineating the LV especially at the apex. Having calculated the cardiac volume for every chunk, the total volume can be then calculated as,

$$Vol = \sum_{i=1}^{N} V_i \tag{9}$$

Oblique LAX

In practice, the plane of the LAX slice is not perfectly selected perpendicular to the acquired stack of the SAX slices (as shown in Fig. 3). This oblique orientation results in a larger apparent area of the LAX slice and thus the calculated area of the LAX contour, $A_{LAX}^{i}(0)$, should be compensated to account for this factor. One simple solution is to replace $A_{LAX}^{i}(0)$ with a corrected area, $A_{LAX}^{\prime i}(0)$ given by,

$$A_{LAX}^{\prime i}(0) = A_{LAX}^{i}(0) \cos(\Phi_i) \tag{10}$$

where Φ_i is the angle between the line connecting the center-of-mass points of the SAX contours forming the chunk and the LAX image plane.

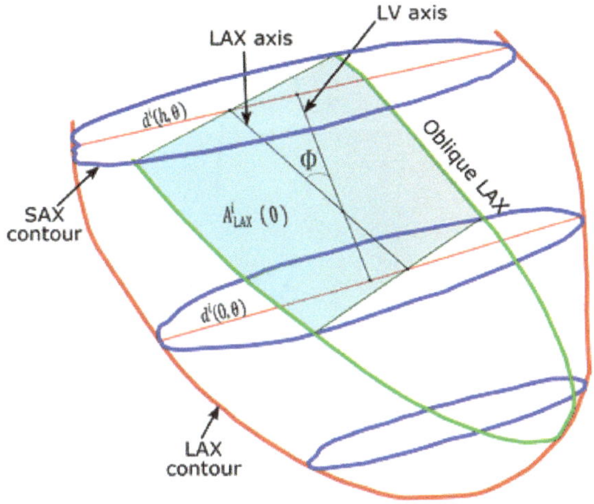

Figure 3: Oblique LAX contour (in green) generates a larger intersection area with the cardiac chunk. The correction factor of such area depends on the inclination angle (Φ) between the axis of LV and the oblique LAX plane.

Model validation using CT-based phantoms

In order to validate the developed model, the actual surface geometry of five human hearts have been constructed from data acquired using Computed Tomography (CT) as described in [18]. The dataset (publicly available on the internet [19]) contains single breath-hold cardiac-gated CT acquisitions with resolution 0.43 × 0.43 mm. Rendering of the 3D volume for each heart has been done and the volume is calculated and recorded as the ground truth. Then, each reconstructed volume was re-sliced to create cross-sectional images (matrix size: 512 × 512; voxel size: 0.43 × 0.43 × 3.5 mm) in the SAX and LAX directions as shown in Fig. 4. All processing was done using 3D-Slicer software tool [20]. First, a stack of twelve SAX slices covering the LV from base to apex was reconstructed. Secondly, a set of four LAX image slices with different orientations was reconstructed. The epicardium and endocardium contours of all acquired images have been manually delineated and used to calculate the difference LV volumes using the different methods.

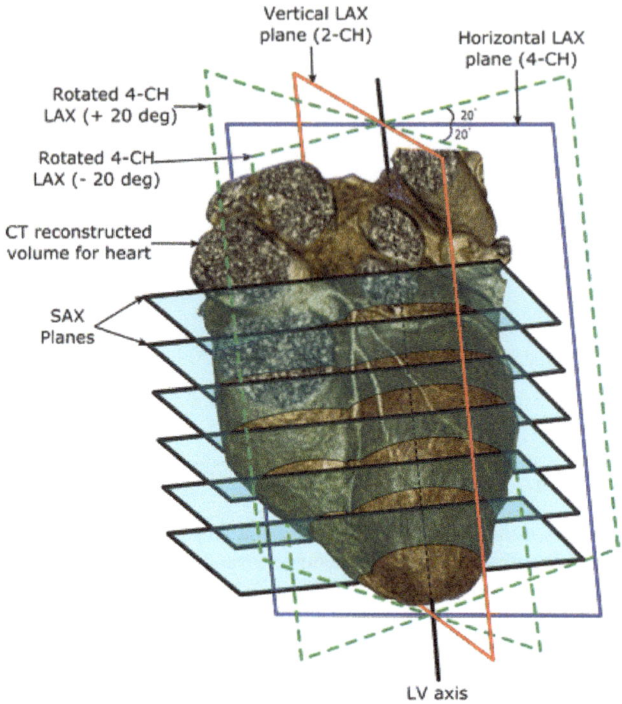

Figure 4: Cardiac CT reconstructed volume re-sliced to generate different cardiac cross-sections: SAX, horizontal LAX (i.e. 4-chamber), vertical LAX slice (i.e. 2-chamber), and two LAX slices (rotated ± 20° from the horizontal LAX plane).

Two sets of experiments have been done to test the performance and the robustness of the proposed method. The first experiment was done to quantify the error resulting from decreasing the number of SAX slices. In this experiment, the proposed model and mSimp method has been used to calculate the cardiac volume from one (4CH) LAX slice combined with different number of SAX slices ($n = 4, 6, 8, 10, 12$). The reduced set of SAX slices was selected such that we include the most basal slice in which the LV SAX contour appears as a complete ring. In addition, the set includes the most apical slice where the blood pool can barely be differentiated at end-systole phase. The remaining slices are selected to uniformly cover the distance between the already selected basal and apical slices. The volume estimated by each method was recorded and the mean and standard deviation of the error (relative to the ground truth) was calculated.

The second set of experiments was done to assess the robustness and reproducibility of the proposed method. First, the proposed method was tested to report its reliability in presence of misregistration among the LAX and SAX contours caused by respiratory motion. This was done by simulating different levels of breath-holds by randomly changing the location of the heart in the 3D space prior to the re-slicing operation described above. The breathing-induced motion was assumed to be in the superior-inferior direction with maximum displacement of 18 mm and in the anterior-posterior direction with maximum displacement of 2.5 mm [21]. The whole experiment is repeated 10 times with random displacement and the mean and standard deviation have been recorded for the different number of slices as above. Another experiment was done to test the reproducibility of the proposed model at different selections of LAX imaging planes. For this purpose, a set of LAX image planes was used to reconstruct: one horizontal LAX slice (i.e. 4-chamber or 4CH); one vertical LAX slice (i.e. 2-chamber or 2CH); and two rotated horizontal LAX slices (±20°) around the axis of the LV. Each of these four LAX images was combined with different numbers of SAX slices (n = 4, 6, 8, 10, 12) to calculate the volume.

Model validation using real MRI data

A database of MRI images for 25 human subjects with symptoms of ischemic heart disease to test and evaluate the proposed model. Ten patients were scanned using 1.5T Siemens scanner, and 15 patients were scanned using 3T Philips scanner. The number of slices for each dataset was (9–12) SAX slices and one LAX slice. The pixel size was in the range of (1.116–1.406 mm) and the slice thickness ranges from 5 to 8 mm. Only the end-diastole and end-systole timeframes were considered for processing and analysis. In general, all slices are assumed to be acquired while the patient is holding his/her breath at the same level. To quantify the volume calculation error, the ground truth volume for a given heart was calculated by mSimp method applied to all available SAX slices. Then, the proposed model was applied to compute the volume using one LAX slice and different numbers of SAX slices: 1 (mid-cavity), 2 (most basal and most apical), 3, 5, 7, 9 and 11. For a number of slices >2, the slices are selected to include and uniformly cover the distance between the selected basal and apical slices. After calculating the volumes enclosed by the cardiac contours, two functional parameters, namely ejection fraction and stroke volume, have been estimated by the two methods and the error was calculated. Due to the anticipated inadequate performance of the mSimp method at very low number of SAX slices (<4), other model-based methods described in literature have been investigated and compared to the proposed method. These model-based methods approximate the shape of the heart using simple geometries such as single plane ellipsoid, Biplane ellipsoid, Teichholz model, Hemisphere cylinder (for more details about these models, please refer to [14]).

RESULTS AND DISCUSSION

Validation using CT-based phantoms

Figure 5 shows the results of the first phantom experiment, which measures the error in calculating the LV surface volume (LVV_s) while increasing the number of slices from 4 to 12. As expected, the error of both the mSimp method (using n SAX slices) and the proposed trapezoidal model (using n − 1 SAX slices and one LAX slice) decreases with the number of slices. However, for the same number of slices, the error of the trapezoidal model is lower than that of the mSimp. At a small number of slices (<7), the figure shows that the error of the trapezoidal model (<−2.5 %) is much lower error than that of the mSimp (<10 %). At a higher number of slices, the error of the mSimp becomes less than 5 % and converges to 0.4 % error at maximum number of slices. On the other hand, the error of the proposed method remains almost constant for a number of slices more than seven with an overestimation of less than 0.5 %. Statistical analysis showed a statistically-significant difference (p value <0.01) between the errors of the two methods at all number of slices below eight.

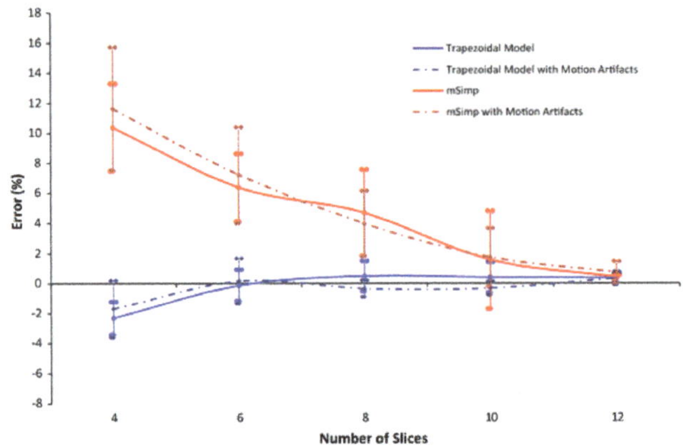

Figure 5: Error (mean ± SD) of the estimated volume at different number of SAX slices using the proposed method and the mSimp method (phantom experiment).

Table 1 summarizes the results of the second set of experiments which measures the reproducibility of the proposed model when changing orientation of the LAX slice. It can be shown that no orientation leads to an error that is substantially and consistently lower than the errors of the other orientations. This might indicate that the proposed method is reliable to the specific selection of the LAX orientation. From another perspective, this shows that the proposed method has a lower bound on the error that cannot be further improved by changing the LAX slice orientation. Table 2 shows the error of both methods caused by simulated respiratory motion artifacts. Comparing these values to those reported in Fig. 5, it could be observed that the standard deviation of the error has increased due to the simulated movement. Nevertheless in both techniques, there was no significant difference between the reported errors before and after applying the respiratory motion.

Table 1: Percentage error (mean ± SD) of LV surface volume due to the reproducibility experiments

LAX orientation\#slices	4	6	8	10	12
4-CH	−2.3 ± 1.09	−0.13 ± 1.04	−0.48 ± 1.00	0.39 ± 1.01	0.34 ± 0.29
2-CH	−1.72 ± 1.14	0.11 ± 0.76	0.43 ± 1.15	0.57 ± 0.93	0.47 ± 1.14
+20 deg.	−1.2 ± 4.1	0.04 ± 1.01	0.32 ± 1.21	0.48 ± 0.98	0.63 ± 1.01
−20 deg.	−2.24 ± 1.4	−0.03 ± 0.95	0.34 ± 1.03	0.34 ± 0.89	0.03 ± 0.65

Table 2: Percentage error (mean ± SD) of LV surface volume due to the motion artifacts of the different simulated breath-holds experiments

Method\#slices	4	6	8	10	12
mSimp	11.63 ± 4.1	7.21 ± 3.2	3.96 ± 2.17	1.72 ± 1.93	0.72 ± 0.96
Trapezoidal model	−1.7 ± 1.9	0.16 ± 1.5	−0.35 ± 0.55	−0.33 ± 0.45	0.33 ± 0.43

Validation using real MRI data

The results of the real data experiment show that the volume calculated by the trapezoidal model is generally lower than that of the mSimp method with statistically-significant lower error at number of slices less than 7. As can be shown in Fig. 6, the error of the trapezoidal model at 4 slices equals to −1.5 ± 2.56 % and keeps decreasing until it converges to 0.36 ± 2.04 % at higher number of slices. Similar to the phantom study, statistical analysis showed that the error of the proposed method in calculating the LV volumes is significantly lower than that of the mSimp with p value <0.01 for a number of slices less than eight.

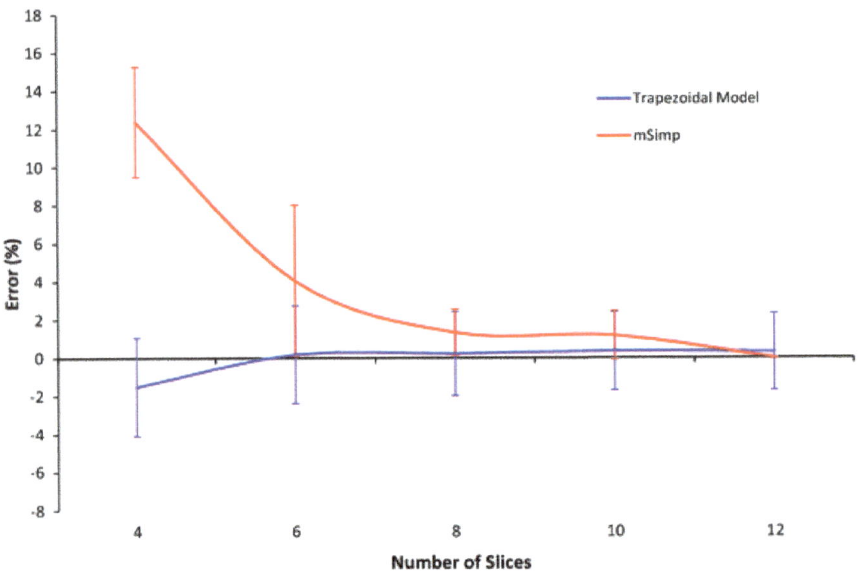

Figure 6: Error (mean ± SD) of the estimated volume at different number of slices using the proposed method and the mSimp method (real MRI data).

To further illustrate the difference among the estimated volumes at low number of slices, Fig. 7 shows the Bland–Altman plot of the calculated LV volume using the different methods compared to the ground truth at 4 and 6 slices. As mentioned above, the ground truth is calculated by applying the mSimp method on the entire set of available SAX contours. As can be shown in Fig. 7a, b, the volume calculated by the proposed method comes in agreement with the ground truth with constant bias (independent of the LV volume) of −8.1 ± 9.9 ml at 4 slices and −1.6 ± 3.6 ml at 6 slices. On the other hand, as shown in Fig. 7c, d, the difference between the LV volume calculated by the mSimp and the ground truth depends on the LV volume. In particular, the mSimp has a mean bias of 29 ± 19.3 ml compared to the ground truth volume at 4 slices and 11 ± 13.1 ml at 6 slices. This indicates the accuracy of the proposed method, relative to the mSimp method, to calculate the LV volume when only a small number of slices are acquired.

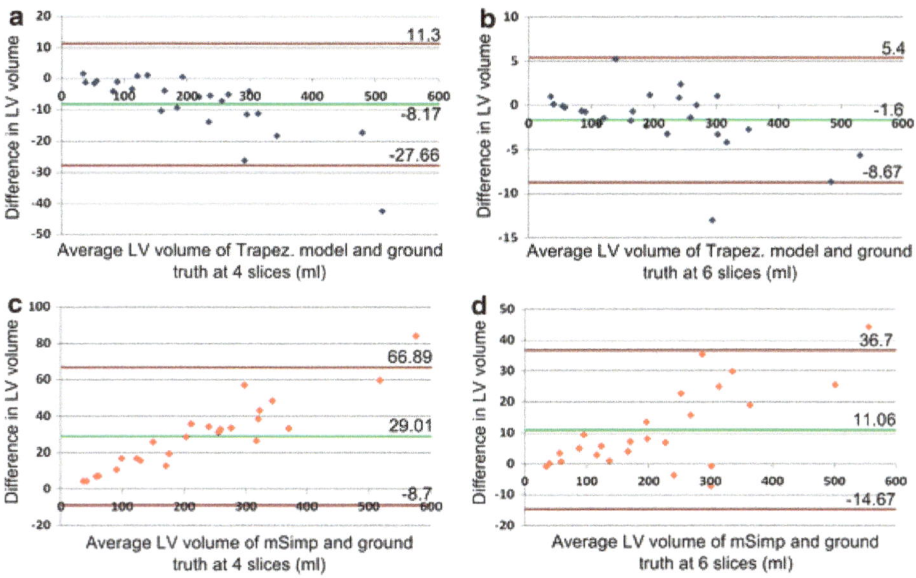

Figure 7: Bland-Altman plot for the LV volume calculation showing the agreement between the trapezoidal model and the ground truth at 4 and 6 slices (a and b respectively); and between the mSimp and the ground truth at 4 and 6 slices (c and d respectively).

The calculations of the ejection fraction (EF), stroke volume (SV), and myocardial LV mass (LVM) of each dataset are listed in Table 3. As can be seen in the table, the average error of calculating the EF error in both methods is less than 1.55 % for all number of slices with a SD value which decreases with increasing the number of slices. Analysis showed no statistically-significant difference between the two methods. On the other hand, the error of calculating the SV and myocardial LVM was found significantly lower (p value ≈ 0) in the proposed method at number of slices less than seven.

At extremely small number of slices (three slices or less), the performance of the proposed method was compared to different models that were proposed in literature to handle the problem of severely reducing the number of slices. Table 4 shows the percentage error of calculating the LV surface volume using these models compared to the proposed model at the same number of slices. As can be seen in the table, using two SAX slices, the Biplane ellipsoid and Hemisphere cylinder models resulted in an error of -9.9 ± 5.88 % and 3.6 ± 7.4 % respectively. This error is significantly higher than that of the proposed trapezoid model ($=1.92 \pm 5.96$ %) using one LAX and one SAX slice. At three slices (2 SAX and 1 LAX), the modified Simpson method resulted in an error of -5.73 ± 8.95 % compared to -2.28 ± 4.38 % resulting from the proposed method. Nevertheless, it was found that at such very small number of slices, the error of the other functional parameters increases significantly relative to the error at 4 slices. For example, the LVM and SV were found to be -18.1 ± 11.9 and -16.68 ± 10.1 respectively at 2 slices, which may not be appropriate for accurate estimation of the cardiac function.

Table 3: Percentage error (mean ± SD) of LV surface volume (LVV_s), EF, SV and myocardial LV mass (LVM) computed by the proposed Trapezoidal and the mSimp methods calculated at different numbers of slices 4, 6, 8, 10 and 12

Method	# slices	4	6	8	10	12
Trapezoidal model	LVV_s	−2.3 ± 1.09	−0.13 ± 1.04	−0.48 ± 1.00	0.39 ± 1.01	0.34 ± 0.29
	EF	0.44 ± 4.1	0.77 ± 1.7	−0.25 ± 1.44	0.2 ± 0.9	0.21 ± 0.87
	SV	−2.7 ± 9.1	−0.16 ± 2.7	−0.7 ± 2.5	0.18 ± 0.83	0.21 ± 0.92
	LVM	−3.46 ± 7.8	0.86 ± 3.57	0.79 ± 3.2	0.98 ± 2.59	0.92 ± 2.38
mSimp	LVV	12.4 ± 2.8	4.1 ± 3.9	1.4 ± 1.3	1.19 ± 1.26	0.0 ± 0.0
	EF	−0.98 ± 7.31	1.53 ± 2.17	−0.67 ± 1.45	−0.018 ± 0.07	0.0 ± 0.0
	SV	7. 8 ± 12.53	4.24 ± 5.64	0.69 ± 2.35	−0.06 ± 0.22	0.0 ± 0.0
	LVM	16.8 ± 5.07	5.57 ± 4.99	2.47 ± 2.43	2.42 ± 2.56	0.0 ± 0.0

Table 4: Percentage error (mean ± SD) of LV surface volume using different models that using either two, or three slices, and the corresponding Trapezoidal model at the same number of slices

Number of slices	Type of slices	Model name	Error (mean ± SD)	Trapezoidal model
2 slices	2 LAX	Biplane ellipsoid	−9.9 ± 5.88	1.92 ± 5.96
	1 SAX + 1 LAX	Hemisphere cylinder	3.6 ± 7.4	
3 slices	2 SAX + 1 LAX	Modified Simpson rule	−5.73 ± 8.95	−2.28 ± 4.38

One advantage of the proposed method is the simplicity of the computations given by Eq. (7). The equation involves only a computation of the area of three contours (or polygons) in addition to the length of two line segments. That is, combining the information from the LAX and SAX s does not involve actual handling of the 3D positions of the SAX or the LAX contour points. However, it is worth mentioning that an implicit step is required to compute the intersection line between the LAX plane and each SAX plane. The overall average computation time on a PC (Dual-core 3 GHz processor, 4 GB RAM) using Matlab implementation (Mathworks, Inc.) is 32 ms per imaging cross-section.

CONCLUSION

In this work, a method for estimating the left ventricular volume from segmented MRI images has been presented. The method incorporates cardiac long axis and short axis cross-sectional s to accurately estimate the myocardium volume. A simple trapezoidal model was used to approximate the myocardium LAX cross-section between pairs of SAX slices. This allowed accurate estimation of the volume compared to the traditional techniques. Results on simulated and real MRI datasets showed the superiority of the proposed method compared to other available methods at small number of slices.

DECLARATIONS

Authors' contributions

ASF and HE contributed to developing the idea, assessment of the results, and interpretation of the findings. HE contributed to the implementation of the algorithm. All authors contributed to writing and revising the manuscript. Both authors read and approved the final manuscript.

Acknowledgements

This work is fully supported by a research and development Grant (CFP59-PDP2012. R12.4) from ITIDA agency, Ministry of Communication and Information Technology, Egypt. The authors would like to thank Dr. Ayman Khalifa at Diagnosoft, Inc. for the useful discussion and support. This work is protected by a provisional patent US 62/106,314.

REFERENCES

1. Messroghli DR, Bainbridge GJ, Alfakih K, Jones TR, Plein S, Ridgway JP, Sivananthan MU. Assessment of regional left ventricular function: accuracy and reproducibility of positioning standard short-axis sections in cardiac MR imaging. Radiology. 2005;235:229–36.
2. Koskenvuo JW, Karra H, Lehtinen J, Niemi P, Pärkkä J, Knuuti J, Hartiala JJ. Cardiac MRI: accuracy of simultaneous measurement of left and right ventricular parameters using three different sequences. Clin Physiol Funct Imaging.

2007;27:385–93.

3. White HD, Norris RM, Brown MA, Brandt PW, Whitlock RM, Wild CJ. Left ventricular end-systolic volume as the major determinant of survival after recovery from myocardial infarction. Circulation. 1987;76:44–51.
4. Sanz G, Castañer A, Betriu A, Magriña J, Roig E, Coll S, Paré JC, Navarro-López F. Determinants of prognosis in survivors of myocardial infarction: a prospective clinical angiographic study. N Engl J Med. 1982;306:1065–70.
5. Dewey M, Müller M, Eddicks S, Schnapauff D, Teige F, Rutsch W, Borges AC, Hamm B. Evaluation of global and regional left ventricular function with 16-slice computed tomography, biplane cineventriculography, and two-dimensional transthoracic echocardiography. Comparison with magnetic resonance imaging. J Am Coll Cardiol. 2006;48:2034–44.
6. Bellenger NG, Burgess MI, Ray SG, Lahiri A, Coats AJS, Cleland JGF, Pennell DJ. Comparison of left ventricular ejection fraction and volumes in heart failure by echocardiography, radionuclide ventriculography and cardiovascular magnetic resonance. Are they interchangeable? Eur Heart J. 2000;21:1387–96.
7. Alattar MA, Osman NF, Fahmy AS. Myocardial segmentation using constrained multi-seeded region growing. Lect Notes Comput Sci. 2010;6112:89–98.
8. Pennell DJ. Ventricular volume and mass by CMR. J Cardiovasc Magn Reson. 2002;4:507–13.
9. Cheng-Baron J, Chow K, Khoo NS, Esch BT, Scott JM, Haykowsky MJ, Tyberg JV, Thompson RB. Measurements of changes in left ventricular volume, strain, and twist during isovolumic relaxation using MRI. Am J Physiol Heart Circ Physiol. 2010;298:H1908–18.
10. Sharma R, Sharma A, Williams CD. A simple assessment of left ventricular function and mass with cine MRI. Inform Medica Slov. 2007;12:22–8.
11. Semelka RC, Tomei E, Wagner S, Mayo J, Caputo G, O'Sullivan M, Parmley WW, Chatterjee K, Wolfe C, Higgins CB. Interstudy reproducibility of dimensional and functional measurements between cine magnetic resonance studies in the morphologically abnormal left ventricle. Am Heart J. 1990;119:1367–73.
12. Fortun NJ, Hood WP, Sherman ME, Craige E. Determination of left ventricular volumes by ultrasound. Circulation. 1971;44:575–84.
13. Folland ED, Parisi AF, Moynihan PF, Jones DR, Feldman CL, Tow DE. Assessment of left ventricular ejection fraction and volumes by real- time, two-dimensional echocardiography. A comparison of cineangiographic and radionuclide techniques. Circulation. 1979;60(4):760–6.
14. Thiele H, Paetsch I, Schnackenburg B, Bornstedt A, Grebe O, Wellnhofer E, Schuler G, Fleck E, Nagel E. Improved accuracy of quantitative assessment of left ventricular volume and ejection fraction by geometric models with steady-state free precession. J Cardiovasc Magn Reson. 2002;4:327–39.
15. Linhart JW, Mintz GS, Segal BL, Kawai N, Kotler MN. Left ventricular volume measurement by echocardiography: fact or fiction? Am J Cardiol. 1975;36(1):114–

8.

16. Elen A, Hermans J, Ganame J, Loeckx D, Bogaert J, Maes F, Suetens P. Automatic 3-D breath-hold related motion correction of dynamic multislice MRI. IEEE Trans Med Imaging. 2010;29:868–78.
17. Swingen C, Seethamraju RT, Jerosch-Herold M. An approach to the three-dimensional display of left ventricular function and viability using MRI. Int J Cardiovasc Imaging. 2003;19:325–36.
18. El-Rewaidy H, Khalifa A, Fahmy AS. Accurate estimation of the myocardium global function from reduced magnetic resonance image acquisitions. In: Engineering in medicine and biology society (EMBC), 36th annual international conference of the IEEE, Chicago, IL; 2014. p. 6728–31.
19. DICOM sample image sets. http://www.osirix-er.com/datasets/.
20. Pieper S, Halle M, Kikinis R. 3D slicer. 2004 2nd IEEE international symposium on biomedical imaging: macro to nano (IEEE Cat No. 04EX821); 2004.
21. Wang Y, Riederer SJ, Ehman RL. Respiratory motion of the heart: kinematics and the implications for the spatial resolution in coronary imaging. Magn Reson Med. 1995;33:713–9.

9
CHAPTER

NEURAL NETWORK MODEL OF VESTIBULAR NUCLEI REACTION TO ONSET OF VESTIBULAR PROSTHETIC STIMULATION

Jack DiGiovanna, T. A. K. Nguyen, Nils Guinand, Angelica Pérez-Fornos and Silvestro Micera

Keywords: Vestibular prosthesis, electrical stimulation, functional models, adaptation, physiological, synapses, vestibular ocular reflex

INTRODUCTION

Vestibular prosthetics are designed to restore sensory information in chronic and severe loss of natural vestibular organ function. Overall, the number of persons with reduced vestibular function is estimated to be about 35% (Agrawal et al., 2009). In particular, vestibular loss can be debilitating in cases of severe bilateral vestibular loss (BVL). In these cases, adaptive mechanisms such as central compensation fail to improve the patient's condition, despite intensive physical therapy (Zingler et al., 2007). Patients are both restricted in activities of daily life (Guinand et al., 2012) and have a poor outlook on recovery (Sun et al., 2014). This highlights the urgent need for new treatment options (Van De Berg et al., 2011).

One treatment option currently in the prototype stage is vestibular prosthetics. These prosthetics are designed to mimic the afferent firing rates that would be generated by healthy semicircular canals (SCCs). A configuration that has been used both in animal models (Gong and Merfeld, 2002; Della Santina et al., 2007) and humans (Van De Berg et al., 2011; Perez Fornos et al., 2014) achieves this via monopolar stimulation from electrodes in close proximity to the ampullae or vestibular

Citation: DiGiovanna J, Nguyen TAK, Guinand N, Pérez-Fornos A and Micera S (2016) Neural Network Model of Vestibular Nuclei Reaction to Onset of Vestibular Prosthetic Stimulation. Front. Bioeng. Biotechnol. 4:34. doi: 10.3389/fbioe.2016.00034.

afferents. This electrical stimulation engages afferents from the SCCs and establishes a clear relationship between the delivered simulation and sensory response, and this relationship is possible due to the homogeneous organization of these sensory organs. In contrast, the peripheral vestibular organs that sense linear acceleration (the otoliths) have a heterogeneous organization (Lewis, 2015). Prosthetic designers have thus far only attempted to restore canal function and not otolithic function because of (i) the relatively simple organization (and accessibility) of SCC afferents and (ii) the complex anatomo-physiology of the otoliths. Given these constraints, current prototypes aim to restore rotational, but not translational, information.

In a healthy animal, changes in firing rate of SCC afferents correlate well with the rotational velocities around axes aligned with that canal (Fernandez and Goldberg, 1971). Modulating electrical stimulation parameters, e.g., pulse rate or pulse amplitude, applied to these afferents can similarly induce corresponding eye movements (Suzuki and Cohen, 1964; Merfeld et al., 2007; Davidovics et al., 2012). Detailed finite element models have been developed to simulate recruitment of vestibular afferents based on the applied electrical stimulation; then changes in eye movements can be calculated as a function of the number of afferents recruited (Marianelli et al., 2015). That model predicted symmetrical changes in eye velocities when pulse rate modulation (PRM) was applied, but sharply non-linear changes when pulse amplitude modulation (PAM) was applied. Overall, it well approximated the literature and also highlighted a range of comodulation possibilities (Marianelli et al., 2015), as experimentally demonstrated in Davidovics et al. (2012).

We build on experimental and modeling work discussed in the prior paragraph but study a different time point in prosthetic use. The existing literature evaluates modulation relative to a baseline stimulation rate. Importantly, at the onset of this baseline rate, there is a discontinuity in stimulation from 0 pps (pulses per second) to a baseline rate (e.g., 200–400 pps). Since stimulation can overwrite residual resting firing rate, there is a corresponding discontinuity in afferent activity. This discontinuous and sharp step from resting rate imposes a transient nystagmus that must attenuate before the prosthetic can be used. This strategy is reflected in common experimental paradigms, e.g., "baseline stimulation was applied and after*N* minutes nystagmus attenuated; we then modulated stimulation and measured eye-movement output." The timeframe *N* is species- and time-dependent [e.g., Merfeld et al. (2006), Guyot et al. (2011), andDavidovics et al. (2012)]. Our focus is on that often-skipped timeframe.

Specifically, could synaptic plasticity between the afferents and the vestibular nuclei accommodate this transient nystagmus attenuation? Arnold and Robinson (1997) built a six-layer neural network composed of four different types of neurons connecting the SCCs with the ocular movements. We model the synaptic strength between each afferent (two types) and the vestibular nuclei as in Arnold and Robinson (1997), instead of a global function between afferent firing and stimulation parameters to eye movements (Marianelli et al., 2015). We start from healthy SCCs with afferents having a distribution of resting firing rates, variances, and response magnitude to rotation. There is a corresponding distribution of synaptic strengths. We then simulate BVL, baseline prosthetic stimulation, and finally pulse modulation. The onset of baseline stimulation is a "perturbation" and the model adapts the synaptic strengths to reduce error (no aberrant eye movements). Any subsequent changes in stimulation, either modulation or a change in baseline rate, will induce eye movements. We examine how synaptic strength adaptation affects subsequent VOR to modulation of stimulation. Specifically, how does adaptation of a portion of the synapses affect the efficacy of subsequent PRM or PAM? Additionally, are there non-obvious characteristics of prosthetic stimulation exposed through this model?

We abstract a simple neural network model from biological principles to model the pathway including the electrode, afferents, vestibular nuclei, and eyes. Model inputs are electrical pulse stimulation amplitude and rate. The model output is eye velocity around a single axis (e.g., horizontal, vertical, or torsional); these three axes comprise the space of eye movements (Haslwanter, 1995). Conceptually, the model could produce velocity around three axes to accommodate current spread or "cross talk." However, we will discuss in Section "Results" why we restricted our analysis to a single axis.

Simulations of acute (short-duration trials within the clinic in humans) vestibular prosthetic modulation after this adaptation predict eye movements that followed the same trends as acute clinical testing for PAM and PRM[1]. Searching over a spectrum of resting firing rate distributions showed minimal influence on relative stimulation efficacy. Finally, we simulated a comodulation of pulse rate and pulse amplitude that was previously used in animals (Davidovics et al., 2012). The model predicts both boosted outputs for combined stimulation and equipotent outputs using less PAM, an important factor in reducing current spread and misalignment of eye-movement responses.

MATERIALS AND METHODS

The model is divided into two main components: electrode–nerve interface and nerve–nuclei interface. The model has one layer of free parameters, specifically the synaptic strengths. These are adapted during the onset of prosthetic stimulation. We describe the model components below. Experiments were performed in accordance with the Declaration of Helsinki and approved by the ethics committees of the University Hospitals Geneva (NAC 11-080).

Electrode–Nerve Interface

Rotation is normally sensed by hair cells within the ampulla; it results in modulated firing rates of vestibular nerve fibers. In patients with BVL, these cells are significantly less sensitive or non-responsive to rotational stimuli or may be lost. The electrode–nerve interface is built upon existing physics of electrical stimulation (McIntyre et al., 2002; Capogrosso et al., 2013; Marianelli et al., 2015). An electrical field generated by injected current will spread spherically through a space of uniform conductance. Injecting more or less current will change the radius of this sphere. Any afferents within this sphere can be depolarized above the threshold voltage, which will generate an action potential if the cell is not in the refractory period. Resting firing rate statistics were extrapolated based on animal models, including (Fernandez and Goldberg, 1971) squirrel monkeys with 91.3 ± 36.3 spikes/s; (Sadeghi et al., 2007) macaque monkeys population afferent firing rate was approximately 95 spikes/s; (Baird et al., 1988) chinchilla had an afferent population firing rate of 70.9 ± 1.1 spikes/s for regular units, respectively; (Bronte-Stewart and Lisberger, 1994) rhesus monkey had a distribution of resting afferent firing rates from 29 to 158 spikes/s with a peak around 100 spikes/s; and (Hullar et al., 2005) chinchilla population afferent resting firing rate of 42 ± 21.5 spikes/s, However, note that detailed characterizations of this nerve have not been performed in humans or after BVL.

The model will have N afferents within the sphere of delivered charge:

$$N = n(A_b + A_m) \quad (1)$$

where n is a ratio between the number of recruited afferents vs. injected current. This weighting is dependent on electrode placement and impedance. Here, we set n such that $N = 40\%$ of afferents (400 afferents out of the 1000 afferents simulated) at baseline (A_b) current while modulated (A_m) stimulation is 0. This reflects the procedure used in patient trials to set the baseline current amplitude in the middle between the threshold current amplitude and the upper comfortable level (Perez Fornos et al., 2014). It is challenging to generalize "typical" values for A_b and A_m, as the effect of stimulation is dependent on patient anatomy, surgical placement, and electrode condition. Detailed dynamic ranges for a group of 11 patients are given in Guinand et al. (2015). We use 1000 afferents per SCC for this paper. Results are consistent, simulating different numbers of afferents; only runtime and resolution are affected (unpublished).

We assume that afferents continuously generate action potentials, according to probability distributions of firing rates. Multiple distributions were tested, but for this paper, all mean firing rates were sampled from the lognormal distribution (mean = 26.3 spikes/s and SD = 6.6 spikes/s), as shown in Figure 1A. Each afferent also had a variance in firing rate, depending on whether it was irregular [33% of afferents, coefficient of variation (CV) >0.1] or regular (67% of afferents, CV <0.1), these variances were sampled from the uniform distribution for each type shown in Figure 1B. The percentages of regular and irregular afferents (and CV ranges for each type) were extrapolated based on animal models, including (Fernandez and Goldberg, 1971) squirrel monkeys that had a 1:2 ratio of regular (CV <0.058) to non-regular (CV >0.238) afferents; (Sadeghi et al., 2007) macaque monkeys that had a 3:2 ratio of regular (CV* <0.15) to irregular (CV* >0.15) afferents; (Baird et al., 1988) chinchilla that had 3:1 ratio of regular (CV* <0.1) to irregular (CV* >0.2) afferents; (Bronte-Stewart and Lisberger, 1994) rhesus monkey that had a nearly 6:1 ratio of regular (CV* <0.1) to irregular (CV* >0.2) afferents; and (Hullar et al., 2005) chinchilla had a 1:3 ratio of regular (CV* <0.1) to irregular (CV* >0.2) afferents. For the sub ensemble of N afferents influenced by the electrical stimulation, the firing rate is locked to the stimulation rate if it exceeds the residual resting firing rate.

$$fr_i = \max\left(\mathrm{PR}_b + \mathrm{PR}_m, p(s_i, u_i)\right) \quad (2)$$

where PR_b and PR_m are pulse rates of baseline and modulated stimulation, i is the afferent index, and u and s are the mean and variances of the residual resting firing rates, respectively. The difference between the stimulation modalities (PAM and PRM; Figure 1C) that influence on vestibular nerve activity (Figure1D) is captured with A_m and PR_m in Eqs 1 and 2.

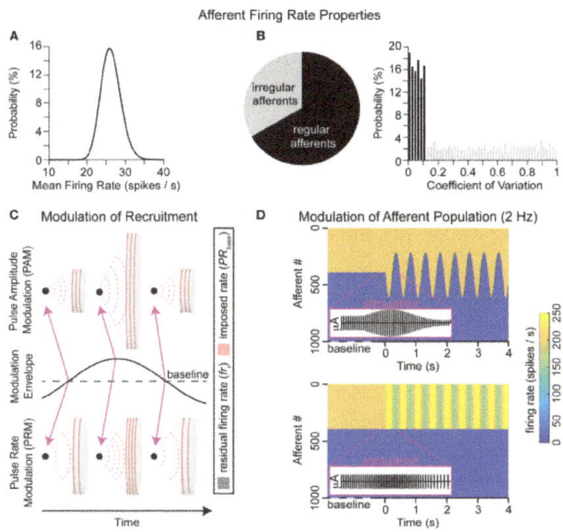

Figure 1: Electrode–nerve interface. (A) Distributions of resting mean firing rates for the population. (B) The percentage of regular (67%) and irregular (33%) afferents is illustrated in the pie plot; the distribution of CVs for each afferent type is also shown. Each afferent will have a mean residual firing rate sampled from (A) and a variance sampled from (B). (C) Concept of stimulation from a monopolar electrode (black dot) in an environment with uniform conductance. The area stimulated depends on pulse amplitude, while the frequency of action potentials depends on pulse rate. A sinusoidal envelope modulates both modalities from baseline to ± maximum values. This modulation envelope is a 2-Hz sine wave. At baseline, there is no modulation (e.g., A_m and/or PR_m go to 0). Positive (negative) values of the modulation envelope correspond to delivering higher (lower) values of pulse amplitude and/or pulse rate than baseline (e.g., A_m and/or PR_m are non-zero). Pink arrows show that the first and last examples here are at baseline stimulation, while the middle example is a peak positive modulation. (D) Simulated vestibular afferent populations during baseline stimulation followed by PAM or PRM. In purple, we overlay the zoom into brief section of the applied stimulation pulses, including baseline, maximum, and minimum modulation values.

Nerve–Nuclei Interface

The vestibular nuclei are innervated by multiple components of the nervous system, one of which is partially composed of the afferents within the vestibular nerve. Each afferent synapses onto the nuclei, with the influence of delivered action potentials determined by the synaptic strength (Arnold and Robinson, 1997). Afferents within this vestibular nerve synapse directly onto position-vestibular-pause neurons (Cullen and McCrea, 1993; Sadeghi et al., 2009, 2011) within the vestibular nuclei in the brainstem. Each nucleus receives bilateral input from afferents within the vestibular nerves. We model the strengths of these synapses with linear weight terms. The nuclei sum the weighted firing rates from all afferents and then apply a saturating non-linearity, which encapsulates both non-linearity in the nucleus and in eye muscle contractions [for a detailed model of the individual non-linear elements, see Arnold and Robinson (1997)]. The synaptic strengths are plastic, i.e., they adapt to minimize retinal slip. Prior research has shown that adaptation similar to long-term depression (LTD) (Markram et al., 1997) may account for reduced sensitivity to unilateral afferent inputs at supra-physiological rates (Mitchell et al., 2014). The final output of these nuclei is an eye velocity command (Figure 2A), which will pass through the abducens nucleus, trochlear nucleus, oculomotor nuclei, and the ocular muscles (Purves et al., 2004). We make three additional assumptions to model these nuclei: (a) inputs (represented as weighted firing rates) from each synapse are summed, (b) an "offset" that can globally attenuate inputs (e.g., rely on vision for slow movement in good lighting), and (c) other inputs are grouped into a single term *P*. Thus, the equation for the model is

$$v = f\left(\sum_{i} w_i fr_i - b, P\right) \tag{3}$$

where v is the observed eye velocity (around a single axis), w_i is the synaptic strength for each afferent, i, $b$is the offset, and P represents all other inputs to the vestibular nuclei. These inputs are known to influence gains of the VOR, but the exact methods for achieving this are disputed (Loeb and Tsianos, 2015). For the remainder of this work, we assume P is independent of stimulation modality (PRM or PAM) and can be removed from the model, as it will cancel out in any differential comparisons. A non-linear hyperbolic tangent function was used for the mapping $f()$ between the nuclei and eye movements; it was selected based on the relationship between firing rate and eye movement previously detailed in monkeys (Fernandez and Goldberg, 1971). This mapping and the removal of P reduces Eq. 3 to a standard single-layer perceptron, as described in Haykin (1994).

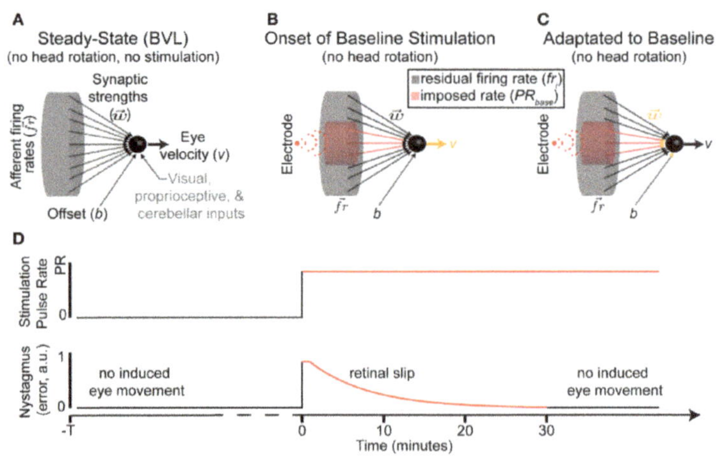

Figure 2: Nerve–nucleus interface. (A) Model of primary afferents in BVL without prosthetic stimulation. There is no eye movement despite residual afferent activity. (B,C) The onset of baseline

stimulation introduces imbalances between the synaptic strengths, self-regulation, and induced firing rates within stimulated afferents. Any changes are color coded in orange. (D) Nystagmus occurs immediately after baseline stimulation onset, but attenuated in all tested patients within a maximum of 30 min. We model this as a change in synaptic strengths and/or self-regulation in (C).

Acute Adaptation

After vestibular injury or loss, the vestibular nerve does not provide useful information. The hair cells that normally modulate afferent firing either die or become non-responsive to rotational stimulation. Thus, the population of afferents is no longer modulated by the hair cells and instead reverts to a residual resting discharge that is independent of head rotation. The vestibular nuclei must attenuate the influence of afferent's residual resting discharge, which may be lower than the healthy resting discharge rate, to minimize retinal slip. Retinal slip (*e* in Eq. 4) is the difference between the appropriate (i.e., perfectly compensating for head rotations) and actual eye movements; this slip induces aberrant percepts of image motion. Experimentally, nystagmus (an eye movement consisting of a slow movement in one direction followed by a rapid movement in the opposite direction, conceptually a series of retinal slips) induced by abrupt onsets of electrical stimulation attenuated to negligible values within a maximum of 30 min while the patient was sitting in a dark room (Guyot et al., 2011). To achieve this attenuation in the model is possible *via* Eq. 5.

$$e = v_{\text{eye}} + v_{\text{head}} \tag{4}$$

$$0 = v_{\text{eye}}$$
$$0 = f\left(\sum_{\text{i}} w_{\text{i}} fr_{\text{i}} - b\right) \tag{5}$$

Setting the sum of weighted firing rates equal to the offset will minimize error. We do not reintroduce *P*from Eq. 3, as we assumed that within the timescale of adaptation to baseline stimulation onset, while the patient is seated in a dark room, the contribution of *P* is constant. Thus, nuclei adaptation is restricted to*w* and *b* (Figures 2B,C).

Mean squared error is back propagated, according to Eqs 6 and 7 (Eq. 7 includes a Fahlman constant; is the error, back propagated through the output node), where d_{v} is the desired eye velocity, i.e., opposite of head movement to keep the gaze focused. The synaptic strengths, here represented as a vector, and offset are updated with Eqs 8 and 9.

$$e = d_{\text{v}} - v \tag{6}$$

$$\delta = e \times (1.1 - v^2) \tag{7}$$

$$\Delta w = \alpha_{\text{s}} \delta fr \tag{8}$$

$$\Delta b = \alpha_{\text{b}} \delta \tag{9}$$

Here, there are different learning rates for the synaptic strengths (α_s) and offset term (α_b). This feature was added to address the uncertainty of the nuclei attenuating all afferent input ($\alpha_b \gg \alpha_s$), attenuating only the stimulated afferents ($\alpha_s \gg \alpha_b$), or a hybrid approach in response to the discontinuity introduced by the onset of baseline stimulation. This spectrum of relative learning rates was chosen to emulate heterosynaptic and homosynaptic LTD, respectively. Homosynaptic LTD is a Hebbian-type learning that decreases the synaptic strength if both the pre- and postsynaptic neurons are active (Purves et al., 2004). In contrast, heterosynaptic LTD attenuates synapses independently of neuron activity.

Modulation

The prosthetic modulates eye velocity commands (Eq. 3), based on the changing afferent firing rates, as described by Eqs 1 and 2. The relationship between actual head rotations and afferent firing rates in healthy monkeys (Fernandez and Goldberg, 1971) is shown in Figure 3A. Similarly, the mapping between detected rotations and prosthetic stimulation is given in Figure 3B for PRM. Equivalently, PAM can be achieved by swapping PR_m with A_m.

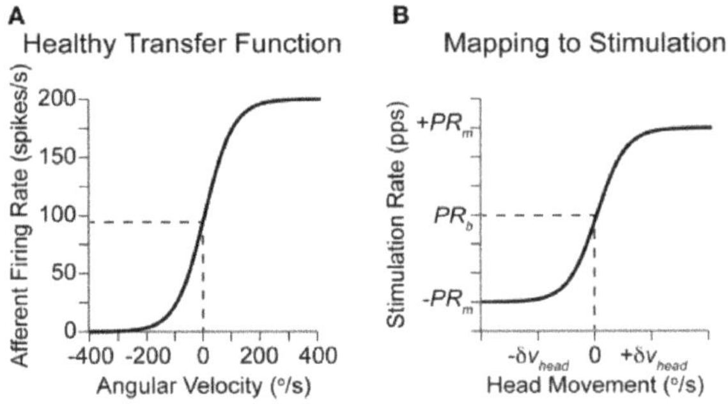

Figure 3: Relationship between head rotation and afferent activity. (A) Approximate transfer function between head rotations along a single axis and afferent firing rates in healthy monkeys (Fernandez and Goldberg, 1971). (B) Imposed transfer function for each axis in a vestibular prosthetic using PRM. The width of the linear region can be set based on the observed patient-specific head rotations or the maximal range of possible rotations (Gong and Merfeld, 2000; Della Santina et al., 2007).

For this paper, we apply only a fixed sinusoidal (2 Hz) modulation of stimulation parameters (see Figure1B) between $A_b + A_m$ and $A_b - A_m$ independently of any actual head rotations of the vestibular prosthetic user (or between $PR_b + PR_m$ and $PR_b - PR_m$). This modulation frequency (2 Hz) was selected because it is a prevalent head frequency in everyday tasks, such as walking (Grossman et al., 1989; Guinand et al., 2015). The desired outcome is to evoke maximal eye velocity. This configuration mimics the acute clinical testing of a prosthetic as shown by Guyot et al. (2010). Outputs for PAM and PRM using common clinical settings are shown in Figures 4A,B. The metric for evaluating performance is the positive peak eye velocity (PEV) shown in Figure 4C. Using only positive, PEV hides the imbalance between positive and negative eye velocities in this model with PAM (Figures 4A,C). However, real eye-movement data (Figure 4D) is noisy, particularly in the measured eye positions during the negative portion of the cycle. Differentiating this signal to calculate velocity compounds the problem, so we first applied a 5-Hz low-pass filter (third order, non-causal Butterworth) to the position (Figure 4D). This creates the expected periodic modulation in the velocity signals, in this example, it is obvious for times >2 s (Figure 4E). However, compiling and averaging these modulation cycles reveals a sinusoid with different phase amplitudes and frequencies (Figure 4F). Alternatively, eye position can be fit for each cycle, as in Perez Fornos et al. (2014), and then differentiated (Figure 4G). This generates a much cleaner output, but the necessary detail (positive vs. negative velocity) for model fitting is lost. Given the noise in the eye velocity calculations (Figure 4F) and the dependency on the cut-off frequency of the low-pass filter, we only consider one portion (PEV) of the model output.

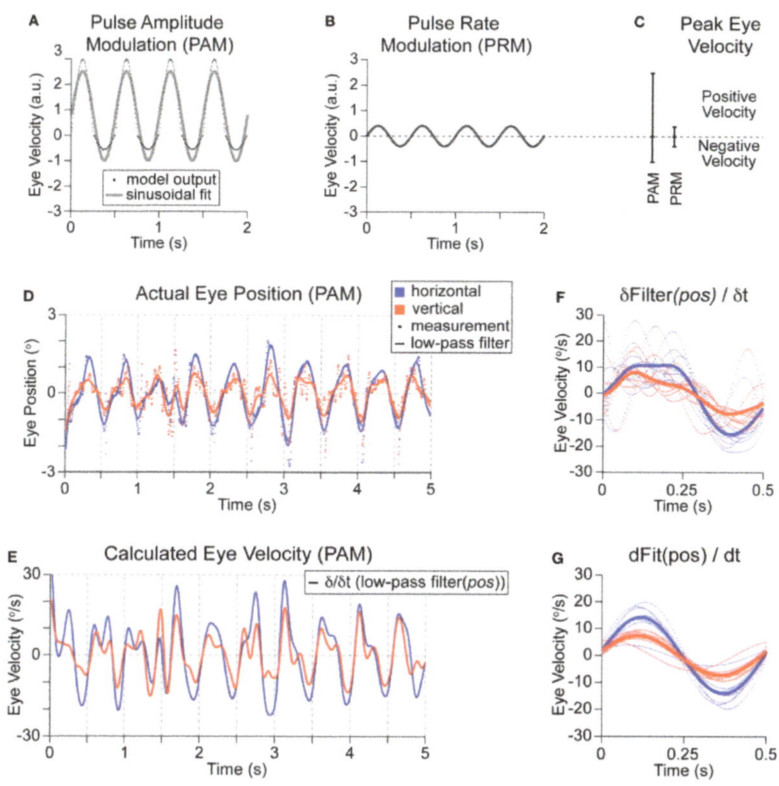

Figure 4: Model outputs and patient measurements. Models were trained using clinical settings of 200-pps baseline stimulation and then ±25% modulation depth was applied. (A) PAM generated relatively large positive eye velocities with muted negative eye velocities. Applying a sinusoidal fit shows a peak positive eye velocity of 2.5 in arbitrary units. (B) Applying PRM to the same model generates much smaller eye velocities, but without any imbalance in positive and negative outputs. There is complete overlap of the model outputs on the sinusoidal fit. (C) The

peak eye velocities for each modality are shown. (D) Representative PAM recording from a single patient during stimulation of the lateral ampullary nerve (which should elicit purely horizontal eye velocities) shows a 2-Hz modulation of eye position (dots) in the horizontal (red) and vertical (blue) dimensions. Traces are generated with a 5-Hz low-pass filter. (E) Differentiating these traces estimates eye velocity. (F) Compiling all cycles of modulation reveals a broad and uneven positive velocity peak followed by a more sinusoidal shaped and larger magnitude negative velocity peak. (G) Alternatively, each cycle of the position signal in (D) is fitted with a sinusoid, then differentiated. This dramatically cleans up the velocity outputs but obscures any imbalance in positive and negative outputs or modulation shapes.

These representative eye positions also highlight another challenge for vestibular prosthetics. In this patient, the lateral SCC was stimulated, which should have evoked purely horizontal eye movements. Instead, there are both horizontal and vertical eye movements. This is an example of the common phenomena of current spread; here, the unwanted movements (vertical) are nearly two thirds as large as the desired (horizontal) movements. Using PAM accesses the horizontal SCC as desired but also spreads to stimulate the anterior SCC (and potentially other unintended targets), which generates unwanted eye movements. Current spread may be reduced by changing the maximal change in PAM; however, this will also reduce the desired horizontal movement magnitude. In the model, the maximal change in stimulation for PRM and PAM was balanced for any comparisons. Specifically, the multiplier from A_b to A_m was the same as from P_b to P_m. We labeled this "charge-balanced." This multiplier was often 1.25 (or 25%), which has been a common upper bound in current acute clinical PAM testing.

Hybrid comodulation of stimulation was also modeled. All three stimulation modes are summarized by the change in charge in Eq. 10. (Note that the A_m component also has a geometric multiplier based on Eq. 1. We also removed the pulse-width term, as this is common over methods). In PAM or PRM, only the first or second terms, respectively, are non-zero. In contrast, for hybrid stimulation all three terms are non-zero. We do not restrict hybrid stimulation to be charge-balanced with PAM or PRM. Instead, we characterize possible hybrid model outputs across possible percentages of PRM and PAM.

$$\Delta Q = \mathrm{PR_b} A_m + \mathrm{PR_m} A_b + \mathrm{PR_m} A_m \qquad (10)$$

RESULTS

This simple model of vestibular prosthetic and vestibular–ocular interaction exposed two important relationships. First, there may be a large discontinuity between the induced pulse rate and the residual resting discharge of the population of non-recruited afferents. This discontinuity is exacerbated, as higher baseline pulse rates are used. Second, the adaptation to baseline stimulation tends to attenuate the weight of the recruited afferents (e.g., afferents #1–#400 in Figure 1C). Both of these relationships disproportionally degrade the efficacy of PRM.

Influence of Baseline Pulse Rate and Residual Resting Discharge

The most influential relationship exposed by this model is the discontinuity between baseline pulse rate and residual resting discharge. In Figure 5A, we compare the average firing rate within the ensemble of afferents for PAM (22.5–62.5% afferents stimulated, 200 pps) and PRM (40% afferents stimulated, 200 ± 50 pps) at 25% modulation for both methods. Note that this average includes many non-modulated afferents (for either PAM or PRM), which lowers the value toward the residual resting firing rates as shown in Figure 1A. For example, afferent #500 (Figure 1C) switches from a mean firing rate of approximately 27 to 200 pps during the positive modulation half-cycle of PAM. The subpopulation of neurons with this discontinuity contributes to the sharp increase in ensemble firing rate. This dependency is described in Eqs 10 and 11, where Δfr is the change in the afferent ensemble firing rate, and all other variables are from Eqs 1 and 2.

$$\Delta fr_{\mathrm{PAM}} = \sum_{i=nA_b+1}^{n(A_m+A_b)} \mathrm{PR_b} - fr_i \qquad (11)$$

$$\Delta fr_{\mathrm{PRM}} = nA_b(\mathrm{PR_m} - \mathrm{PR_b}) \qquad (12)$$

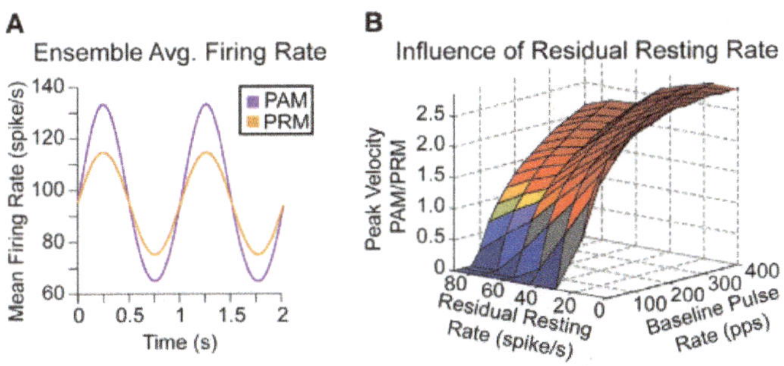

Figure 5: Ensemble and residual firing rates. (A) Given changes in pulse rate or pulse amplitude, there is a larger modulation in firing rate for PAM. Here, the baseline recruitment (A_b) is fixed to 40% of afferents, modulation (pulse rate or pulse amplitude) is fixed to 25%, and we scan over all residual firing rates and baseline pulse rates. (B) There is higher peak eye velocity for PAM (red) over a large region of this space. However, PRM does generate higher peak eye velocities (blue) for low baseline pulse rates, especially if the residual firing rate is also low.

The baseline population ($n \times A_b$) of stimulated neurons subjected to the modulated pulse rate (Eq. 12) is larger than the modulated population [$n \times (A_m - A_b)$], i.e., afferents stimulated only during the positive sine wave of PAM. However, the discrepancy between baseline pulse rate and residual resting discharge in Eq. 11 during the positive sine wave of PAM causes a larger overall change in ensemble firing rate.

In the first acute tests with proof of concept prosthetics (Perez Fornos et al., 2014), 25% modulation depth (i.e., stimulation intensity ranged from 25 to 75% of the dynamic range, where 100% is the upper comfortable level) corresponded to a typical clinical case. Fixing the modulation depth of PR to ±25% of baseline PR, it is clear that PAM will generate eye movements with greater magnitude throughout a majority of possible combinations (Figure 5B).

Influence of Stimulated Afferents and Learning Rates

The differences in outputs can be understood through the synaptic strengths in the model. In the healthy situation, synapses are organized such that increasing firing rates in afferents from a SCC on one side are weighted positively while inputs from the opposite SCC are weighted negatively (Figure 6A). Conceptually, one could consider positive synaptic strengths excitatory while negative strengths are inhibitory. Alternatively, positive and negative may be defined relative to the direction that the eyes are moved. Either interpretation combines the push–pull mechanism of vestibular sensory function to create a single eye movement in the correct direction. After BVL, there is no more natural modulation in afferents from either SCC; instead, all afferents fall to a distribution of residual resting rates (Figure 1A). The synapses in the model are all evenly adapted to accommodate this lower input rate. Later, a unilateral prosthetic is implanted and afferents from a single canal are stimulated tonically at a baseline frequency for approximately 30 min (Figure 2D). We assumed that 40% of afferents would be recruited at this current amplitude. This means 400 afferents (shown in gray in Figure 6B) suddenly went from a low residual firing rate (normally distributed around approximately 27 pps) to the baseline stimulation rate of 200 pps. The model again adapts the weights, according to Eqs 8 and 9; however, there is a sharp difference in the firing rate for this subpopulation of afferents. Thus, synapses for these afferents are adapted more rapidly than the non-stimulated afferents. Figure 6B shows the impacts of this adaptation, many synapses within the recruited population (in gray) become negative and overall the mean value of these synapses is lower than other afferents. This means that increases in firing rate within certain afferents in the recruited population actually contribute to attenuate positive eye movements. It also highlights the subpopulation of afferents (in purple) only influenced during PAM, which have a higher mean synaptic strength. Given the same change in firing rate between two afferents, the afferent with the higher synaptic strength contributes more to generate positive eye movement. The different changes in ensemble firing rates (inputs) and synaptic strengths combine to generate a much higher velocity from PAM than from PRM (Figures 4A,B and 6C).

The ratio of bias vs. synaptic learning rates also affects the model output. At extreme values of bias learning rate (heterosynaptic, solid lines in Figure 6C), the magnitude of model output for PRM increases, and the imbalance between PEV and negative peak eye velocity (NEV) for PAM decreases. Both of these effects are due to adaptation of the bias term completely offsetting any errors at high learning rates. That strategy preserves the afferent weights at nearly the original values (Figure 6A), which boosts PRM output. Not adapting the afferent weights also avoids the discontinuity between baseline and PAM stimulated afferents (Figure 6B); this correspondingly reduces PEV vs. NEV imbalance for PAM. Scanning over possible learning rate ratios in Figure 6D shows that these positive changes occur at bias learning rates that are 3×10^4 times larger than the learning rate for a synapse (or 30 times larger than the combined change in all afferents). Such rapid bias learning rates mitigate the problematic synaptic properties shown in Figure 6B for lower bias learning rates.

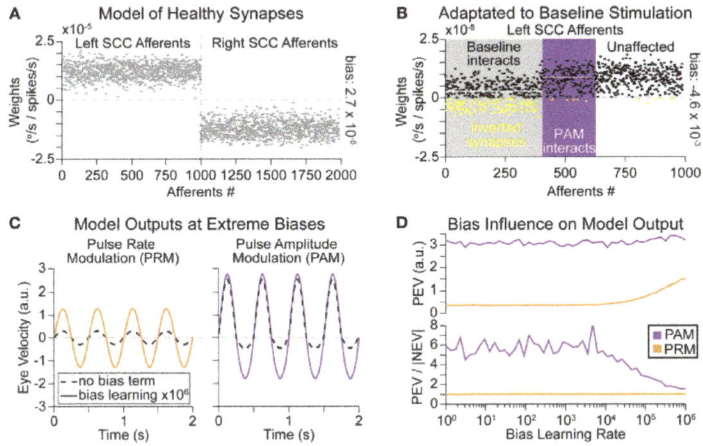

Figure 6: Synaptic strengths and learning rate ratios. (A) Modeled healthy afferent strength values connecting to the vestibular nuclei. Increased firing rates from left SCC afferents cause positive eye movement (move to right); decreased firing rates from right SCC afferents have the same effect as they are multiplied by a negative strength (B) During baseline adaptation to left SCC stimulation by a vestibular implant, there is a population (shown in gray) of afferents entrained to 200-pps activity. This excess activity causes nystagmus (error). To correct this error, the network increases the bias term and adapts the other strengths. Here, the bias strength was 2×10^3. Now, there are strengths in the incorrect region of space (inverted synapses are colored yellow), and increasing firing rates in these afferents would yield negative eye movement. Additionally, the mean strength value is lower in the gray area compared to the rest of the population (mean values shown as white overlay lines for each region). This creates an advantage for PAM, which interacts with a subpopulation of afferents (shown in purple) with larger strengths during the positive phase of modulation. (C) The ratio of learning rates between the bias term and neurons is adapted to simulate heterosynaptic (bias rate very high) vs. homosynaptic (synapse rate very high) LTD. The ratio of learning rates affects the magnitude of PRM and the symmetry of PAM. Relatively faster bias term adaptation increases both the factors. (D) Simulation of different bias rates showing the increase in PEV for PRM, as bias learning rate increased above 3×10^4. The increase in symmetry (PEV/|NEV| goes toward 1.0) for PAM occurs around the same learning rate.

Modulation Efficacy

Precise modulation of eye velocity is important for vestibular prosthetic function. All prior sections focused on peak output using a 200-pps baseline with ±25% modulation depth. We also checked other modulation strengths from 10 to 50%. For two baseline pulse rates, 100 and 200 pps, PAM generated larger eye velocities (Figure 7A). However, we see a large drop in PAM output at the 100-pps baseline due to the PR_b term in Eq. 11. This change in baseline does not affect PRM. Normalizing by eye velocity at 10% modulation depth, we see that both PAM and PRM created an approximately unity increase in eye velocity for each additional 10% change in modulation (Figure 7B), indicating similar modulation efficacy.

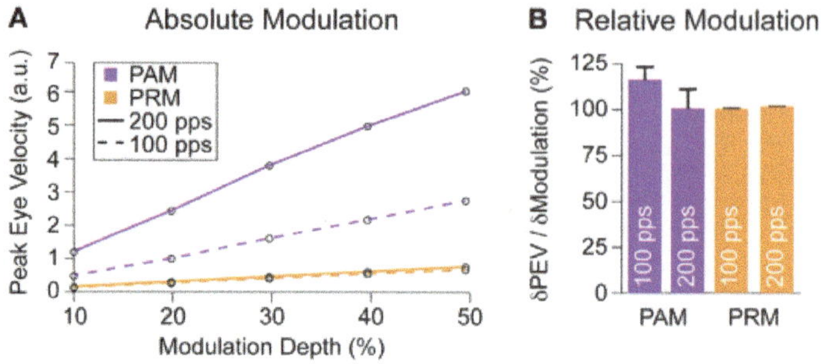

Figure 7: Modulation efficacy. (A) Peak eye velocity over different modulation strengths for PAM and PRM at 100- and 200-pps baseline stimulation. There is a clear attenuation of PAM at lower baseline stimulation while PRM remains unaffected. (B) Normalizing to the change in output at 10% modulation, we see both PAM and PRM increase PEV about 100% per 10% change in modulation.

Finally, we combined the two methods to simulate comodulation. Specifically, both A_m and PR_m were varied together at a 200-pps baseline stimulation rate and 2×10^3 bias learning rate ratio. Adding PRM on top of PAM creates a non-linear multiplier (see Eq. 10) on the eye velocity output (Figure 8A). For example, adding 100% PRM to 25% PAM increases the model output by a factor of 2. Alternatively, we assume that eye velocity at 25% modulation depth for PAM is sufficient for prosthetic function. To reduce current spread and avoid reaching the upper level, there are equipotent contours in hybrid stimulation space (Figure 8B) that can achieve the same eye velocity output with less PAM.

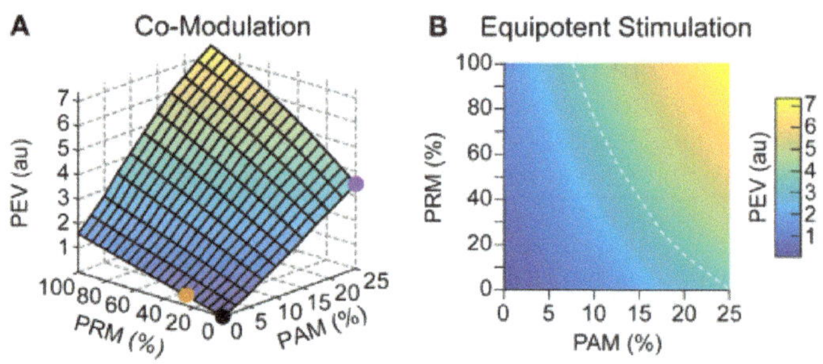

Figure 8: Comodulation. An alternative stimulation strategy to PAM and PRM is to modulate both the pulse amplitude and rate of stimulation. (A) The orange and purple dots represent pure PAM and PRM, respectively, as previously presented. Combining these modulation methods further increases the possible PEV output. (B) Similarly, there are multiple combinations of stimulation methods which are equivalent to 25% PAM. For example, the white dashed line shows that the same output can be achieved with 12.5% PAM combined with 55% PRM.

DISCUSSION

We have presented a simple, functional model of the interaction between vestibular prosthetic stimulation and induced eye velocity. The novelty of this model is the adaptation of vestibular nuclei synaptic strengths to emulate neural plasticity in the processing of afferent activity. We specifically focus on the tonic baseline stimulation period of vestibular prosthetic onset, which initially causes a nystagmus that attenuates after 30 min (Guyot et al., 2011). Since there has been no change in the input, we focused on the synapses to explain the change in the output. LTD was proposed as a physiological mechanism for synaptic adaptation, including both hetero- (all synapses are adapted independently of activity) and homo- [only active (stimulated) synapses are adapted] synaptic components. Spike-time-dependent plasticity, which LTD is a subset of, appears rapid enough to allow such error attenuation. It has been shown to occur with approximately 100 action potential pairings repeated at fixed frequencies (Markram et al., 1997; Bi and Poo, 1998; Sjöström et al., 2001). There is no consensus of the optimal baseline prosthetic stimulation rate; however, even 100 pps already delivers an abundance of action potentials to the stimulated afferents. This adaptation was modeled as back propagation of error with a bias term serving to model homosynaptic components. Specifically, adaptation of the bias term has a relative impact on the contribution of all synapses, regardless of their activity level.

Importantly, we did not focus on model fitting to clinical data. Such patient-specific models have been evaluated (unpublished), but the data were insufficient to test for robust generalization. To date, there are only 12 total patients implanted with some variant of a 1- to 3-branch vestibular prosthetic (Guinand et al., 2015). This makes it impossible to pool data across patients to train the models. Further, eye velocity data are extremely noisy (see Figures 4D,E) (Perez Fornos et al., 2014), and only the positive half of the modulation cycle is reliably present in the recordings. Without a measurement of the PAM output imbalance, there is no reference point to set the ratio of bias to synaptic learning rates beside a very wide range of relative differences in PEV in Figure 6D. There were also modulation frequency dependent gains (Van De Berg et al., 2015) and current spread during PAM to adjacent vestibular structures that caused eye velocities along unwanted axes. These were not addressed in this paper but further diluted the available data. Despite these strong caveats, we were able to reproduce the relative differences in PEV for PAM and PRM at 2 Hz for a 200-pps baseline stimulation as shown in Nguyen et al. (2016)[1] across a spectrum of residual firing rates and learning rate ratios. We also reproduced the drop in PAM output for 100-pps baseline stimulation without any significant change in PRM output[1]. Interestingly, our model predicts that the same *normalized* modulation is possible using either PAM or PRM. However, since PRM is modulating relative to such a small absolute output, it may be obscured by measurement noise.

This simplified model not only replicated the higher efficacy of PAM of electrical stimulation compared to PRM observed in acute clinical testing (Guyot et al., 2011; Pelizzone et al., 2014; Perez Fornos et al., 2014) but also presented two non-intuitive relationships that may explain this phenomenon. First, physics dictate that PAM will cause a larger overall change in afferent ensemble firing rate than PRM, given the same amount of relative modulation. The charge spreads spherically to recruit a larger population of afferents, and there is a discontinuity between these afferents' residual resting discharge rates and the (usually much higher) baseline simulation rates. Second, the model sharply attenuates the synaptic strengths for the subpopulation of afferents recruited during baseline stimulation to reduce nystagmus. Synapses for non-recruited afferents are less sharply attenuated. PRM only interacts with the subpopulation of afferents with sharply attenuated synaptic strengths. Combining these relationships, it is clear that PRM is less efficient in enacting a change in ensemble afferent activity and further restricted by lower amplitude synapses. Although this model is limited to synaptic strengths, those parameters are sufficient to predict multiple behaviors. Thus, those parameters may serve an important role in the actual circuit (Loeb and Tsianos, 2015).

Finally, we explored the comodulation of PA and PR, because this strategy had shown good results in chinchilla experiments (Davidovics et al., 2012). By incorporating non-zero PAM, any PRM partially accessed the less-attenuated synapses normally solely available to PAM. Adding a PRM component to the stimulation boosts the eye velocity output of a given PAM percentage. One way to think about this is generating larger total eye velocity that is useful for prosthetics. Alternatively, it is important to consider current spread and misalignment of eye-movement responses shown in Figure 4. This is a limiting factor that prevents prosthetic controllers from using high magnitudes of PAM. As amplitude grows too large, the charge spreads to adjacent canals and begins to generate eye velocities along incorrect axes. To avoid this, the model suggests following an equipotent hybrid stimulation contour to find a comodulation that can avoid current spread or user discomfort while maintaining velocity magnitudes.

If more high-quality data become available, it will be valuable to emulate chronic adaptation to vestibular prosthetic use. A chronic model of vestibular prosthetic function is critically missing. Specifically, there are multiple *chronic* animal studies that demonstrate effective control of eye movements using PRM (Gong and Merfeld, 2002; Wall et al., 2003; Della Santina et al., 2007; Merfeld, 2008; Fridman et al., 2010); this was not captured by any possible parameter combination in our *acute* model. Furthermore, prosthetic designers could rapidly scan different stimulation parameter combinations to minimize adaptation time and error, all the way from acute prosthetic onset in the clinic to chronic outside-the-clinic use.

AUTHOR CONTRIBUTIONS

JD designed and implemented the model. JD and TAKN revised the model. TAKN, AP-F, and NG performed the clinical recordings. TAKN and AP-F analyzed the data. All authors conceived aspects of the experiments and analysis. JD and TAKN prepared the figures with the help of the other authors. JD and TAKN wrote the manuscript, and all the authors contributed to its editing. SM and AP-F supervised all aspects of the work.

CONFLICT OF INTEREST STATEMENT

The authors declare that the research was conducted in the absence of any commercial or financial relationships that could be construed as a potential conflict of interest.

FUNDING

This work was funded by the European Commission (FP7 CLONS, Project 225929). Med-El supported TN's salary during the period this manuscript was being written.

REFERENCES

1. Agrawal, Y., Carey, J. P., Della Santina, C. C., Schubert, M. C., and Minor, L. B. (2009). Disorders of balance and vestibular function in US adults: data from the National Health and Nutrition Examination Survey, 2001-2004. *Arch. Intern. Med.* 169, 938–944. doi:10.1001/archinternmed.2009.66
2. Arnold, D., and Robinson, D. (1997). The oculomotor integrator: testing of a neural network model. *Exp. Brain Res.* 113, 57–74. doi:10.1007/BF02454142
3. Baird, R., Desmadryl, G., Fernandez, C., and Goldberg, J. (1988). The vestibular nerve of the chinchilla. II. Relation between afferent response properties and peripheral innervation patterns in the semicircular canals. *J. Neurophysiol.* 60, 182–203.
4. Bi, G.-Q., and Poo, M.-M. (1998). Synaptic modifications in cultured hippocampal neurons: dependence on spike timing, synaptic strength, and postsynaptic cell type. *J. Neurosci.* 18, 10464–10472.
5. Bronte-Stewart, H., and Lisberger, S. G. (1994). Physiological properties of vestibular primary afferents that mediate motor learning and normal performance of the vestibulo-ocular reflex in monkeys. *J. Neurosci.* 14, 1290–1308.
6. Capogrosso, M., Wenger, N., Raspopovic, S., Musienko, P., Beauparlant, J., Luciani, L. B., et al. (2013). A computational model for epidural electrical stimulation of spinal sensorimotor circuits. *J. Neurosci.* 33, 19326–19340. doi:10.1523/JNEUROSCI.1688-13.2013
7. Cullen, K. E., and McCrea, R. A. (1993). Firing behavior of brain stem neurons during voluntary cancellation of the horizontal vestibuloocular reflex. I. Secondary vestibular neurons. *J. Neurophysiol.* 70, 828–843.
8. Davidovics, N., Fridman, G., and Della Santina, C. (2012). Co-modulation of stimulus rate and current from elevated baselines expands head motion encoding range of the vestibular prosthesis. *Exp. Brain Res.* 1–12. doi:10.1007/s00221-012-3025-8
9. Della Santina, C. C., Migliaccio, A. A., and Patel, A. H. (2007). A multichannel semicircular canal neural prosthesis using electrical stimulation to restore 3-D vestibular sensation. *IEEE Trans. Biomed. Eng.* 54, 1016–1030. doi:10.1109/TBME.2007.894629
10. Fernandez, C., and Goldberg, J. M. (1971). Physiology of peripheral neurons innervating semicircular canals of the squirrel monkey. II. Response to sinusoidal stimulation and dynamics of peripheral vestibular system. *J. Neurophysiol.* 34, 661–675.

11. Fridman, G. Y., Davidovics, N. S., Dai, C., Migliaccio, A. A., and Della Santina, C. C. (2010). Vestibulo-ocular reflex responses to a multichannel vestibular prosthesis incorporating a 3D coordinate transformation for correction of misalignment. *J. Assoc. Res. Otolaryngol.* 11, 367–381. doi:10.1007/s10162-010-0208-5

12. Gong, W., and Merfeld, D. M. (2000). Prototype neural semicircular canal prosthesis using patterned electrical stimulation. *Ann. Biomed. Eng.* 28, 572–581. doi:10.1114/1.293

13. Gong, W., and Merfeld, D. M. (2002). System design and performance of an unilateral semicircular canal prosthesis. *IEEE Trans. Biomed. Eng.* 49, 175–181. doi:10.1109/10.979358

14. Grossman, G. E., Leigh, R. J., Bruce, E. N., Huebner, W. P., and Lanska, D. J. (1989). Performance of the human vestibuloocular reflex during locomotion. *J. Neurophysiol.* 62, 264–272.

15. Guinand, N., Boselie, F., Guyot, J.-P., and Kingma, H. (2012). Quality of life of patients with bilateral vestibulopathy. *Ann. Otol. Rhinol. Laryngol.* 121, 471–477. doi:10.1177/000348941212100708

16. Guinand, N., van de Berg, R., Cavuscens, S., Stokroos, R. J., Ranieri, M., Pelizzone, M., et al. (2015). Vestibular implants: 8 years of experience with electrical stimulation of the vestibular nerve in 11 patients with bilateral vestibular loss. *ORL* 77, 227–240. doi:10.1159/000433554

17. Guyot, J.-P., Sigrist, A., Pelizzone, M., Feigl, G. C., and Kos, M. I. (2010). Eye movements in response to electrical stimulation of the lateral and superior ampullary nerves. *Ann. Otol. Rhinol. Laryngol.* 120, 81–87. doi:10.1177/000348941112000202

18. Guyot, J.-P., Sigrist, A., Pelizzone, M., and Kos, M. I. (2011). Adaptation to steady-state electrical stimulation of the vestibular system in the human. *Ann. Otol. Rhinol. Laryngol.* 120, 143–149. doi:10.1177/000348941112000301

19. Haslwanter, T. (1995). Mathematics of three-dimensional eye rotations. *Vision Res.* 35, 1727–1739. doi:10.1016/0042-6989(94)00257-M

20. Haykin, S. (1994). *Neural Networks: A Comprehensive Foundation*. New York, Toronto: Macmillan; Maxwell Macmillan Canada.

21. Hullar, T. E., Della Santina, C. C., Hirvonen, T., Lasker, D. M., Carey, J. P., and Minor, L. B. (2005). Responses of irregularly discharging chinchilla semicircular canal vestibular-nerve afferents during high-frequency head rotations. *J. Neurophysiol.* 93, 2777–2786. doi:10.1152/jn.01002.2004

22. Lewis, R. F. (2015). Advances in the diagnosis and treatment of vestibular disorders: psychophysics and prosthetics. *J. Neurosci.* 35, 5089–5096. doi:10.1523/JNEUROSCI.3922-14.2015

23. Loeb, G. E., and Tsianos, G. A. (2015). Major remaining gaps in models of sensorimotor systems. *Front. Comput. Neurosci.* 9:70. doi:10.3389/fncom.2015.00070

24. Marianelli, P., Capogrosso, M., Bassi Luciani, L., Panarese, A., and Micera, S. (2015). A computational framework for electrical stimulation of vestibular nerve. *IEEE Trans. Neural Syst. Rehabil. Eng.* 23, 897–909. doi:10.1109/TNSRE.2015.2407861

25. Markram, H., Lübke, J., Frotscher, M., and Sakmann, B. (1997). Regulation of synaptic efficacy by coincidence of postsynaptic APs and EPSPs. *Science* 275, 213–215. doi:10.1126/science.275.5297.213

26. McIntyre, C. C., Richardson, A. G., and Grill, W. M. (2002). Modeling the excitability of mammalian nerve fibers: influence of afterpotentials on the recovery cycle. *J. Neurophysiol.* 87, 995–1006.

27. Merfeld, D. M. (2008). "Spatial orientation and the vestibular system," in *Sensation and Perception* (Sunderland, MA: Sinauer Associates, Inc).

28. Merfeld, D. M., Gong, W., Morrissey, J., Saginaw, M., Haburcakova, C., and Lewis, R. F. (2006). Acclimation to chronic constant-rate peripheral stimulation provided by a vestibular prosthesis. *IEEE Trans. Biomed. Eng.* 53, 2362–2372. doi:10.1109/TBME.2006.883645

29. Merfeld, D. M., Haburcakova, C., Gong, W., and Lewis, R. F. (2007). Chronic vestibulo-ocular reflexes evoked by a vestibular prosthesis.*IEEE Trans. Biomed. Eng.* 54, 1005–1015. doi:10.1109/TBME.2007.891943

30. Mitchell, D. E., Della Santina, C. C., and Cullen, K. E. (2014). Plasticity at the vestibular afferent to the central neuron synapse: effects of vestibular prosthetic stimulation. *Soc. Neurosci. Abstr. 157.10. 2014.*

31. Pelizzone, M., Fornos, A. P., Guinand, N., van de Berg, R., Kos, I., Stokroos, R., et al. (2014). First functional rehabilitation via vestibular implants. *Cochlear Implants Int.* 15, S62–S64. doi:10.1179/1467010014Z.000000000165

32. Perez Fornos, A., Guinand, N., Van De Berg, R., Stokroos, R., Micera, S., Kingma, H., et al. (2014). Artificial balance: restoration of the vestibulo-ocular reflex in humans with a prototype vestibular neuroprosthesis. *Front Neurol.* 5:66. doi:10.3389/fneur.2014.00066

33. Purves, D., Augustine, G. J., Fitzpatrick, D., Hall, W. C., LaMantia, A.-S., McNamara, J. O., et al. (eds) (2004). *Neuroscience.* Sunderland, MA: Sinauer Associates, Inc.

34. Sadeghi, S. G., Chacron, M. J., Taylor, M. C., and Cullen, K. E. (2007). Neural variability, detection thresholds, and information transmission in the vestibular system. *J. Neurosci.* 27, 771–781. doi:10.1523/JNEUROSCI.4690-06.2007

35. Sadeghi, S. G., Minor, L. B., and Cullen, K. E. (2011). Multimodal integration after unilateral labyrinthine lesion: single vestibular nuclei neuron responses and implications for postural compensation. *J. Neurophysiol.* 105, 661–673. doi:10.1152/jn.00788.2010

36. Sadeghi, S. G., Mitchell, D. E., and Cullen, K. E. (2009). Different neural strategies for multimodal integration: comparison of two macaque monkey species. *Exp. Brain Res.* 195, 45–57. doi:10.1007/s00221-009-1751-3

37. Sjöström, P. J., Turrigiano, G. G., and Nelson, S. B. (2001). Rate, timing, and cooperativity jointly determine cortical synaptic plasticity. *Neuron* 32, 1149–1164. doi:10.1016/S0896-6273(01)00542-6

38. Sun, D. Q., Ward, B. K., Semenov, Y. R., Carey, J. P., and Della Santina, C. C. (2014). Bilateral vestibular deficiency: quality of life and economic implications. *JAMA Otolaryngol. Head Neck Surg.* 140, 527–534. doi:10.1001/jamaoto.2014.490

39. Suzuki, J.-I., and Cohen, B. (1964). Head, eye, body and limb movements from semicircular canal nerves. *Exp. Neurol.* 10, 393–405. doi:10.1016/0014-4886(64)90031-7

40. Van De Berg, R., Guinand, N., Nguyen, K., Ranieri, M., Cavuscens, S., GUYOT, J. P., et al. (2015). The vestibular implant: frequency-dependency of the electrically evoked vestibulo-ocular reflex in humans. *Front. Syst. Neurosci.* 8:255. doi:10.3389/fnsys.2014.00255

41. Van De Berg, R., Guinand, N., Stokroos, R. J., Guyot, J.-P., and Kingma, H. (2011). The vestibular implant: quo vadis? *Front. Neurol.*2:47. doi:10.3389/fneur.2011.00047

42. Wall, C., Merfeld, D. M., Rauch, S. D., and Black, F. O. (2003). Vestibular prostheses: the engineering and biomedical issues. *J. Vestib. Res.* 12, 95–113.

43. Zingler, V. C., Cnyrim, C., Jahn, K., Weintz, E., Fernbacher, J., Frenzel, C., et al. (2007). Causative factors and epidemiology of bilateral vestibulopathy in 255 patients. *Ann. Neurol.* 61, 524–532. doi:10.1002/ana.21105

10
CHAPTER

ULTRASOUND GUIDED DOUBLE INJECTION OF BLOOD INTO CISTERNA MAGNA: A RABBIT MODEL FOR TREATMENT OF CEREBRAL VASOSPASM

Yongchao Chen, Youzhi Zhu, Yu Zhang, Zixuan Zhang, Juan Lian, Fucheng Luo, Xuefei Deng and Kelvin KL Wong

Keywords: Cerebral vasospasm, Double injection of blood into cisterna magna, Animal model, Ultrasound guided puncture

BACKGROUND

Despite the advances in diagnosis and treatment of subarachnoid hemorrhage, effective therapeutic interventions are still limited and clinical outcomes remain disappointing [1]. There is substantial evidence that delayed cerebral vasospasm contributes to the significant mortality and morbidity rates following subarachnoid hemorrhage [1, 2, 3, 4, 5, 6, 7, 8, 9]. Cerebral vasospasm can lead to cerebral hypoperfusion, culminating in delayed ischemic neurological deficit, which has been considered a major cause of high mortality and poor outcome. In the last several decades, many researchers have been primarily focused on vasospasm and its sequelae [1, 2, 3, 4, 5, 6, 7, 8, 9, 10, 11, 12, 13, 14, 15, 16]. However, the success rate with regard to improved outcome is also limited [1]. For a better understanding of the pathogenic mechanism of cerebral vasospasm and to develop efficacious therapeutic strategies, many animal models have been stimulated [17, 18, 19, 20].

Choosing an appropriate animal model is a critical step in the productive cerebral vasospasm research [21]. Primates may be the most preferred species, as the time course of delayed cerebral vasospasm is similar to that observed in humans and the

Citation: Yongchao Chen, Youzhi Zhu, Yu Zhang, Zixuan Zhang, Juan Lian, Fucheng Luo, Xuefei Deng and Kelvin KL Wong, Ultrasound guided double injection of blood into cisterna magna: a rabbit model for treatment of cerebral vasospasm, DOI: 10.1186/s12938-016-0123-z.

angiography is relatively easy to perform [20]. However, drawbacks with these species include high costs, limited availability, and difficulties in inducing subarachnoid hemorrhage. Canines are another suitable species, especially when used in the molecular biology research [22]. However, the canines are too small and the angiography is hard to perform. Therefore, rabbits are the alternative species of choice, as they offer many advantages [22, 23, 24, 25, 26]. First, the time course of cerebral vasospasm shows a biphasic pattern of early and delayed vasospasm as found in humans. Second, the morphological changes in arteries and ventricles observed in rabbit models are similar to those observed in humans. Third, rabbit models are available in larger numbers with relatively low costs, and intubation and respiratory support are not required in anesthesia. Finally, rabbits are relatively easy to restrain when using an appropriate restraining device, given their relatively docile nature.

In the 1980s, rabbits emerged as a new species in delayed cerebral vasospasm research. Since Liszczak et al. presented models of blood injection into cisterna magna [27], this technique became the standard for subarachnoid hemorrhage induction in rabbits. It can generate a pathologic condition similar to that seen after the rupture of an intracranial aneurysm and it is easy to perform with a high success rate. The frequency of blood injection ranges from 1 to 3 times. Double injection method induces a more severe and prolonged vasospasm than single injection method, and is well established in dog and rat models [17, 19, 20, 22]. In rabbits, double injection method reportedly produces a vasospasm that is more severe and persistent. The vasospasm peaks approximately 5 days after first injection and persists for up to the next 2 days [21]. However, due to the unacceptably high mortality rate, reported by Baker et al. (41 %) [28], Spallone and Pastore (20 %) [29], double injection method is not popular in rabbit models.

Deaths of animal occurring during the procedure are mainly caused by a failure to the brainstem needling or intraparenchymal blood injection [26]. Various methods have been used to avoid puncture failure such as having an appropriate posture, not evacuating too much cerebrospinal fluid, directing the needle slightly rostrally [25, 26]. However, deaths of animal were inevitable as the cisterna magna is small and the location of needle tip cannot be confirmed. Moreover, double injection method tends to increase the risk of death [25]. Ultrasound guided puncture is a widely used interventional technique in the clinic, which provides real-time imaging guidance for all kinds of puncture [30, 31, 32, 33, 34, 35, 36]. The present study was designed to use ultrasound guided puncture in the establishment of cerebral vasospasm model so as to provide a safe and effective rabbit model of cerebral vasospasm after subarachnoid hemorrhage.

METHODS

Experimental animal grouping and development of subarachnoid hemorrhage model

This study was approved by the Ethics Committee of Anhui Medical University (Hefei,

China, 2012238). All animal use and care protocols including the operation procedures were carried out in strict accordance with the recommendation in Guide for the Care and Use of Laboratory Animals of the National Institutes of Health.

A total of 160 adult male New Zealand white rabbits that weigh from 2.5 to 3.2 kg were supplied by the experimental animal center of Anhui Medical University. All rabbits were randomly divided into four groups of 40 each: (1) manual control group, (2) manual model group, (3) ultrasound guided control group, and (4) ultrasound guided model group. We established and detailed the groups as follows:

Manual model group. After rabbits were fixed on the operating table, they were anesthetized using 3 % sodium pentobarbital (1 ml/kg) after an intravenous injection through auricular vein. The occipital hair was shaved, and the skin was sterilized with 75 % alcohol. A 5 ml-syringe with a 22-gauge needle was inserted into cisterna magna through atlano-occipital fascia (Fig. 1). Once the dura mater was perforated, a small amount of cerebrospinal fluid (about 0.4 ml/kg) was removed. The autologous non-heparinized fresh auricular arterial blood (about 0.6 ml/kg) was injected into cisterna magna slowly. The rabbits were kept in head-down position for 30 min, whereby the blood would distribute into other subarachnoid spaces with cerebrospinal fluid circulation. The second injection was accomplished 48 h after the first injection, and 0.4 ml/kg blood was injected into cisterna magna using the same procedure as first injection.

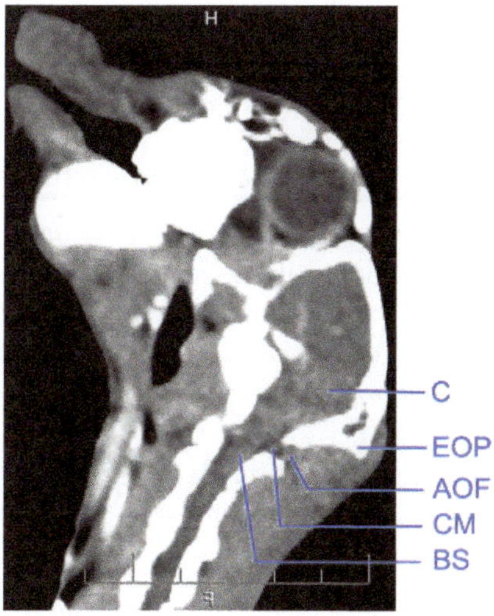

Figure 1: Cisterna magna and atlano-occipital fascia in CT sagittal image. *C* cerebellum, *EOP* external occipital protuberance,*AOF* atlano-occipital fascia, *CM* cisterna magna, *BS* brain stem.

Manual control group. All the procedures were the same as model group, except normal saline was used instead of autologous blood.

Ultrasound guided model group. Before puncture, the depth of cisterna magna was measured by ultrasound. The best puncture direction was designed according to the relationship between atlano-occipital fascia and the deepest part of cisterna magna (Fig.

2). If the cisterna magna was found to be too small (the depth was less than 0.23 cm, which is the length of inclined plane of needle tip), the amount of autologous blood injected into cisterna magna would be decreased. Guided by ultrasound, the needle was inserted into cisterna magna. Other procedures remained the same as manual model group.

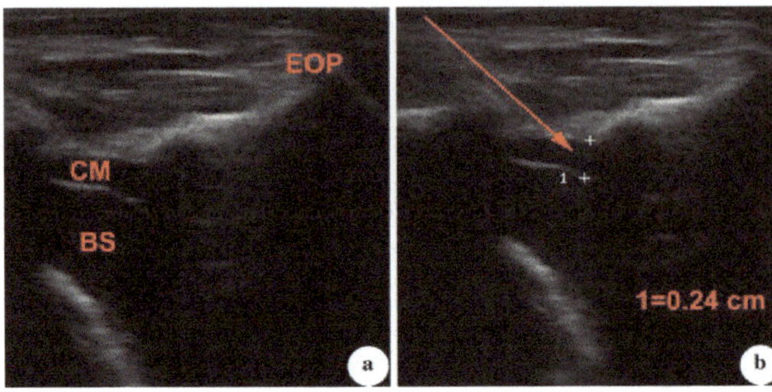

Figure 2: Measurement and observation of cisterna magna that is guided by ultrasound. **a** Cisterna magna and adjacent structures were displayed by ultrasound. **b** Depth of cisterna magna was measured at its optimal part. The puncture direction was designed based on the *line* from atlano-occipital fascia to the deepest part of cisterna magna. *CM* cisterna magna, *BS* brain stem, *EOP* external occipital protuberance.

Ultrasound guided control group. All the procedures were the same as model group except that normal saline was used instead of autologous blood.

Observation of the rabbit subarachnoid hemorrhage model under CT

The rabbits underwent CT scanning 1 day after modeling, to determine whether there was blood in the subarachnoid space. All CT images were obtained using a 16-MDCT unit (Siemens Healthcare). The scanning parameters were as follows: 80 kV, 100 mA, 1.25-mm section thickness, 1-mm intersection gap, 0.7 cm/s table speed, 9.6-cm FOV, and 512 × 512 matrix.

Observation of cerebral vasospasm with magnetic resonance angiography

Next, the rabbits underwent MR scanning before modeling and 5 days after modeling, to determine whether cerebral vasospasm occurred. MR scanning was performed with a 3.0 T MR unit (Siemens Healthcare) using a knee joint coil. After a T2-weighted sequence with a TR/TE of 2000/96 ms was performed to display the loose connective tissue, the time of flight magnetic resonance angiography (TOF-MRA) was performed to display cerebral artery. The scanning parameters were as follows: 256 × 256 matrix, 0.5-mm section thickness, 11-cm FOV, TR 25 ms, and TE 5.72 ms. The data were translated to post-processing workstation after scanning. The basilar artery diameters were measured by two radiologists independently, and their mean values were calculated.

The vasospasm severity was calculated based on the basilar artery diameters before modeling and 5 days after modeling. The calculation formula was modified from Laslo et al. [37] in Eq. (1) as follows:

$$\text{Vasospasm severity} = (BA_0 - BA_5) \times 100\% / BA_0 \tag{1}$$

In this formula, BA_0 represents the basilar artery diameter before modeling, while BA_5 represents the basilar artery diameter 5 days after modeling in the same rabbit.

Statistical analysis

All the statistical analyses were performed with SPSS software for Windows, and are presented as the mean ± standard deviation (SD). Statistical comparisons of the basilar artery diameter before and after modeling were made using paired *t* test. Statistical comparisons of the mortality rate and the vasospasm severity were made using Chi square test. Here, $P < 0.05$ was considered to indicate a significant difference.

RESULTS

Operation based on ultrasound guided puncture

The cisterna magna was a dilated subarachnoid space between cerebellum and medulla oblongata (Fig. 3). Before the puncture procedure, the cisterna magna, brain stem and external occipital protuberance were displayed by ultrasound. The depth of the cisterna magna was (0.42 ± 0.06) cm (Fig. 2). According the line from atlano-occipital fascia to the deepest part of cisterna magna, the best puncture direction was designed. The angle between puncture needle and vertical line was (56 ± 11)°, while the depth of puncture was (2.38 ± 0.81) cm (Fig. 3).

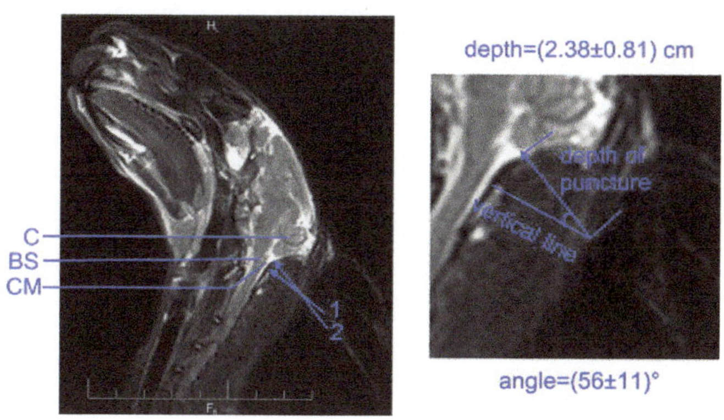

Figure 3: Illustration of puncture direction in MR sagittal image. *C* cerebellum, *CM* cisterna magna, *BS* brain stem, *Arrow 1* puncture direction in manual model group (*vertical line*), *Arrow 2* puncture direction in ultrasound guided model group.

During ultrasound guided puncture procedure, the whole process of the needle entering into cisterna magna was observed directly. The depth of needle tip entering into cisterna magna and the distance between tip and brain stem were controlled by operator (Fig. 4a). When blood was injected into cisterna magna, the signal of flow blood was monitored by ultrasound (Fig. 4b). At 1 day after modeling, the blood was observed in subarachnoid space in CT images (Fig. 4c), which illustrated that the injection was successful.

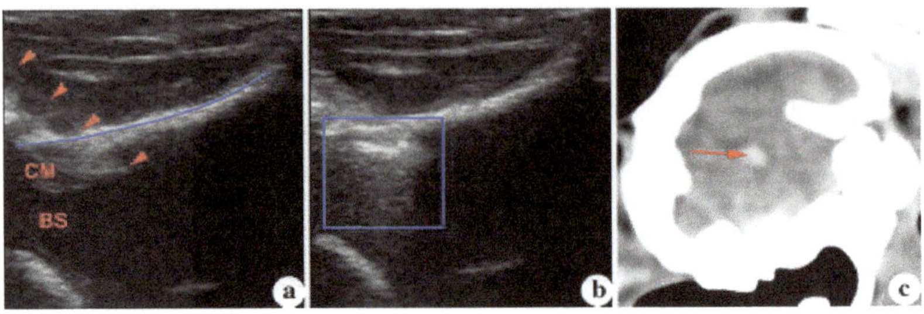

Figure 4: Ultrasound guided puncture procedure. a Needle was showed in the puncture procedure. b When blood was injected, the signal of flow blood was monitored by ultrasound, and boundary between cisterna magna and brain stem was disturbed by the high signal. c Blood in subarachnoid space at 1 day after modeling. *CM* cisterna magna,*BS* brain stem, *Blue line* dura mater, *Red arrowhead* puncture needle, *Blue block* blood signal, *Red arrow* blood in subarachnoid space.

Safety considerations of puncture

For the manual control group (40 rabbits), six rabbits died within 30 min after puncture. Two died in the first puncture, while the other four died during the second puncture. The mortality rate in manual control group was 15 %. For the manual model group (40 rabbits), nine rabbits died within 30 min after puncture, while six rabbits died during the second puncture. The mortality rate in manual model group was 23 %. There was no statistical difference between the mortality rate of manual control group and manual model group ($x^2 = 0.738, P = 0.390$).

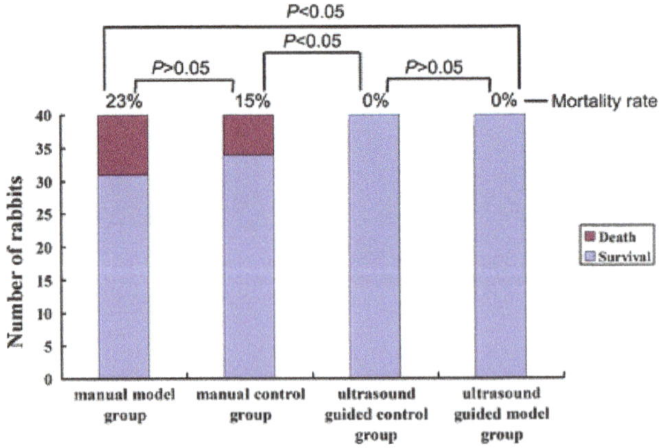

Figure 5: Comparison of mortality rates among four groups.

There were no deaths among all 80 rabbits in ultrasound guided control group and model group. Compared with manual model group, the mortality rate in ultrasound guided model group was significantly lower (x^2 = 10.141. P = 0.002). The same difference was observed between manual control group and ultrasound guided control group (x^2 = 6.486. P = 0.026). Comparison of the mortality rates between all four groups was shown in Fig. 5.

Effectiveness of rabbit cerebral vasospasm model

In both the manual and ultrasound guided control groups, there were no statistical differences in basilar artery diameter between the day before and after modeling. Before modeling, the basilar artery diameter in manual model group was (0.66 ± 0.05) mm, while the diameter was (0.67 ± 0.06) mm in ultrasound guided model group. Five days after modeling, the diameter changed to (0.49 ± 0.13) and (0.36 ± 0.02) mm in manual model group and ultrasound guided model group, respectively. Compared with the diameter before modeling, the basilar artery was significantly narrower after modeling, in both the manual and ultrasound guided model groups. However, the change in ultrasound model group was larger than that in manual guided model group (Figs. 6 and 7).

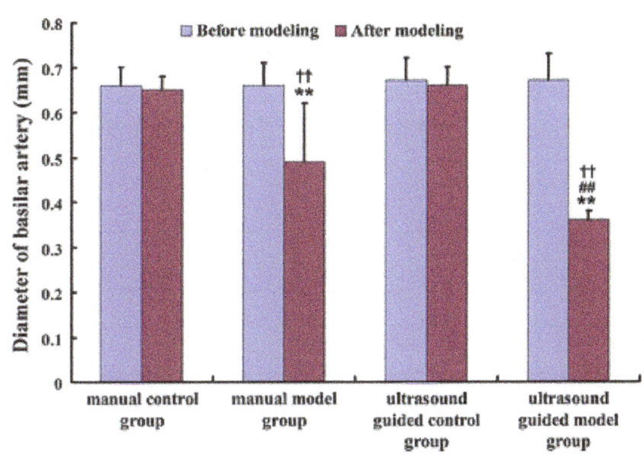

Figure 6: Comparison of basilar artery diameter among four groups. **Compare with the diameter before modeling,$P < 0.05$. ##Compare with the diameter in the manual group, $P < 0.05$. ††Compare with the diameter in the control group, $P < 0.05$.

After calculating the vasospasm severity, the mean severity in manual model group and ultrasound guided model group was 26 and 46 %, respectively. The proportions of the severe (≥30 %), moderate (20 ~ 29 %), mild (10 ~ 19 %) and little (<10 %) were shown in Table 1. The proportion of severe vasospasms was more in ultrasound guided group than that of manual group (x^2 = 12.917, P = 0.001). In the ultrasound guided group, the depth of cisterna magna in two rabbits was 0.22 and 0.20 cm, respectively. The cisterna magna was too small and not enough blood was injected, and the vasospasm severity was 14 and 16 %, respectively, while in other rabbits, the severity was higher than 30 %. In the manual group, no obvious vasospasm was found in three (8 %) rabbits, which indicates the failure of model's establishment (Table 1).

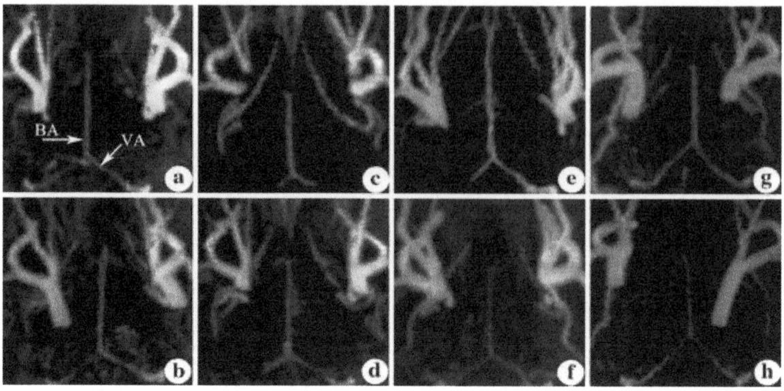

Figure 7: Observation of basilar artery in MRA before and after modeling. a, b Manual control group. c, d Ultrasound guided control group. e, f Manual model group. g, h ultrasound guided model group. a, c, e, g Before modeling. b, d, f, h5 days after modeling. *BA* basilar artery, *VA* vertebral artery.

Table 1: Vasospasm severity of basilar artery before and after modeling (number/ %)

Severity of vasospasm	Manual puncture		Ultrasound guided puncture	
	Control group	Model group	Control group	Model group
Severe (≥30 %)	0/0	26/65	0/0	38/95
Moderate (20 ~ 29 %)	0/0	7/18	0/0	0/0
Mild (10 ~ 19 %)	0/0	4/10	0/0	2/5
Small (<10 %)	40/100	3/8	40/100	0/0

DISCUSSION

There are two basic requirements in the establishment of cerebral vasospasm model: one is subarachnoid hemorrhage, and the other is sufficient stimulation of blood. The methods are varied for different subarachnoid hemorrhage models, they are usually as follows [38]: (1) Let the blood coagulate around the blood vessels by pricking intracranial arteries. (2) After surgical exposure of the experimental arteries, the blood from other parts of the body is injected around the vessels. (3) Autologous blood is injected into cerebral cistern, ventricle or subarachnoid space percutaneously, and the blood coagulates around blood vessels with the flow of cerebrospinal fluid. These three methods have their inherent advantages and disadvantages. The former two methods have many disadvantages such as their associated major trauma and high mortality rates. Double injections of blood into cisterna magna allow high-precision control of injection volume, velocity and time. Due to its low mortality rate, this method has good repeatability, which is suitable for single factor analysis under the stable conditions. Due to the importance of pathogenesis of cerebral vasospasm, double injections of blood into cisterna magna were used to establish the cerebral vasospasm model successfully in rats [39, 40], rabbits [25, 26] and dogs [22].

In the process of establishing cerebral vasospasm model, the death of experimental animals seems inevitable in traditional double injections of blood into cisterna magna. This study showed that even when the blood injected into cisterna magna was replaced with normal saline (manual control group), 15 % of the New Zealand rabbits died during the puncture procedure. The mortality rate was slight higher (23 %) in manual model group. However, no significant difference was found between the manual control and model groups, which indicates that the death of rabbits was caused by the puncture procedure itself, not the blood. The cisterna magna is located behind brain stem. Thus, it is easy to damage the vital center inside brain stem, as the entry depth of needle tip is hard to control in the puncture. The rabbits may die as a result of respiratory arrest. In ultrasound guided puncture procedure, the cisterna magna was found to be too small in two rabbits. Because the depth of cisterna magna was less than the length of inclined plane of needle tip, the brain stem would be damaged in traditional manual model group.

Considering the safety of puncture process, a new technology that can monitor entire puncture process is needed to reduce the mortality rate of rabbits. This study modified puncture technology combined with an interventional ultrasound technique. With ultrasound guidance, the cisterna magna, brain stem and external occipital protuberance were displayed. The brain stem remained undamaged because the depth of needle tip entering into cisterna magna was controlled by the operator. To ensure the safety of puncture process, the best puncture direction was designed according the relationship between atlano-occipital fascia and the deepest part of cisterna magna. As the inclined course in cisterna magna increased the activities of needle tip, the tip would not be able to touch brain stem. Before operation, the angle and the depth of puncture can be detected and calculated by ultrasound. The angle was (56 ± 11) degree, while the depth was (2.38 ± 0.81) cm. These data vary in different rabbits and therefore, a uniform puncture scheme is not sufficient for injection of blood into cisterna magna. With ultrasound guidance, no deaths occurred in 80 cases of New Zealand rabbits and the mortality rate was significantly lower than manual group, which confirmed the safety of this new puncture technology.

The next problem to solve is the validity of model pertaining to whether cerebral vasospasm occurs. Cerebral vasospasm is easier to occur as there are two stimulations in double injections of blood into cisterna magna. In this study, no obvious vasospasm was found in three rabbits in the manual group (8 %), which indicated the failure of model's establishment. In the ultrasound guided control group, cerebral vasospasm occurred in all experimental animals 5 days after modeling, and the proportion of severe vasospasm was as high as 95 %, which was more than that of manual group (65 %).

Two questions should be considered in ultrasound real-time observation. First, the cisterna magna was too small in 5 % of the rabbits. Insufficient blood was injected to prevent intracranial hypertension. In these rabbits, mild vasospasm was found in MRA images 5 days after modeling. This study suggests that the operator should give up modeling when they find a small cisterna magna. Second, in most of second punctures, adhesion was found near the cisterna magna. It is hard to feel the perforation of dura mater when the needles enter into cisterna magna. If traditional manual puncture were selected, the operator may choose a shallow needle, to prevent damage of brain stem. No blood enters into cisterna magna leading the lack of second stimulation of vessels, reducing the incidence of cerebral vasospasm. This may be the most important reason for the lack of vasospasm in 8 % of rabbits in manual model group.

CONCLUSIONS

In summary, the ultrasound guided double injection of blood into cisterna magna not only has a low animal mortality rate, but it also ensures the occurrence of cerebral vasospasm. This method should be further popularized and applied as a safe and effective rabbit model of cerebral vasospasm.

DECLARATIONS

Authors' contributions

YCC contributed to the experimental design, analysis and interpretation of data. YZZ and YZ participated in acquisition of the CT and MR data. ZXZ, JL and FCL carried out part of the experiments and of the statistical analysis. XFD was involved in all aspects of study conception, design, analysis and interpretation and provided final approval of the version of the submitted manuscript. KKLW participated in the design of the study and helped draft and revise the manuscript. All authors read and approved the final manuscript.

Acknowledgements

The project was funded by the National Natural Science Foundation of China (Reference No: 81200895) and the Medical and Health Foundation of Nanjing Military Area (Reference No: 12z12).

REFERENCES

1. Ciurea AV, Palade C, Voinescu D, Nica DA. Subarachnoid hemorrhage and cerebral vasospasm—literature review. J Med Life. 2013;6(2):120–5.
2. Dabus G, Nogueira RG. Current options for the management of aneurysmal subarachnoid hemorrhage-induced cerebral vasospasm: a comprehensive review of the literature. Interv Neurol. 2013;2(1):30–51. doi:10.1159/000354755.
3. Bar B, MacKenzie L, Hurst RW, Grant R, Weigele J, Bhalla PK, et al. Hyperacute vasospasm after aneurysmal subarachnoid hemorrhage. Neurocrit Care. 2015. doi:10.1007/s12028-015-0177-y.
4. Przybycien-Szymanska MM, Ashley WW Jr. Biomarker discovery in cerebral vasospasm after aneurysmal subarachnoid hemorrhage. J Stroke Cerebrovasc Dis Off J Natl Stroke Assoc. 2015;24(7):1453–64. doi:10.1016/j.jstrokecerebrovasdis.2015.03.047.

5. Dusick JR, Gonzalez NR. Management of arterial vasospasm following aneurysmal subarachnoid hemorrhage. Semin Neurol. 2013;33(5):488–97. doi:10.1055/s-0033-1364216.

6. Izzy S, Muehlschlegel S. Cerebral vasospasm after aneurysmal subarachnoid hemorrhage and traumatic brain injury. Curr Treat Options Neurol. 2014;16(1):278. doi:10.1007/s11940-013-0278-x.

7. Gross BA, Lin N, Frerichs KU, Du R. Vasospasm after spontaneous angiographically negative subarachnoid hemorrhage. Acta Neurochir (Wien). 2012;154(7):1127–33. doi:10.1007/s00701-012-1383-4.

8. Velat GJ, Kimball MM, Mocco JD, Hoh BL. Vasospasm after aneurysmal subarachnoid hemorrhage: review of randomized controlled trials and meta-analyses in the literature. World Neurosurg. 2011;76(5):446–54. doi:10.1016/j.wneu.2011.02.030.

9. Pluta RM, Hansen-Schwartz J, Dreier J, Vajkoczy P, Macdonald RL, Nishizawa S, et al. Cerebral vasospasm following subarachnoid hemorrhage: time for a new world of thought. Neurol Res. 2009;31(2):151–8. doi:10.1179/174313209x393564.

10. Brathwaite S, Macdonald RL. Current management of delayed cerebral ischemia: update from results of recent clinical trials. Transl Stroke Res. 2014;5(2):207–26. doi:10.1007/s12975-013-0316-8.

11. Budohoski KP, Guilfoyle M, Helmy A, Huuskonen T, Czosnyka M, Kirollos R, et al. The pathophysiology and treatment of delayed cerebral ischaemia following subarachnoid haemorrhage. J Neurol Neurosurg Psychiatry. 2014;85(12):1343–53. doi:10.1136/jnnp-2014-307711.

12. Rowland MJ, Hadjipavlou G, Kelly M, Westbrook J, Pattinson KT. Delayed cerebral ischaemia after subarachnoid haemorrhage: looking beyond vasospasm. Br J Anaesth. 2012;109(3):315–29. doi:10.1093/bja/aes264.

13. Mortimer AM, Steinfort B, Faulder K, Harrington T. Delayed infarction following aneurysmal subarachnoid hemorrhage: can the role of severe angiographic vasospasm really be dismissed? J Neurointerv Surg. 2015. doi:10.1136/neurintsurg-2015-011854.

14. Brown RJ, Kumar A, Dhar R, Sampson TR, Diringer MN. The relationship between delayed infarcts and angiographic vasospasm after aneurysmal subarachnoid hemorrhage. Neurosurgery. 2013;72(5):702–7. doi:10.1227/NEU.0b013e318285c3db

15. Caner B, Hou J, Altay O, Fujii M, Zhang JH. Transition of research focus from vasospasm to early brain injury after subarachnoid hemorrhage. J Neurochem. 2012;123(Suppl 2):12–21. doi:10.1111/j.1471-4159.2012.07939.x.

16. Crowley RW, Medel R, Dumont AS, Ilodigwe D, Kassell NF, Mayer SA, et al. Angiographic vasospasm is strongly correlated with cerebral infarction after subarachnoid hemorrhage. Stroke J Cerebral Circ. 2011;42(4):919–23. doi:10.1161/strokeaha.110.597005.

17. Dudhani RV, Kyle M, Dedeo C, Riordan M, Deshaies EM. A low mortality rat

model to assess delayed cerebral vasospasm after experimental subarachnoid hemorrhage. J Vis Exp JoVE. 2013;71:e4157. doi:10.3791/4157.

18. Marbacher S, Fandino J, Kitchen N. Characteristics of in vivo animal models of delayed cerebral vasospasm. Acta Neurochir Suppl. 2011;110(Pt 1):173–5. doi:10.1007/978-3-7091-0353-1_30.

19. Marbacher S, Fandino J, Kitchen ND. Standard intracranial in vivo animal models of delayed cerebral vasospasm. Br J Neurosurg. 2010;24(4):415–34. doi:10.3109/02688691003746274.

20. Megyesi JF, Vollrath B, Cook DA, Findlay JM. In vivo animal models of cerebral vasospasm: a review. Neurosurgery. 2000;46(2):448–60

21. Zhou ML, Shi JX, Zhu JQ, Hang CH, Mao L, Chen KF, et al. Comparison between one- and two-hemorrhage models of cerebral vasospasm in rabbits. J Neurosci Methods. 2007;159(2):318–24. doi:10.1016/j.jneumeth.2006.07.026.

22. Mori K. Double cisterna magna blood injection model of experimental subarachnoid hemorrhage in dogs. Transl Stroke Res. 2014;5(6):647–52. doi:10.1007/s12975-014-0356-8.

23. Raslan F, Albert-Weissenberger C, Westermaier T, Saker S, Kleinschnitz C, Lee JY. A modified double injection model of cisterna magna for the study of delayed cerebral vasospasm following subarachnoid hemorrhage in rats. Exp Transl Stroke Med. 2012;4(1):23. doi:10.1186/2040-7378-4-23.

24. Guresir E, Schuss P, Borger V, Vatter H. Experimental subarachnoid hemorrhage: double cisterna magna injection rat model–assessment of delayed pathological effects of cerebral vasospasm. Transl Stroke Res. 2015;6(3):242–51. doi:10.1007/s12975-015-0392-z.

25. Kikkawa Y. A rabbit cisterna magna double-injection subarachnoid hemorrhage model. Acta Neurochir Suppl. 2015;120:331–5. doi:10.1007/978-3-319-04981-6_57.

26. Kikkawa Y, Kurogi R, Sasaki T. The single and double blood injection rabbit subarachnoid hemorrhage model. Transl Stroke Res. 2015;6(1):88–97. doi:10.1007/s12975-014-0375-5.

27. Liszczak TM, Black PM, Tzouras A, Foley L, Zervas NT. Morphological changes of the basilar artery, ventricles, and choroid plexus after experimental SAH. J Neurosurg. 1984;61(3):486–93. doi:10.3171/jns.1984.61.3.0486.

28. Baker KF, Zervas NT, Pile-Spellman J, Vacanti FX, Miller D. Angiographic evidence of basilar artery constriction in the rabbit: a new model of vasospasm. Surg Neurol. 1987;27(2):107–12.

29. Spallone A, Pastore FS. Cerebral vasospasm in a double-injection model in rabbit. Surg Neurol. 1989;32(6):408–17.

30. Zhong X, Hamill M, Collier B, Bradburn E, Ferrara J. Dynamic multiplanar real time ultrasound guided infraclavicular subclavian vein catheterization. Am Surg. 2015;81(6):621–5.

31. Chacko J, Gagan B, Kumar U, Mundlapudi B. Real-time ultrasound guided

percutaneous dilatational tracheostomy with and without bronchoscopic control: an observational study. Minerva Anestesiol. 2015;81(2):166–74.

32. Sadahiro H, Nomura S, Goto H, Sugimoto K, Inamura A, Fujiyama Y, et al. Real-time ultrasound-guided endoscopic surgery for putaminal hemorrhage. J Neurosurg. 2015. doi:10.3171/2014.11.jns141508.

33. Menace C, Choquet O, Abbal B, Morau D, Biboulet P, Bringuier S, et al. Real-time ultrasound-guided epidural anaesthesia technique can be improved by new echogenic Tuohy needles: a pilot study in cadavers. Br J Anaesth. 2014;113(2):299–301. doi:10.1093/bja/aeu247.

34. Sobolev M, Slovut DP, Lee Chang A, Shiloh AL, Eisen LA. Ultrasound-guided catheterization of the femoral artery: a systematic review and meta-analysis of randomized controlled trials. J Invasive Cardiol. 2015;27(7):318–23.

35. Stolz LA, Stolz U, Howe C, Farrell IJ, Adhikari S. Ultrasound-guided peripheral venous access: a meta-analysis and systematic review. J Vasc Access. 2015;16(4):321–6. doi:10.5301/jva.5000346.

36. Tan LA, Lopes DK, Fontes RB. Ultrasound-guided posterolateral approach for midline calcified thoracic disc herniation. J Korean Neurosurg Soc. 2014;55(6):383–6. doi:10.3340/jkns.2014.55.6.383.

37. Laslo AM, Eastwood JD, Pakkiri P, Chen F, Lee TY. CT perfusion-derived mean transit time predicts early mortality and delayed vasospasm after experimental subarachnoid hemorrhage. AJNR Am J Neuroradiol. 2008;29(1):79–85. doi:10.3174/ajnr.A0747.

38. Zhou Y, Martin RD, Zhang JH. Advances in experimental subarachnoid hemorrhage. Acta Neurochir Suppl. 2011;110(Pt 1):15–21. doi:10.1007/978-3-7091-0353-1_3.

39. Guresir E, Schuss P, Borger V, Vatter H. Experimental subarachnoid hemorrhage: double cisterna magna injection rat model-assessment of delayed pathological effects of cerebral vasospasm. Transl Stroke Res. 2015;6(3):242–51. doi:10.1007/s12975-015-0392-z.

40. Hu N, Wu Y, Chen BZ, Han JF, Zhou MT. Protective effect of stellate ganglion block on delayed cerebral vasospasm in an experimental rat model of subarachnoid hemorrhage. Brain Res. 2014;1585:63–71. doi:10.1016/j.brainres.2014.08.012.

11
CHAPTER

DYNAMIC EXPRESSIONS OF MONOCYTE CHEMO ATTRACTANT PROTEIN-1 AND CC CHAMOMILE RECEPTOR 2 AFTER BALLOON INJURY AND THEIR EFFECTS IN INTIMAL PROLIFERATION

Zhigang Huang, Yuebing Li, Lili Niu, Yang Xiao, Xiaodong Pu, Hairong Zheng and Ming Qian

Keywords: Balloon injury, Intima proliferation, Monocyte chemoattractant protein-1, CC chemokine receptor 2

INTRODUCTION

Ever since percutaneous transluminal coronary angioplasty (PTCA) was performed by the Swiss physician, Gruentzig [1] in 1977, it has been proven to have many advantages such as resulting in small trauma, ease of implementation, ability to relieve symptoms, and is rapid and reliable [2,3]. As such, it rapidly popularize and partially replace coronary artery bypass graft (CABG), and now it has become one of the more simple and effective methods, which are used to treat cardiovascular disease. But many clinical researchers find that acute coronary occlusion and restenosis easily occur after PTCA and the rate of restenosis is as high as 30% to 50%, which affect its long-term effect and clinical application [4]. From 1987 till now, stent placement, which is regarded as a new technology, is used in clinic all the time. Based on the supporting role of stents, it can significantly prevent and treat vascular remodeling which is caused by vascular elastic recoil and can effectively reduce the incidence of restenosis after PTCA [5].

Citation: Zhigang Huang, Yuebing Li, Lili Niu, Yang Xiao, Xiaodong Pu, Hairong Zheng and Ming Qian, Dynamic expressions of monocyte chemo attractant protein-1 and CC chamomile receptor 2 after balloon injury and their effects in intimal proliferation, DOI: 10.1186/s12938-015-0030-8.

Restenosis refers to a repair response that occurs after local vascular injury. Restenosis is reconstruction and remodeling of partial vascular that is mediated by a variety of cytokines and growth factors; it is caused by the migration, proliferation and apoptosis of vascular smooth muscle cells (VSMC) and secretion and accumulation of extracellular matrix (ECM). It is also responsible for the changes of structures and functions of vascular wall, which are caused by abnormal expressions of a series of genes [6]. The gold standards of diagnosis of restenosis are coronary angiography and ultrasound inspection in coronary arteries. When loss of diameter of lumen is more than 50% after coronary dilatation, it related to restenosis occurrence in vessels [7,8].

In simple angioplasty of balloon expansion, the mechanism of restenosis mainly may be vascular elastic recoil in early stage, proliferation of VSMC and secretion of ECM in metaphase and tardive and contractile vascular remodeling, which is caused by repair of damaged vessels in advanced stage. But the occurrence of restenosis after stent placement is mainly related with proliferation of VSMC and secretion of ECM.

There are injuries and exfoliation of endotheliums in each PTCA. Injuries of endothelium are the initial factors of the occurrence of restenosis [9,10]. In recent years, large numbers of studies have proved that inflammatory response is a key part of the occurrences and developments of many cardiovascular diseases. Many cytokines take part in inflammatory response and constitute complex networks of cytokines. Some inflammatory markers may be predictive factors of cardiovascular diseases, among the markers, MCP-1 plays a significant role in inflammatory cells, especially in the chemoattractant and activation of monocytes in inflammatory responses of cardiovascular diseases [11-13].

In this experiment, we used model of balloon injury of rats to observe expressions of monocyte chemoattractant protein-1 (MCP-1), CC chemokine receptor 2 (CCR2) and MCP-1 proteins at different times after balloon injury. The purpose of the experiment is investigating their possible roles in intimal hyperplasia.

MATERIALS AND METHODS

Instruments and reagents

A number of instruments and reagents were used, including Super-clean Bench (SuJing VS-1300 V), Gel Imaging Instrument (PHARMACIA UDS-CL), Analytic Apparatus of Protein and Nucleic Acid (BECKMAN DU640), PCR Instrument (Eppendorf-personal, Gradient), Low-temperature and High-speed Centrifuge (Heraeus-Biofuge), Balloon Catheter (Cordis 2.0 × 15 mm), Pressure Pump (Cordis), Electrophoresis Apparatus, Cryopreservation Refrigerator (from MDF392 Sanyang Company), Microscope (Olympus), Ultraviolet Spectrophotometer (Shanghai Analysis Instrument Factory Type 751-GW), TRIZOL (Invitrogen), Reverse Transcription Kit (Promega A3500), PCR Reagents (Takara Company), Immune Tissue Staining Kit, and Elastic Fiber Staining Kit.

Animal specimens

Forty-eight rats were used in this study. The rats were provided by Shanghai Animal Center Laboratory of China Medical Sciences Academy. The rats' weights ranged from 350 to 450 grams, with an average age of 12 to 14 weeks. These rats were divided randomly into six groups, and formed one sham group and five balloon injury groups. The sham group consists of 8 rats and the balloon injury group was evenly divided into 5 subgroups, which were respectively named as 1st day group, 4th day group, 7th day group, 14th day group, 28th day group.

Production of animal model and drawing materials

Rats were raised and used in the Animal Laboratory of Peking University Shenzhen Hospital. Two rats were placed into each cage which were considered as one group, then put all cages into laminar flow rack which was placed in the room whose temperature was 21 to 23°C. Rats were fed normal diets for 7 days at a dose of 20 grams per day and fed with water freely. Before operation, rats were restricted from eating and drinking for 24 hours. Subsequently, 2% Sodium Pentobarbital whose dose was 2 ml/kg (0.04 g/kg) was injected into their abdominal cavity to anesthetize the rats.

The rat's limbs and heads were fixed. Its fur was sheared off at the middle of the neck and was conventionally disinfected using a spread towel. An incision with length of about 2.5 cm were cut in the middle of the neck above the sternum about 1 cm. The subcutaneous tissues were separated, and the sternocleidomastoid was removed. The common carotid sheath was opened to separate the left common carotid artery (CCA). Later on, the distal end of CCA was ligated with silks, and pulled up in the proximal end with silks to prevent blood flow. Also a few drops of 2% Lidocaine Hydrochloride were dripped on the common carotid artery to dilate vessels. A small incision was cut in the CCA and the guide wires and balloon (2.0 mm × 15 mm) were inserted into the distal end of abdominal aorta from the proximal end of the left CCA. The balloon was filled at 8 atmospheric pressures and rotated for 120 degrees, in order to peel artery endothelial. This procedure was repeated for three times. Then, the balloon was pumped to negative pressure and removed the guide wire with balloon out of the abdominal aorta. In the end, the rat was put into a cage living freely. The operators executed the rats respectively on the operating day, 1st, 4th, 7th, 14th and 28th days for experiment. Treatment measures of sham group were identical to balloon injury group without inserting the guide wire and balloon. When the phenomenon of denudation and hyperplasia of intima appeared in histopathological examination, it indicated that the model was developed.

Indicators and measurements

Formalin with concentration of 10% was used to fix the abdominal aorta that was above 2 to 3 cm from iliac artery bifurcation in the rats. The specimen was embedded with paraffin, and routine pathological serially section was performed. The slice was 4 μm thick. After that, H&E staining and Elastic Fiber staining were performed. Finally, a vascular morphological detection on the section was made. The procedure for the morphological observation and image analysis of vascular hyperplastic intima was as following. The condition of intimal hyperplasia was observed with microscopy. The images within sections and in the images vascular cross-sectional was recorded. Then the images were processed by an Computer Image Analysis System and the intimal thickness, media thickness were measured and the ratio of intimal thickness and media thickness was calculated.

The remaining aorta was put into a liquid nitrogen pot immediately, and was stored in ultralow refrigerator at a temperature below minus 80°C. The stored aorta was used for detecting the expressions of genes (MCP-1, CCR2mRNA) by RT-PCR. The mRNA sequences of target genes MCP-1 and CCR2 (Serial number respectively is M57441and NM021866) and internal gene GAPDH were obtained from Genbank, Subsequently upstream and downstream primers of target genes were designed by Primer Express and specific analysis was made on each primer using BLAST engine to ensure that each primer had no homology to other known genes in the gene pool of rats. Primer sequences were respectively showed in below. Upstream of MCP-1 (288 bp) was 5′—CAATGAGTCGGCTGGAGAAC —3′ and downstream of MCP-1 (288 bp) was 5′—CAGAAGTGCTTGAGGTGGTTG—3′, upstream of CCR2 (236 bp) was 5′—GAGGCATAGGGCTGTGAGG—3′ and downstream of CCR2 (236 bp) was 5′—GATACCTTCGGAACTTCTCACC—3′, upstream of GAPDH (143 bp) was 5′—GGCTGAGAATGGGAAGCTGGTCAT—3′ and downstream of GAPDH (143 bp) was 5′—CAGCCTTCTCCATGGTGGTGAAGA—3′. The design of primer was completed by Medical Molecular Biology Center of Fujian Medical University, and the synthesis of primers was performed by the Shanghai Boya Corporation.

The total RNA was extracted referring to the process of instructions of extraction of RNA kit that was provided by Gibco Company, and the steps were as below. First, the frozen aorta was taken from ultra-low refrigerator, weighed, and rinsed with sterilizing water. Then it was cut into pieces and transferred into glass tubes. Subsequently Trizol was added at a dose of 100 mg per ml and speeded the tubes. After that, the tubes were put into ice bath for 10 to 15 minutes. Second, the slices were put into a new EP tube whose volume was 1.5 ml, and was then spun at 3000 g at 4 centigrade for 10 minutes. The supernatant fluid was removed to another EP tube and placed at indoor temperature for 10 to 15 minutes. After that, Chloroform was added at a dose of 0.2 ml per ml of Trizol. The tube was shook for 15 s and placed the tube for 5 minutes at room temperature. Later on it was spun at 12000 g at 4 centigrade for 15 minutes. The upper aqueous phase was carefully drawn and put into a new EP tube. Third, Isopropanol was added into the new tube and the tube was rolled slowly and then placed at room temperature for 10 minutes. It was spun again at 12000 g at 4 centigrade for 10 minutes. Then, white precipitate can be seen on the bottom of EP tube. Fourth, the supernatant liquid was discarded and 1 ml 75% Ethanol was added. The tube was shook to wash precipitate adequately, and was subsequently spun at 11000 g at 4 centigrade for 5 minutes. Fifth, the Ethanol was absorbed and dried the tube for 10 minutes with air. DEPC water was added into the tube. Sixth, the RNA was dissolved in water whose volume was 50 μl and whose nuclease was removed. Next it was placed in minus 20°C to cryopreservation and standby. Seventh, the total extracted RNA was taken to estimate the quantitative and purity of the RNA using ultraviolet spectrophotometer and the value of OD260 and

OD280 were measured. Eighth, the ratio value of OD260 and OD280 were measured. If the values of all specimens were 1.7 to 2.0, the RNA purity was considered to be good. Finally, electrophoresis was made with 1% Agarose Gel on total extracted RNA. Subsequently two clear bands of rRNA could be observed which respectively were 28S and 18S, suggesting that extracted RNA was not degraded.

The semi-quantitative reverse transcription - polymerase chain reaction (RT-PCR) was performed referring to the instructions of reverse transcription kit and PCR reagents which were provided by Promega and Takara Corporation. First, we compound the first chain of cDNA. The reaction systems had total RNA of 2 μg, 10 × buffer of 2 μl, 25 mmol/L MgC12 of 4 μl, 10 mmol/L dNTPs of 2 μl, random primers of 100 ng, Rnasin (RNA enzyme inhibitor) of 20 U, AMV reverse transcriptase of 15 U and ddH2O of 20 μl. The reaction conditions were 70°C for 10 minutes, amplification at 42°C for 60 minutes, inactivating AMV at 95°C for 5 minutes. Products of cDNA were placed in subzero 20°C. Secondly, we performed PCR amplification. The reaction systems had cDNA of 3 μl, 10 × PCR Buffer of 2.5 μl, 25 mmol / L MgC12 of 1.5 μl, 10 mmol/L dNTP of 0.5 μl, EXTaq enzyme of 1.5 U and deionized water of 25 μl. The reaction conditions were predenaturation at 4°C for 5 minutes, denaturation at 94°C for 30 s, annealing at 60°C for 30 s and extension at 72°Cfor 60 s, total cycles of 30 and further extension at 72°C for 5 minutes.

Finally, the electrophoresis and image scanning were implemented and the steps were assessed as follows. First, we took PCR products of 10 μl to make electrophoresis with 2% Agarose Gel whose voltage dropped 5 V per cm. Here, the process lasted for 60 minutes. Second, we stained them with Ethidium Bromide. Third, we scanned the products by the Image Master VDS-CL of Gel Imaging System. At the fourth step, we calculated gray integral of electrophoresis bands of PCR products and did standard correction by using gray integral of GAPDH. Relative quantities of PCR products of target genes was the ratio value of gray integral of electrophoresis bands of target genes and gray integral of GAPDH.

The immunohistochemical detection was performed and semi-quantitative analysis of immunohistochemical results. Referring to the instructions of UltraSensitiveTM SP hypersensitivity kit (Kit-9701) of Fujian Maixin Biotechnology Development Limited Company, we uniformly sliced 6 to 10 slices on the already embedded vessels and the thickness of each slice was 4 μm. After that, we attached slices to object slides which had already been treated by Poly-lysine and grilled slides for 4 hours at 60°C to standby. First, paraffin sections were took off the wax by Xylene for 15 minutes for twice. Later on, we used Gradient Alcohol (100% alcohol for 3 minutes for twice, 95 % alcohol for 3 minutes, 85% alcohol for 3 minutes) to hydrate them.. Second, we used Phosphate Buffered Saline (PBS) whose PH was 7.4 to wash them 3 times, 3 minutes each time. Third, we exposed antigens with high temperature and high pressure of tissue antigen retrieval method: we put a certain amount of citrate buffers whose PH was 6.0 into a pressure cooker, next used fire heat it to boiling, at this time, we placed tissue sections into plastic sliced rack which resists high temperature, later on put the rack into already boiling buffer and covered and fastened the pressure valve, continue heated to jet and lasted this condition for 1.5 minutes, we removed the pressure cooker from heat, let it natural cool to room temperature, finally removed the valve and opened the pressure cooker and took out the object slides. Fourth, we washed the slides with distilled water, then rinsed them for three times with PBS and 3 minutes each time. Fifth, drying the moisture surrounding tissues, we dripped 3% Hydrogen Peroxide of 50 μl to each organization and incubated for 10 minutes at room temperature to block activity of endogenous peroxidase, after that, rinsed three times with PBS, 3 minutes each time. Sixth, we prepared and dripped Rabbit Anti-mouse Antibody (Boster, Rabbit Anti-MCP-1, product number is BA1255) based on a usage of 20 ul whose concentration was 1:50 to each organization and incubated it for 60 minutes at room temperature. After that we rinsed them three times with PBS, 3 minutes each time. Seventh, drying moisture surrounding tissues, we dropwise dripped ready-to-use reagents MaxVision of 50 μl to each organization and incubated for 10 to 15 minutes at room temperature. When this was done, we rinsed them three times with PBS and for 3 minutes each time. Eighth, drying moisture surrounding tissues, we used fresh DAB solution, and following that, observed color development for about 5 minutes by microscopy. Then, we washed the items using tap water and dyed them using Hematoxylin. Finally, we rinsed them using PBS. After all these steps, we dehydrated them using Graded Alcohol, cleared them through Xylene and fixed them via neutral gum. The positive reaction gives a brown cytoplasm.

The semi-quantitative analysis of immunohistochemical results was stated. In the Color Image Analysis System, we randomly selected five high-power fields for each slice and measured the areas and mean grays of positive signals within a certain area for each field, next, calculated the index of positive signals of antigen using average value for each slice. The formula is the multiplication of the index of positive signals of antigen is equal to areas of positive signals with the mean grays of positive signals, and then division by the measured areas and followed by a multiplication of 100. Results of semi-quantitative examination of expressions of MCP-1 proteins are replaced by indices of positive signals.

Ethical approval

All animal experiments were approved by the committees for animal experiments of Shenzhen Institutes of Advanced Technology and conducted according to the 2 institutional ethical guidelines for animal experiments and the safety guidelines for research. The experiments complied with the Basel Declaration, Convention on the Trade in Endangered Species of Wild Fauna and Flora and the IUCN Policy Statement on Research Involving Species at Risk of Extinction. All research performed conforms to the ethical guidelines by the International Council for Laboratory Animal Science (ICLAS).

Statistical processing

The measurement data were expressed using the form of $\xi \pm \sigma$, compared groups with each other using *t* test, and then again performed comparison one more time within groups using variance analysis. The relationship between variable and variable was also researched. All statistical processes were completed with software package whose type was SPSS11.0. If P<0.05, it is considered that there had significant difference. If P<0.01, it is considered that there is a highly significant difference.

RESULTS

The statistics of the specimens' weights were showed in Table 1, which summarized the weights of rats. There was no obvious difference in the weights of rats between the sham group and the groups of balloon injury. Situation of intimal hyperplasia was showed in Table 2. Analysis showed that the ratio value of intimal thickness and media thickness increased significantly after balloon injury.

Table 1: Weights of rats in each group (ξ±ΣΔ)

	Sham groups	First day group	4th day group	7th day group	14th day group	28th day group
Sample No.	8	8	8	8	8	8
Weight (g)	434.15±10.4*	434.68±17.2*	434.17±11.3*	434.28±18.38*	434.37±15.1*	434.24±13.7*

There was no significant difference in body weights of rats in each group (*P>0.05).

Table 2: Changes of ratio of intimal thickness and media thickness (ξ±ΣΔ)

	Sham group	4th day group	7th day group	14th day group	28th day group
Sample No.	8	8	8	8	8
Intimal thickness/ media thickness	0.03±0.01	0.19±0.04*	0.35±0.05*	0.66±0.07*	0.91±0.15*

On 4, 7, 14 and 28 days after balloon injury, ratios of intimal thickness and media thickness were higher compared with the sham group and the differences were significant (*P<0.05).

Both H&E staining and elastic fiber staining were performed to all the animals. The results of HE staining of vascular pathology morphological examination were divided into sham group and balloon injury group and were demonstrated in Figure 1. As shown in Figure 1A and B, in the sham group, the intima was smooth, the internal elastic lamina was intact, and endothelial cells were visible. In the subgroup of 4 days after balloon injury, elastic plate fractures were visible and medial smooth muscle cells migrated to the intima (Figure 1C). In the subgroup of 7 days after balloon injury, a few of neointimals grew into the lumen (Figure 1D). In the subgroup of 14 days after balloon injury, hyperplasia of intima was faster and the lumen began to narrow (Figure 1E). Also, hyperplasia of intima was faster and there were more vascular smooth muscle cells and extracellular matrix in neointimal (Figure 1F). In the subgroup of 28 days after balloon injury, intimal hyperplasia was significant and lumen reduced significantly (Figure 1G), and there were many vascular smooth muscle cells and extracellular matrix in neointimal (Figure 1H).

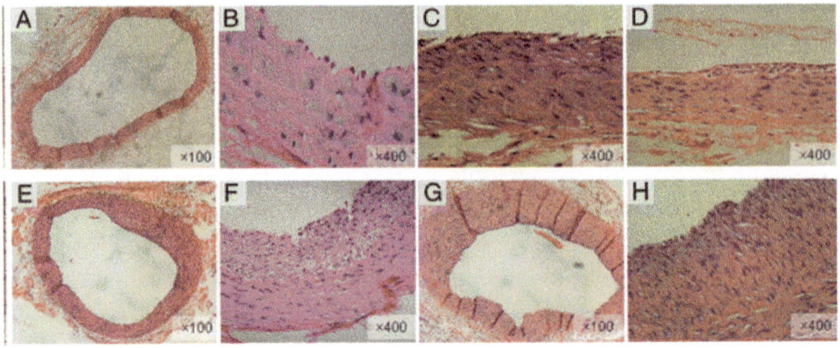

Figure 1: The results of H&E staining of pathology morphological examination of vascular in sham group and in the balloon injury group. A, B In the sham group, the intima was smooth, the internal elastic lamina was intact (H&E staining × 100), and endothelial cells were visible (H&E staining × 400); (C): 4 days after balloon injury, elastic plate fractures were visible and medial smooth muscle cells migrated to the intima (H&E staining × 400); (D): 7 days after balloon injury, a few of neointimals grew into the lumen (H&E staining × 400); (E): 14 days after balloon injury, hyperplasia of intima was faster and the lumen began to narrow (H&E staining × 100); (F): 14 days after balloon injury, hyperplasia of intima was faster and there were more vascular smooth muscle cells and extracellular matrix in neointimal (H&E staining × 400); (G): 28 days after balloon injury, intimal hyperplasia was significant and lumen reduced significantly (H&E staining × 100); (H): 28 days after balloon injury, there were many vascular smooth muscle cells and extracellular matrix in neointimal (H&E staining × 400).

The results of Elastic Fiber staining were showed in Figure 2. In the sham group, there was no intimal hyperplasia in sham group (Figure 2A). In the subgroup of 14 days after balloon injury, intimal hyperplasia was significant (Figure 2B). In the subgroup of 28 days after balloon injury, intimal hyperplasia was significant (Figure 2C).

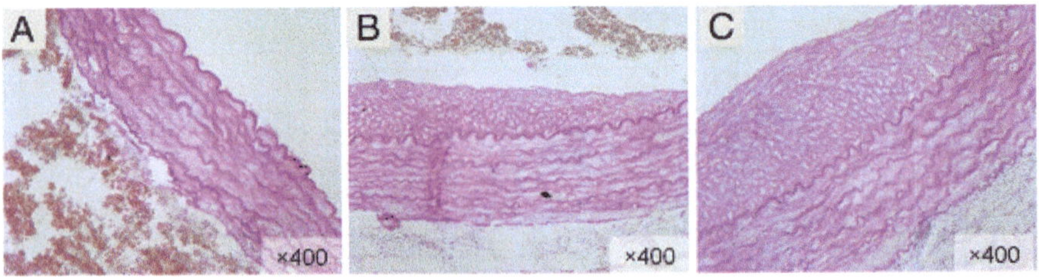

Figure 2: The Results of elastic fiber staining of pathology morphological examination of vascular in sham group and in the balloon injury group. A: Sham group, there was no intimal hyperplasia in sham group (elastic fiber staining × 400);(B): 14 days after balloon injury, intimal hyperplasia was significant (elastic fiber staining × 400); (C): 28 days after balloon injury, intimal hyperplasia was significant (elastic fiber staining × 400).

The results of PCR and identification of product were showed in Figure 3. Corresponding to the electrophoretogram of MCP-1 PCR amplification products (Figure 3A), there was no expression of MCP-1 mRNA in sham group. The expressions of MCP-1 mRNA were detected in all balloon injury groups. As shown in Figure 3C, the expression of MCP-1 mRNA decreased with time. Compared with the sham group, expressions of MCP-1 mRNA increased in the balloon injury group (*P<0.01, **P<0.05). Corresponding to the results of electrophoretogram of CCR2 PCR amplification products, trace expressions of CCR2 mRNA could be detected in both sham group and balloon injury group (Figure 3B). Much larger amounts of expressions of CCR2 mRNA can be detected in the balloon injury groups. As shown in Figure 3D, the expressions of CCR2 mRNA gradually increased and maximized at the 7th day, and then began to decrease. By the 28th day, large amounts of expressions of CCR2 mRNA can still be detected. Compared with the sham group, expressions of MCP-1 mRNA increased in the balloon injury group (*P<0.01, **P<0.05).

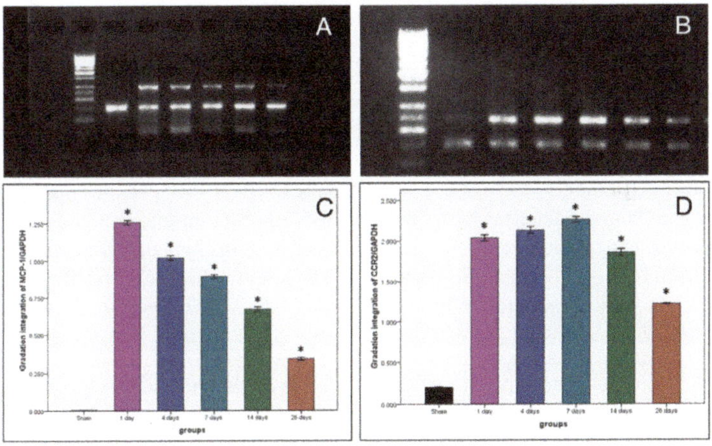

Figure 3: Results of PCR and identification of products. A: electrophoretogram of MCP-1 PCR amplification products at different time points. From left to right respectively were: M: 50 bp DNA Marker, 1: sham group, 2: first day group, 3: 4th day group, 4: 7th day group, 5: 14th day group, 6: 28th day group; (B): trend diagram of gradation integration of MCP-1/GAPDH, from left to right respectively represented sham group, first day group, 4th day group, 7th day group, 14th day group and 28th day group; (C): electrophoretogram of CCR2 PCR amplification products at different time points. From left to right respectively were: M: 50 bp DNA Marker, 1: sham group, 2: first day group, 3: 4th day group, 4: 7th day group, 5: 14th day group, 6: 28th day group; (D): trend diagram of gradation integration of CCR2/GAPDH, from left to right respectively represented sham group, first day group, 4th day group, 7th day group, 14th day group and 28th day group.

The results of immunohistochemistry of MCP-1 proteins in the vessel walls were shown in Figure 4. There was no expression of MCP-1 proteins in sham group (Figure 4A). After balloon injury, expressions of MCP-1 proteins gradually increased and the expressions in cytoplasm of vascular smooth muscle cells near the internal elastic plates increased on the 4th day (Figure 4B). On the 7th day, large amounts of expressions of MCP-1 proteins could be detected in cytoplasm of smooth muscle cells in media (Figure 4D). On the 14th day, expressions in neointimal reached to the peak. on the 28th day, large amounts of expressions could be detected in neointimal.

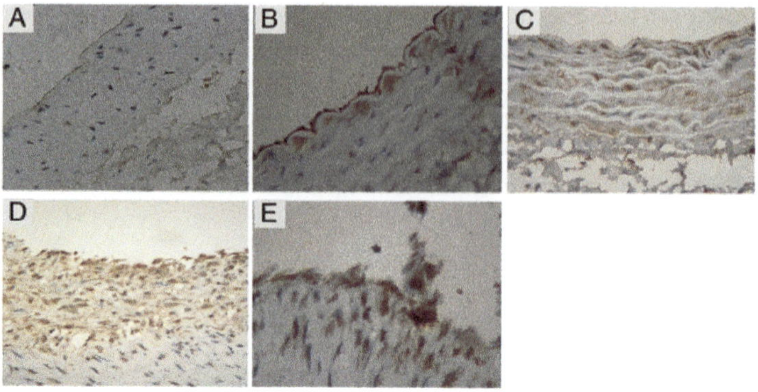

Figure 4: Detection results of immunohistochemistry of MCP-1 proteins in the vessel walls. A: negative expressions of MCP-1 proteins in sham group (Immunohistochemical SP method, DAB color, × 400); (B): positive expressions of MCP-1 proteins in cytoplasm of vascular smooth muscle cells near the internal elastic plates after balloon injury for 4 days (Immunohistochemical SP method, DAB color, × 400); (C): positive expressions of MCP-1 proteins in cytoplasm of smooth muscle cells in media after balloon injury for 7 days (Immunohistochemical SP method, DAB color, × 400);(D): positive expressions of MCP-1 proteins in neointimal after balloon injury for 14 days (Immunohistochemical SP method, DAB color, × 400); (E): positive expressions of MCP-1 proteins in neointimal after balloon injury for 28 days (Immunohistochemical SP method, DAB color, × 400).

Figure 5 shows the index of positive signals of MCP-1 proteins by the semiquantitative method of immunohistochemistry in the arterial tissues of rats in six groups. The expression of MCP-1 were compared with different experimental groups and compared with the sham group, (*P<0.01). The plot shows an increasing trend from the sham group to the 14th day group, and then decreased for the 28th day group (*P<0.05, **P<0.01).

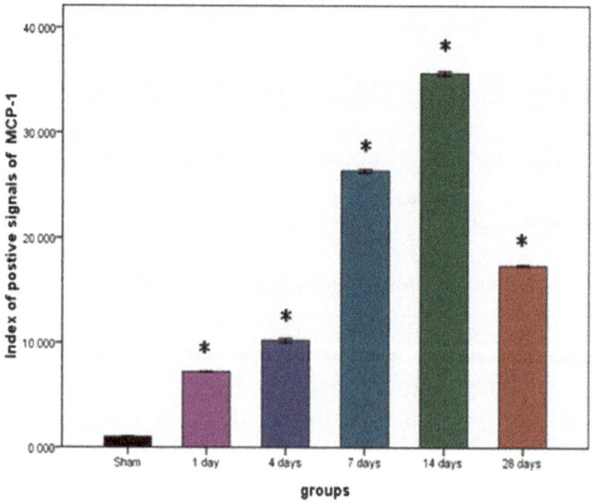

Figure 5: The index of positive signals of MCP-1 proteins by the semiquantitative method of

immunohistochemistry in the arterial tissues of rats in six groups. We compared expression of MCP-1 with different experimental groups and compared with the sham group, (*$P<0.01$).

The correlation of expressions of MCP-1 proteins and index of intimal hyperplasia (the ratio of intimal thickness and media thickness) were plotted and shown in Figure 6. The results of related analysis of Pearson showed that after balloon injury for 4, 7, 14 and 28 days, the related coefficients respectively were 0.831 (P=0.002), 0.869 (P=0.005), 0.880 (P=0.004) and 0.864 (P=0.006). The results showed that the expressions of MCP-1 proteins have an obvious positive correlation to the intimal hyperplasia after balloon injury.

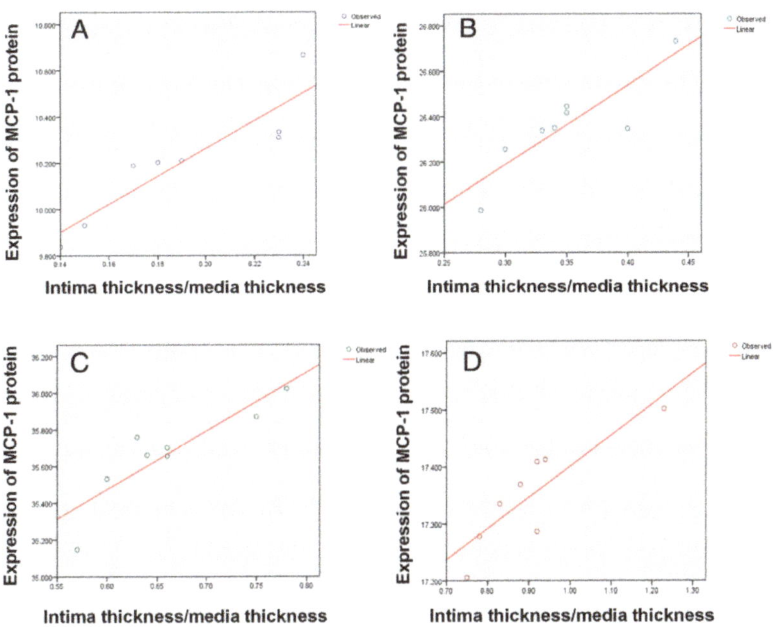

Figure 6: Correlation between expressions of MCP-1 proteins and intimal hyperplasia (the ratio of intimal thickness and media thickness) for 4, 7, 14 and 28 days. The related coefficients respectively were 0.831 ($P=0.002$), 0.869 ($P=0.005$), 0.880 ($P=0.004$) and 0.864 ($P=0.006$) as shown by images A, B, C and D.

DISCUSSIONS

PTCA that is recognized as an effective method for treating stenosis of coronary artery is widely used in clinic, but the high rate of restenosis has already been a thorny and difficult issue which is faced by physicians of cardiovascular intervention [14]. At present, the common method of making animal models of restenosis is that by simulating the process of PTCA which can result in the dilated injury of large and median arteries and pathological changes of intimal hyperplasia and stenosis [15].

In recent years, a large number of studies have shown that inflammatory response in the arterial wall plays an important role in the development of restenosis and chemoattractant and activation of monocyte which located in the arterial wall is an important pathological link in early reaction stage of vascular injury [16]. Chemokines are involved in the migration and activation of leukocytes especially of phagocytes and lymphocytes and play a vital role in inflammatory response [17,18]. According to the distribution and connection types of the two disulfide bonds of cysteine at both ends, they can be divided into CC, CXC, CX3C, C and other 4 sub families. MCP belong to the CC family of chemokine, which are divided into MCP-1, MCP-2, MCP-3, MCP-4, MCP-5, target cells in their respective effects are not the same, wherein MCP-1 is a major role in chemotactic factor of monocytes and macrophages [19,20]. MCP-1 can be secreted by a variety of cells, including osteoblasts, endothelial cells, smooth muscle cells, fibroblasts, monocytes, epidermal cells and some tumor cells. CCR2 is one of CC chemotactic cytokine receptors, mainly expresses in monocytes, kidney, heart, bone marrow, lung, liver and pancreas and other tissues [21]. CCR2 is the physiological receptor of MCP-1, after combining with MCP-1, it can induce activation of monocyte and takes the signal transduction pathway mediated by G protein coupled receptors.

It has been found that in this study 4 days after balloon injury, medial smooth muscle cells began to migrate to intima, on the 7th day, we could see moderate quantities of hyperplasia of vascular smooth muscle, on the 14th day to the 28th day, intima started to thicken obviously. Results of RT-PCR showed that there was no expression of MCP-1 mRNA in sham group and we could see trace expressions of CCR2 mRNA. After balloon injury, expressions of MCP-1 and CCR2 mRNA both significantly increased. The expressions of MCP-1 mRNA reached to the peak on the first day after balloon injury, following that, gradually decreased and it could still be detected on the 28th day. Expressions of CCR2 mRNA increased gradually after balloon injury and reached to the peak on the 7th day. After that, they decreased slowly and we could still detect large amounts of expressions of CCR2 mRNA on the 28th day. Results of immunohistochemistry showed that there was no expression of MCP-1 proteins in sham group. After balloon injury, expressions of MCP-1 proteins increased gradually. On the 4th day, expressions in cytoplasm of vascular smooth muscle cells near the internal elastic lamina increased. On the 7th day, we could detect a relatively large amount of expressions in the cytoplasm of smooth muscle cells in media. By the 14th day, we could detect significant expressions in the hyperplasia endometrium; on the 28th day, we could detect large amounts of expressions in the hyperplasia endometrium, but the expressions in smooth muscle cells in media decreased obviously. These results that expressions of MCP-1 and CCR2 increased in the repair process of vascular injury were consistent with foreign researches.

Currently, although the pathological mechanism of restenosis after PTCA has not yet been fully elucidated, excessive intimal hyperplasia caused by large proliferation of vascular smooth muscle cells and migration to intima which is induced by vascular endothelial injury is still widely considered to be the main pathological mechanism of restenosis after PTCA [22,23]. Our research demonstrates that the expressions of MCP-1 mRNA increased significantly after balloon injury and there were a lot of MCP-1 proteins expressed in the cytoplasm of smooth muscle cells and endometrial tissues, however we did not find the expression in sham group. Relevant analysis showed that the expressions of MCP-1 proteins had more significant positive correlation with intimal hyperplasia. This conclusion suggested that MCP-1 may participate in the migration and proliferation of VSMC and the occurrence and development of intimal hyperplasia. Porreca *et al.* found that MCP-1 is not only chemotactic activator but also the mitogen of vascular smooth muscle cells of rats, DNA analysis, cell count and cell division cycle analysis all have confirmed this conclusion [24]. Spinetti G *et al.*found that MCP-1 and CCR2 can promote the migration and proliferation of vascular smooth muscle cells of rats [25]. Various other researchers discovered that taking intervention measures, which can block the expressions of MCP-1, can inhibit the migration and proliferation of vascular smooth muscle cells after vascular injury, subsequently further reduce intimal hyperplasia. Zuoyun *et al.* found monoclonal antibody of MCP-1 can inhibit proliferation and migration of vascular smooth muscle cells, which mediate by angiotensin (AngII), through culture of cell *in vitro*. Then, Furukawa *et al.* found that antibody which can anti MCP-1can obviously inhibit the proliferation and migration of VSMC in carotid of rats after balloon injury [26]. In addition, Kim *et al.* reported that intimal hyperplasia in nude mice whose MCP-1 genes were knocked out after arterial injury significantly reduce compared with wild-type mice and confirmed that MCP-1 reduce the effect of intimal hyperplasia main through inhibiting the proliferation of vascular smooth muscle cells [27]. Now, 7ND is a variant of MCP-1 and its N-terminal miss 2 to 8 amino acids, it can combine with MCP-1, later on form to 7ND/MCP-1 heterodimer, further combine with CCR2, but lack physiological functions of MCP-1 and commonly is used to block the biological effects of MCP-1 [28]. Emiko *et al.* blocked the combining of MCP-1 and CCR2 by the method of injection 7ND to skeletal muscle, which can obviously inhibit the migration and proliferation of smooth muscle cells after arterial balloon injury caused by hyperlipidemia in rabbit [29]. These results of researches all strongly confirmed the pathway of signal transduction mediated by MCP-1 participated in the migration and proliferation of vascular smooth muscle cells and the occurrence and development of intimal hyperplasia from different angles. MCP-1 promote the migration and proliferation of vascular smooth muscle cells through which mechanism, now be not yet fully elucidated. Porreca *et al.*believed the main mechanisms is that: increasing the number and proportion of vascular smooth muscle cells in the S phase, meanwhile reducing the number of vascular smooth muscle cells in G0/G1 phase. By culturing vascular smooth muscle cells of human in vitro, Craig *et al.* found that MCP-1 lead to the proliferation of vascular smooth muscle cells mainly through increasing expressions of cyclin A and further effecting cell cycles [30]. The study also found that the expressions of CCR2 mRNA significantly increased after balloon injury, CCR2 is the major physiological receptor of MCP-1 and it plays an irreplaceable role in the process of MCP-1 play biological effects, these prompt CCR2 may also be involved in the proliferation of the intima after balloon injury.

So far, the mechanisms of MCP-1 and CCR2 in intimal hyperplasia has not yet been fully elucidated, conclusions that are obtained by interventions of MCP-1 and CCR2 are mostly based on animal models, but pathological environments of animal are not exactly same to human, so the exact mechanism of MCP-1 and CCR2 play a role in intimal hyperplasia and stenosis still need be further studied.

CONCLUSION

In this study, the rat models of balloon injury were developed, the changes of intimal proliferation were observed with optical microscopy, and the expressions of MCP-1 and CCR2 at different times were examined with the methods of RT-PCR and immunohistochemistry. The expressions of MCP-1 and CCR2 in the arterial tissues were detected using reverse transcription polymerase chain reaction (RT-PCR) and analyzed by semi-quantitative method. The results showed that the dynamic expressions of MCP-1, MCP-1 proteins and CCR2 mRNA after balloon injury were shown to play an important role in intimal proliferation.

DECLARATIONS

Acknowledgment

The work was supported by National Science Foundation Grant (11272329), National Key Technology R&D Program of China (2012BAI13B01), Shenzhen International Collaboration Grant (GJHZ20120617111428312).

AUTHORS' CONTRIBUTIONS

Conceived and designed the experiments: ZH, YL, X. Performed the experiments: ZH, YL. Analyzed the data: ZH, YL, LN, YX, MQ. Contributed reagents/materials/analysis tools: XP, HZ, MQ. Contributed to the writing of the manuscript: ZH, LN, YX, MQ. All authors read and approved the final manuscript.

REFERENCES

1. Pak O. The effects of hypoxia on the cells of the pulmonary vasculature. Eur Respir J. 2007;30(2):364–72.
2. Ng C, Wan S, Yim A. Pulmonary ischaemia-reperfusion injury: role of apoptosis. Eur Respir J. 2005;25(2):356–63.
3. Murphy E, Rahimtoola S, Grüntzig A. Transluminal dilatation for coronary-artery stenosis. Lancet. 1978;311(8073):1093.
4. Meijer AJ, Codogno P. Regulation and role of autophagy in mammalian cells. Int J Biochem Cell Biol. 2004;36(12):2445–62.
5. Kuma A. The role of autophagy during the early neonatal starvation period. Nature. 2004;432(7020):1032–6.
6. Galluzzi L. Guidelines for the use and interpretation of assays for monitoring cell death in higher eukaryotes. Cell Death Differ. 2009;16(8):1093–107.
7. Fitzal F. Early capillary no-reflow during low-flow reperfusion after hind limb ischemia in the rat. Ann Plast Surg. 2002;49(2):170–80.
8. Fischell TA, Carter AJ, Laird JR. The beta-particle—emitting radioisotope stent (isostent): animal studies and planned clinical trials. Am J Cardiol. 1996;78(3):45–50.

9. Fareh J. Cellular effects of β-particle delivery on vascular smooth muscle cells and endothelial cells a dose–response study. Circulation. 1999;99(11):1477–84.
10. Okamoto S. Effects of trapidil (triazolopyrimidine), a platelet-derived growth factor antagonist, in preventing restenosis after percutaneous transluminal coronary angioplasty. Am Heart J. 1992;123(6):1439–44.
11. Hiltunen MO. Intravascular adenovirus-mediated VEGF-C gene transfer reduces neointima formation in balloon-denuded rabbit aorta. Circulation. 2000;102(18):2262–8.
12. Hayashi SI. Roles of P-selectin in inflammation, neointimal formation, and vascular remodeling in balloon-injured rat carotid arteries. Circulation. 2000;102(14):1710–7.
13. Epstein FH, Ross R. Atherosclerosis—an inflammatory disease. N Engl J Med. 1999;340(2):115–26.
14. Scherz-Shouval R, Elazar Z. Regulation of autophagy by ROS: physiology and pathology. Trends Biochem Sci. 2011;36(1):30–8.
15. Geary RL. Time course of cellular proliferation, intimal hyperplasia, and remodeling following angioplasty in monkeys with established atherosclerosis a nonhuman primate model of restenosis. Arterioscler Thromb Vasc Biol. 1996;16(1):34–43.
16. de Lemos JA. Association between plasma levels of monocyte chemoattractant protein-1 and long-term clinical outcomes in patients with acute coronary syndromes. Circulation. 2003;107(5):690–5.
17. Waechter C. Role of the double-stranded RNA-activated protein kinase (PKR) in cell regulation. Biochem Soc Trans. 1997;25:509–13.
18. Campbell JJ, Butcher EC. Chemokines in tissue-specific and microenvironment-specific lymphocyte homing. Curr Opin Immunol. 2000;12(3):336–41.
19. Charo IF, Taubman MB. Chemokines in the pathogenesis of vascular disease. Circ Res. 2004;95(9):858–66.
20. Jarvis TC. Inhibition of vascular smooth muscle cell proliferation by ribozymes that cleave c-myb mRNA. RNA. 1996;2(5):419.
21. Scherz Shouval R. Reactive oxygen species are essential for autophagy and specifically regulate the activity of Atg4. EMBO J. 2007;26(7):1749–60.
22. Autieri MV. Antisense oligonucleotides to the p65 subunit of NF-κB inhibit human vascular smooth muscle cell adherence and proliferation and prevent neointima formation in rat carotid arteries. Biochem Biophys Res Commun. 1995;213(3):827–36.
23. Schwartz RS, Henry TD. Pathophysiology of coronary artery restenosis. Rev Cardiovasc Med. 2001;3:S4–9.
24. Porreca E. Monocyte chemotactic protein 1 (MCP-1) is a mitogen for cultured rat vascular smooth muscle cells. J Vasc Res. 1997;34(1):58–65.
25. Spinetti G. Rat aortic MCP-1 and its receptor CCR2 increase with age and

alter vascular smooth muscle cell function. Arterioscler Thromb Vasc Biol. 2004;24(8):1397–402.

26. Furukawa Y. Anti–monocyte chemoattractant protein-1/monocyte chemotactic and activating factor antibody inhibits neointimal hyperplasia in injured rat carotid arteries. Circ Res. 1999;84(3):306–14.

27. Kim WJ. MCP-1 deficiency is associated with reduced intimal hyperplasia after arterial injury. Biochem Biophys Res Commun. 2003;310(3):936–42.

28. Mukaida N, Harada A, Matsushima K. Interleukin-8 (IL-8) and monocyte chemotactic and activating factor (MCAF/MCP-1), chemokines essentially involved in inflammatory and immune reactions. Cytokine Growth Factor Rev. 1998;9(1):9–23.

29. Mori E. Essential role of monocyte chemoattractant protein-1 in development of restenotic changes (neointimal hyperplasia and constrictive remodeling) after balloon angioplasty in hypercholesterolemic rabbits. Circulation. 2002;105(24):2905–10.

30. Kang R. The Beclin 1 network regulates autophagy and apoptosis. Cell Death Differ. 2011;18(4):571–80.

12
CHAPTER

SUB-MILLIMETER DIAMETER POLY(VINYL ALCOHOL) VASCULAR GRAFT PATENCY IN RABBIT MODEL

Marie F. A. Cutiongco, Marek Kukumberg, Jonnathan L. Peneyra, Matthew S. Yeo, Jia Y. Yao, Abdul Jalil Rufaihah, Catherine Le Visage, Jackie Pei Ho and Evelyn K. F. Yim

Keywords: Small diameter vascular graft, *in vivo* testing, compliance matching, off-the-shelf vascular graft, microvascular graft

INTRODUCTION

Microvascular surgery contributes widely to various surgical procedures, such as replantation and free tissue transfer (Griffin and Thornton, 2005), free flap surgery (Shen et al., 1988), orthopedic surgeries (Doi et al., 1977; Judet et al., 1981), and digital reconstruction (Lanzetta, 1995). During these procedures, vascular grafts are required to anastomose blood vessels together, repair vascular defects, and restore blood flow. The gold standard of using autologous venous and arterial grafts, which is valued for their biocompatibility and non-thrombogenicity, is not without fault. Autologous grafts require tedious and time-consuming harvesting processes and may be limited supply due to comorbidities that affect the vasculature. Moreover, venous autologous grafts lack mechanical integrity while autologous grafts have a propensity for aneurysm formation (So, 1998).

Synthetic small diameter vascular grafts (with diameter <6 mm) made of expanded polytetrafluoroethylene (ePTFE) are widely available today as alternatives to autologous vascular grafts. However, ePTFE grafts are plagued by rapid thrombosis and lack of

Citation: Cutiongco MFA, Kukumberg M, Peneyra JL, Yeo MS, Yao JY, Rufaihah AJ, Le Visage C, Ho JP and Yim EKF (2016) Sub-millimeter Diameter Poly(Vinyl Alcohol) Vascular Graft Patency in Rabbit Model. Front. Bioeng. Biotechnol. 4:44. doi: 10.3389/fbioe.2016.00044.

long-term patency and efficacy caused by mechanical mismatch with the native artery (Uchida et al., 1989; Sarkar et al., 2007). The problems of ePTFE grafts are further magnified in the submillimeter scale, where the low shear stress and flow, and high risk of blood stasis can lead to rapid graft thrombosis and failure (Barnes, 1980; Sarkar et al., 2006). ePTFE grafts with 1 mm diameter have all failed after implantation *in vivo*, showing rapid and extensive thrombosis within a few days of implantation (Lidman et al., 1980; Ganske et al., 1982; Harris and Seikaly, 2002). Thus, the development of a new type of off-the-shelf synthetic vascular graft with submillimeter diameter for microvascular surgery is needed.

Poly(vinyl alcohol) hydrogel (PVA) is widely used for various biomedical purposes, including the production of artificial meniscus (Kobayashi et al., 2005), hemodialysis membrane (Barzin and Madaeni, 2007), heart valve (Wan et al., 2002), artificial vitreous fluid (Lamponi et al., 2012; Feng et al., 2013), and cardiac patch with drug delivery capability (Fathi et al., 2013). PVA is an excellent candidate as a small diameter vascular graft due to its non-immunogenic, bio-inert, and mechanically tunable properties (Chaouat et al., 2008; Cutiongco et al., 2015a, 2016). Herewith, we sought to tune the mechanical properties of submillimeter diameter PVA grafts. Characterization of mechanical and thrombogenic properties of the submillimeter PVA grafts will be performed. Demonstration of efficacy of PVA graft in stringent *in vivo* conditions submillimeter diameter will reiterate the potential of this material as a new vascular graft material for microvascular surgical applications.

MATERIALS AND METHODS

Fabricating PVA Vascular Grafts

Fabrication of grafts made from PVA hydrogel (PVA graft) was performed according to previous studies (Cutiongco et al., 2015b, 2016). Hypodermic needle [0.9 mm outer diameter (OD)] and carbon rod (1 mm OD) were used to fabricate PVA vascular grafts. Cylindrical molds were plasma cleaned (60 W, 8 mL/min O_2 gas) for 1 min to improve adherence of PVA. The mold was then immediately immersed in solution of PVA, crosslinker STMP, and NaOH, removed, and dried for 15 min at room temperature. An additional five layers of PVA were added and allowed to dry at 25°C for 3 days or 4°C for 3 days. Afterward, scaffolds were washed several times in phosphate-buffered saline (PBS) and distilled deionized (DI) water before removal from the tubular mold. PVA tubes were gamma irradiated (25 kGy) while immersed in water to obtain sterile PVA vascular grafts.

Mechanical Testing of Submillimeter PVA Grafts

Wall Thickness and Internal Diameter Measurement

Different sections of PVA vascular grafts (n = 5) hydrated in water were cut into ~1 mm cross-sections and imaged using optical microscope (Nikon Eclipse TS100). The images were used to measure wall thickness and ID using ImageJ (NIH).

Radial Compliance Test

At hydrostatic pressures of 80 and 120 mmHg, images of the distended PVA vascular grafts ($n = 6$) were taken using a stereomicroscope (Nikon SMZ745T). Compliance was calculated as the percent change in PVA vascular graft diameter from 80 to 120 mmHg (Chaouat et al., 2008).

Burst Pressure Test

Nitrogen gas was slowly released into closed-ended PVA vascular grafts ($n = 3$) until scaffold rupture. Pressure at failure was denoted as the burst pressure.

Suture Retention Test

A single throw of 6/0 Vicryl suture (Ethicon) was passed through one end of a PVA vascular graft at ~5 mm from the edge. The suture was attached to a receptacle, where water was added until rupture of the PVA graft. The weight of the receptacle and water was taken as suture retention strength ($n = 4$).

Uniaxial Test

PVA vascular grafts (1 cm length, $n = 3$) were tested using a uniaxial testing machine (INSTRON 3345) with a 10-N load cell, 0.1-N preload, and crosshead speed of 10 mm/min. Measurements of various grafts were taken until break. Linear portions of the graphs were used to determine Young's modulus.

Scanning Electron Microscopy of Submillimeter PVA Grafts

PVA vascular graft was air-dried overnight at ambient temperature, sputter coated with 10 nm platinum film (JEOL-JFC 1600 coater), and visualized using scanning electron microscopy (SEM) (JEOL-JSM 6010LV).

Blood Compatibility of PVA

Incubation of PVA Tubes with Platelet Rich Plasma

In vitro blood compatibility assay was performed, as previously described (Cutiongco et al., 2015a). Blood samples were collected from healthy New Zealand White rabbits in polypropylene tubes primed with heparin (5 U/mL blood). Blood was centrifuged at 100 × *g* and 22°C for 12 min to collect platelet rich plasma (PRP). PVA vascular graft (1 mm ID, $n = 3$, internal surface area of 90 mm^2), Silastic tubing (Dow Corning, $n = 3$, internal surface area of 60 mm^2), and ePTFE tubing (Zeus, $n = 3$, internal surface area of 110 mm^2) were weighed and washed in sterile 0.9% NaCl solution (BBraun). Glass beads coated with bovine Collagen I (Invitrogen; 7.15 µg/mg sample) were placed in a polypropylene tube and included as a positive control. PRP was then added to the lumen of each tube or to the beads at 0.75 µL/mg sample. Since the diameters of the tubes and beads used in this test were different, a constant mass of each sample was used. Tubes were sealed at both ends with sterile Luer lock combistoppers (BBraun). Subsequently, all samples were incubated for 1 h at 37°C with bidirectional *X*-axis rotation at 100 rpm. Resting samples of 100 μL PRP were also included. Tubular samples were kept for platelet morphology analysis using SEM (see Preparation of Samples for SEM Visualization), while PRP was then collected for subsequent flow cytometry analysis (see Flow Cytometric Analysis of Platelet Activation). Assay was done in triplicate for each sample.

Preparation of Samples for SEM Visualization

Tubular samples were washed in PBS and fixed using 2.5% glutaraldehyde at 4°C for 2 h. Thereafter, films were dehydrated using a series of increasing ethanol concentration. After complete drying, films were then coated and visualized under SEM, as described in Section "Scanning Electron Microscopy of Submillimeter PVA Grafts."

Flow Cytometric Analysis of Platelet Activation

Aliquots of PRP (10 μL) were diluted with 200 μL of HEPES-Tyrodes buffer (HTB; 137 mM sodium chloride, 2.7 mM potassium chloride, 16 mM sodium bicarbonate, 5 mM magnesium chloride, 3.5 mM HEPES, 1% glucose, 2% bovine serum albumin, and pH 7.4) and incubated with antibodies against CD61/GPIIb/IIIa (Abbiotec). Platelets were then washed with HTB and centrifuged at 21,000 rpm and 4°C for 5 min. Platelets were then resuspended in 100 μL HTB and incubated with fluorescently conjugated secondary antibodies for 1 h. Samples were fixed with 2% paraformaldehyde in HTB. Platelets were analyzed within 24 h for scatter characteristics and expression of platelet markers using BD LSR Fortessa. Flow cytometry data were analyzed using FlowJo 4.0.

PVA Vascular Graft Implantation in Rabbit Femoral Artery with Multi-level Arterial Occlusion

Animal study was done in accordance with approved guidelines of the Institutional Animal Care and Use Committee of the National University of Singapore. Male New Zealand White rabbits (3.5–4.0 kg, ~6 months old) were used in the study. Multilevel arterial occlusion in the left femoral artery was induced through embolization and ligation of the femoral artery before PVA graft anastomosis (Figure S1 in Supplementary Material).

After sedation and exposure of the left femoral artery, papaverine (1.43 mg/mL) was administered topically and intravascularly to facilitate intra-arterial cannulation. Embolic particles (150–250 μm diameter, Boston Scientific) resuspended in equal volume of 0.9% sodium chloride and 4% gelofusine were injected into the left femoral artery. In a pilot study, the minimum dose of embolic particles needed to induce occlusion of the lower saphenous artery was determined by titration (data not shown). The embolic particles were flushed into the femoral artery with 0.9% NaCl solution. The femoral artery was permanently ligated. A 4-mm length, encompassing the site of intra-arterial cannulation and found between the ligatures, was resected to induce macro-vascular occlusion, thereby completing the induction of the multilevel arterial occlusion.

Immediately afterward, PVA vascular grafts with 4-mm length and 0.9- or 1-mm ID were implanted into the left femoral artery (PVA group). The size of graft implanted was chosen to match the caliber of the femoral artery. PVA vascular grafts were anastomosed using simple interrupted sutures (Ethilon, 10-0) under operating stereomicroscope. During anastomosis, heparin (100 IU/kg) was administered intravenously. Ligation and reperfusion of left femoral artery did not exceed 3 h in all surgeries. Postanastomotic patency was confirmed by refill test and observation of pulsation in the postanastomotic vessel. All animals were treated with enrofloxacin (5 mg/kg) and buprenorphine (0.04 mg/kg) for 7 days postoperatively. The contralateral hindlimbs in each animal were included as an internal control (contralateral group, $n = 7$).

Assessment of Hindlimb Perfusion Using Laser Doppler Flowmeter

The perfusion of the skin on the left dorsal foot was measured using laser Doppler flowmeter (Perimed PeriFlux System 5010 with 1 mm diameter fiber-optic probe). Laser Doppler flowmetry measurement of surface paw perfusion was performed immediately after surgery and at intervals afterward. Animals were sedated before measurement. To ensure consistency, laser Doppler probe was placed on the same location on the depilated dorsal foot, as marked by a small circular tattoo (AIMS animal tattoo). Measurements of surface perfusion were obtained from the stable readout of the laser Doppler flowmeter. All dorsal foot perfusion measurements were normalized to that of the contralateral group. For comparison, standard laser Doppler imaging (Perimed PeriFlux PIM 3) was performed and confirmed the validity of the readings obtained from the laser Doppler flowmeter (Figure S2 in Supplementary Material).

Ultrasound Doppler

Examination of vascular graft patency during implantation was performed using ultrasound Doppler (GE Ultrasound Doppler Vivid S6, 8–13 MHz). Animals were lightly sedated and placed in prone position during the examination.

Endpoint Angiography

Digital subtraction angiography (GE Innova 2100) was performed at ~15 days postimplantation of the PVA grafts. Contralateral limbs were included as the internal control. Contrast agent (GE Omnipaque, 350 mg/mL) and 0.9% NaCl solution at a 1:1 ratio were used for imaging. A midline incision was made on the sedated rabbit. The caudal abdominal aorta was cannulated near the iliac bifurcation for direct delivery of contrast agent through each iliac artery. Quantification of angiographic data was performed, as described previously (Silvestre et al., 2000; Iglarz et al., 2001).

Histology

Heparin (100 IU/kg) was administered systemically before euthanization with sodium pentobarbital (150 mg/kg). Muscle from both the implanted and contralateral limbs were harvested and fixed with 4% paraformaldehyde for 48 h. Tissues were embedded in Paraplast (Leica). Sections 15–20 µm thick were stained with standard hematoxylin and eosin (H&E) and Masson's trichrome stain. Assessment of collateral formation and graft endothelialization was performed through detection of CD31 and α-SMA using Novolink kit (Leica).

Statistical Analysis

All data are presented as mean ± SD. Statistical analysis was performed using one-way ANOVA with Tukey's *post hoc* test (GraphPad Prism v6.0). Differences were taken to be statistically significant at $p < 0.05$.

RESULTS

Tuning Mechanical Properties of Submillimeter Diameter Vascular Grafts

The lack of clinically available submillimeter diameter vascular grafts necessitates the creation of a new vascular graft. Thus, PVA submillimeter diameter vascular grafts were fabricated. Matching size and compliance of a synthetic vascular graft to the native recipient vessel is critical to maintain graft patency (Uchida et al., 1989; Sarkar et al., 2006). To better approximate mechanical properties of the rabbit femoral artery, PVA vascular grafts with uniform ID of 0.9 and 1 mm were fabricated at two different cross-linking temperatures of 25 and 4°C (Table 1).

Table 1: Mechanical properties of poly(vinyl alcohol) (PVA) grafts with submillimeter dimensions and reported values for rabbit femoral artery

Tube	Internal diameter (µm, n = 5)	Wall thickness (µm, n = 5)	Compliance (%, n = 6)	Burst pressure (mmHg, n = 3)	Suture retention (g, n = 4)	Young modulus (kPa, n = 3)	Elongation at break (%, n = 3)	Ultimate tensile strength (kPa, n = 3)
Cross-linking at 25°C								
1 mm diameter	1194 ± 29.62[a] (hydrated)	271.2 ± 70.47	4.00 ± 3.41	725 ± 137[c]	102 ± 16.9	553.1 ± 2.695[b,c]	436.0 ± 25.36[c]	84.4 ± 13.4[b,c]
0.9 mm diameter	1093 ± 63.61 (hydrated)	287.6 ± 27.59	3.04 ± 2.56	868 ± 171[c]	76.6 ± 7.33[a]	388.7 ± 34.28[b]	465.8 ± 21.72[c]	53.7 ± 11.7[b]
Cross-linking at 4°C								
1 mm diameter	1185 ± 9.510[a,b] (hydrated)	273.8 ± 50.71	2.87 ± 0.14	269 ± 134[c]	90.3 ± 13.7	256.9 ± 61.34[c]	161.6 ± 41.22[c]	57.1 ± 9.90[c]
0.9 mm diameter	996.6 ± 29.85[b] (hydrated)	285.1 ± 47.74	3.29 ± 0.63	207 ± 104[c]	74.8 ± 5.90[a]	331.9 ± 90.54	130.7 ± 19.84[c]	44.0 ± 2.83
Rabbit femoral artery (Uchida et al., 1989)	938 ± 201	350–710	5.9 ± 0.5	2031–4225	200 ± 119	230	ND	998

[a]*Denotes statistical significance between PVA graft and rabbit femoral artery.*
[b]*Denotes statistical significance between 1 mm internal diameter (ID) PVA graft and 0.9 mm ID PVA graft cross-linked at the same temperature.*
[c]*Denotes statistical significance of PVA graft with similar ID cross-linked at different temperatures.*

The internal diameter (ID) and wall thickness between PVA grafts cross-linked at different temperatures but with similar ID showed minute differences. On the other hand, compliances of grafts cross-linked at 4°C were generally lower than those of tubes cross-linked at 25°C. Furthermore, burst pressure of grafts were significantly improved when grafts were cross-linked at 25°C compared to 4°C, showing at least a 2.7 times increase in magnitude. Both Young's modulus and ultimate tensile strength of 1 mm ID PVA grafts were invariably improved when cross-linking temperature changed from 4 to 25°C. Similar to the observed improvement in burst pressure, the percent elongation at break was also drastically changed when cross-linking temperature was increased from 4 to 25°C.

Due to the compliance more closely approximating the rabbit femoral artery, together with better mechanical integrity as indicated by higher burst pressure and ultimate tensile strength, PVA grafts cross-linked at 25°C were chosen for implantation in the rabbit femoral artery. Under SEM, the PVA vascular grafts cross-linked at 25°C (afterward referred to simply as PVA graft) showed tubular structure with apparent even wall thickness (Figure 1A; Table 1) and random roughness along its luminal surface (Figure1B).

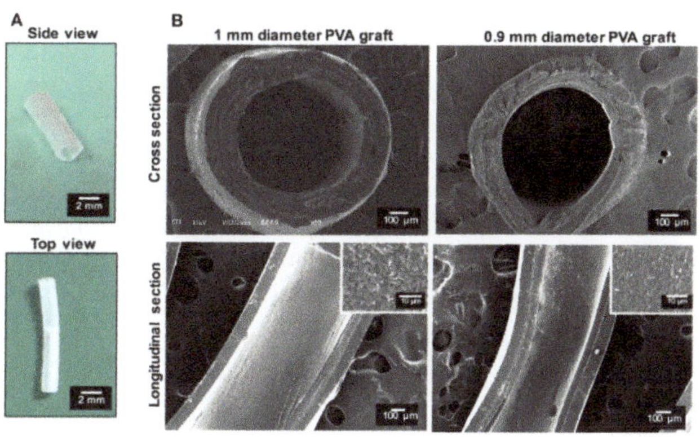

Figure 1: Characterization of submillimeter diameter poly(vinyl alcohol) (PVA) vascular graft. (A) Photomicrograph of PVA vascular graft with 1 mm internal diameter. (B)Scanning electron microscopy (SEM) images show cross section and longitudinal section of 1 and 0.9 mm ID PVA vascular grafts cross-linked at 25°C. The longitudinal section shows surface roughness on lumen.

Blood Compatibility of Submillimeter PVA Vascular Grafts

In vitro blood compatibility assay was performed to determine platelet microparticle release and platelet morphology after contact with PVA grafts (Figure 2). Platelet microparticle release, as measured by the expression of the GPIIb/IIIa marker, is an important indicator of platelet activation (Gemmell et al., 1997). Platelets incubated in PVA grafts showed a statistically similar microparticle release profile with that of ePTFE, a material widely used for vascular grafts (Figure 2A). PVA also showed statistically similar platelet microparticle expression with Silastic, an inert material often used for blood-contacting tubing, and the resting control that did not contact any foreign material. Significantly, both PVA and ePTFE showed significantly lower microparticle release compared with the highly thrombogenic collagen-coated glass. PVA and ePTFE showed statistically similar microparticle release with the rest group, indicative of non-activated platelets (Yim et al., 2007). SEM further indicated the thrombogenic potential of collagen-coated glass through the fibrotic and clumped appearance of adhered platelets (Figure 2B). Meanwhile, platelets were sparse on the PVA surface and less fibrous extensions (Figure 2B). Platelets that contacted ePTFE and silastic surfaces were rounder, indicative of the inactive platelet phenotype.

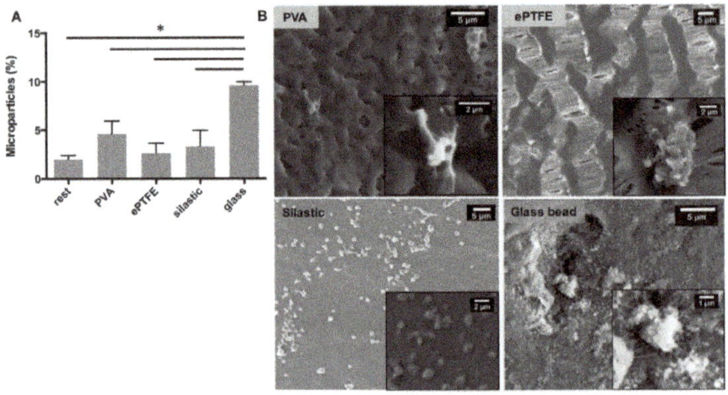

Figure 2: ***In vitro* blood compatibility of PVA vascular grafts. (A)** Percentage of microparticles expressing GPIIb/IIIa receptor released from total platelet count after contacting various surfaces ($n = 3$). *Denotes statistical significance with two-way ANOVA. (B) Morphology of platelets attached to various surfaces observed with SEM. Insets show higher magnification images of platelets.

Implantation of Submillimeter PVA Grafts in Rabbit Femoral Artery

PVA grafts were anastomosed to the left rabbit femoral artery with multilevel arterial occlusion (Figures S3–S5 in Supplementary Material). The multilevel occlusion of the femoral artery was induced to create a challenging environment to test the patency of submillimeter PVA grafts. After implantation of PVA grafts (Table 2), all PVA subjects had normal appearance and mobility 2 days postoperatively. All PVA subjects were alert and responsive with physiological posture and gait at the endpoint. Range of motion of all ankle joints and muscle tone were not affected. No signs of inflammation or infection of the surgical area were seen, indicating the bioinertness of the PVA grafts.

Table 2: Summary of PVA graft implantation

Subject	Endpoint (days after surgery)	Diameter of PVA graft used (mm)	Patency at endpoint
PVA1	15	0.9	Patent
PVA2	17	1	Patent
PVA3	14	1	Occluded

The paw surface perfusion, which represents the overall flow contributed by both graft luminal patency and hindlimb collateral formation, was also measured (Figure 3). A notable minimum of percent perfusion was observed in PVA subjects immediately postoperative (day 0; PVA1 4.24% and PVA2 11.0%), indicative of the occlusion induced in the left femoral artery. More importantly, the percent perfusion on patent PVA grafts achieved or exceeded its preoperative level at endpoint (preoperative: PVA1 69 and PVA2 80%; endpoint: PVA1 101.3 and PVA2 80.0%), indicating arterial recovery through graft patency and collateral network formation. In one instance, percent perfusion exceeded the level of the contralateral group.

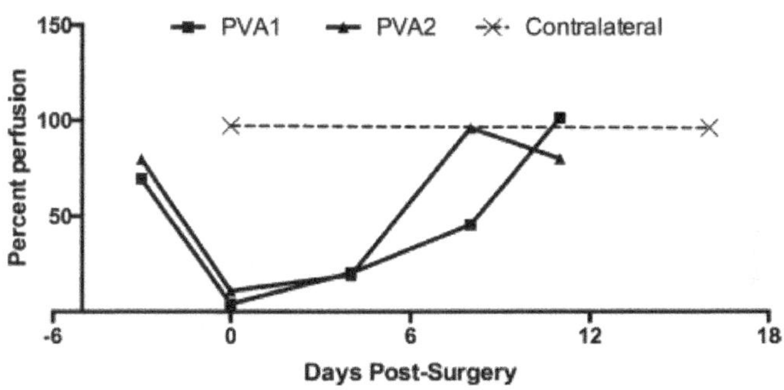

Figure 3: Recovery of hindlimb surface perfusion after PVA graft implantation. Percent perfusion on PVA group given as the ratio of surface perfusion between dorsal foot of implanted limb and contralateral dorsal foot. Percent perfusion was obtained at different timepoints after PVA graft implantation (day 0).

Ultrasound Doppler was used as a means to estimate graft patency *in situ* (Figure 4). Ultrasound Doppler images showed continuous blood flow everywhere for PVA1 at both 4 and 12 days postoperatively. Normal blood flow was observed throughout the femoral artery and the PVA graft. The PVA graft showed no leakage and no dilatation at both days of observation. Endpoint angiography confirmed the patency of two out of three PVA grafts, giving a primary patency rate of 67% (Figure 5A). Significantly, all PVA limbs showed blood flow through the saphenous artery and metatarsal arteries using angiography. Analysis of angiograms showed that PVA limbs exhibited significantly higher pixel occupancy of blood vessels and more extensive collateral network as opposed to contralateral controls (Figure 5B).

Explanted PVA grafts showed that PVA1 showed some residual blood cells in the lumen (Figure 6A). In contrast, luminal tissue in PVA2 graft intensely stained with hematoxylin and its contour was similar to that of the graft wall, while the lumen of graft from PVA3 was completely filled with a thrombus (Figure6A). While an unimplanted PVA graft did not show any positive signal, the entire luminal surface of the patent PVA2 graft indicated the presence of endothelial cells (Figure 6B). Masson's trichrome staining also showed highly organized collagen fibers deposited in the area surrounding the PVA graft (Figure S6A in Supplementary Material).

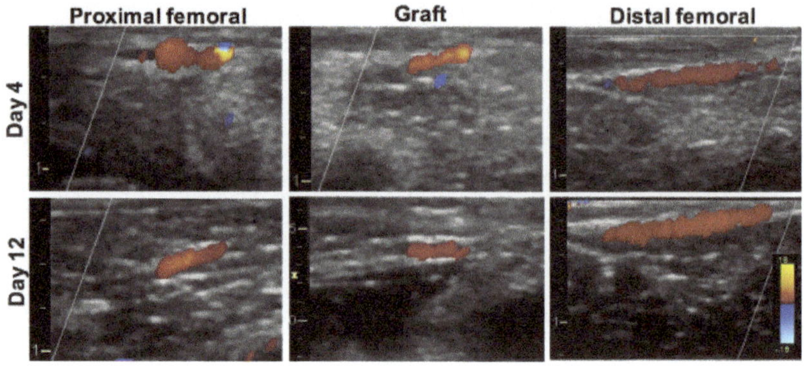

Figure 4: Estimation of PVA graft patency using ultrasound Doppler. Representative ultrasound Doppler images were obtained from PVA1 limb. Ultrasound Doppler images were obtained from various areas of the femoral artery, including the graft, at both 4 and 12 days postsurgery. Color scale represents velocity direction, where red indicates blood flow from left to right of the artery.

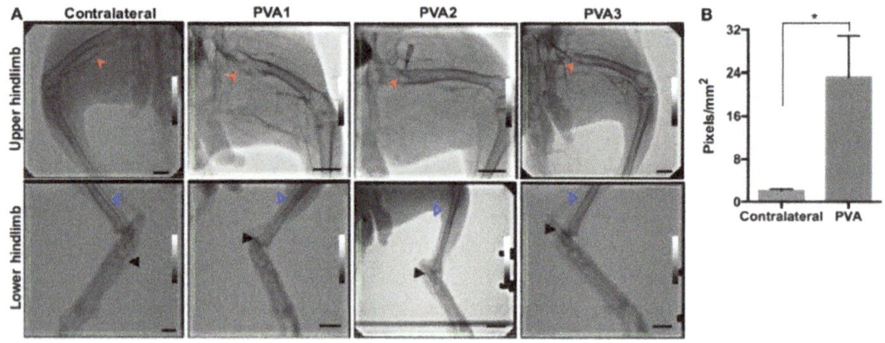

Figure 5: Patency of femoral, saphenous, and metatarsal arteries, and PVA graft in PVA limbs. (A) Hindlimb perfusion was assessed by angiography. All PVA hindlimbs ($n = 3$) showed extensive collateral network proximally, while blood flow through the saphenous artery was maintained distally. Two out of three PVA grafts remained patent after implantation. A representative angiography from contralateral group ($n = 5$) demonstrated full patency of femoral artery and saphenous artery. Red arrow denotes PVA graft. Blue arrow denotes saphenous artery. Black arrow denotes metatarsal artery. Scale bar = 1 cm. (B) Digital examination of angiographs to measure total collateral vessel occupancy in PVA and contralateral group. Collateral vessel occupancy was measured from total pixel area of collaterals normalized to hindlimb area. *Denotes statistical difference using one-way ANOVA.

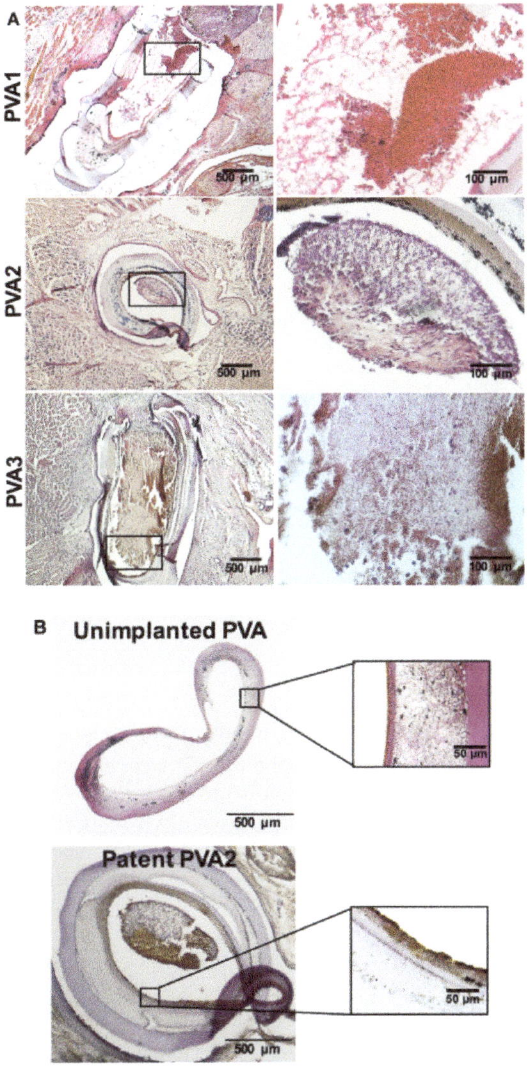

Figure 6: Histological analysis of PVA vascular grafts. (A) Morphology of explanted PVA vascular grafts ($n = 3$). Hematoxylin and eosin (H&E) staining of sections of both patent (PVA1 and PVA2) and occluded PVA (PVA3) grafts (40×). (B) Endothelialization of patent PVA small diameter graft. Positive staining (brown) for CD31 was absent in unimplanted PVA and present in PVA vascular graft after 17 days postimplantation (40×). Insert shows higher magnification (100×).

Hindlimb muscles were also assessed for evidence of arterial recovery. Muscle from PVA2 showed signs of recovery from ischemia, denoted by nuclei in the center of muscle fibers (Figure S6B in Supplementary Material). Hindlimb muscles in PVA limbs were bundled and rounded with uniform size (Figures 7A,B). Capillary density was significantly higher in PVA limbs compared to contralateral controls (Figure 7C). Additionally, mature collaterals surrounded by α-SMA-positive cells were increased in PVA, as opposed to the contralateral group (Figure 7D).

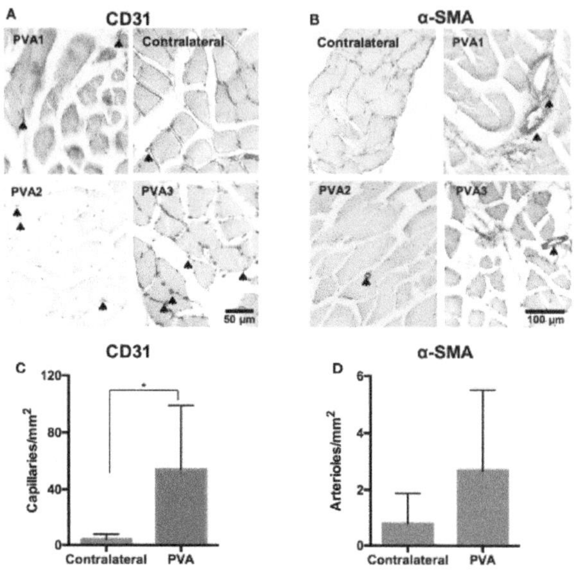

Figure 7: Capillary and arteriole density in hindlimb of PVA group. Sections of hindlimb muscle from PVA group (n = 3) and contralateral group (n = 5) were stained for CD31 [(A), 200×] or α-smooth muscle actin (α-SMA) [(B), 100×] antigen. Vessels positive for antigen are denoted by black arrows and brown staining. (C,D) Quantification of vessel density per unit area. *Denotes statistical significance using one-way ANOVA. No statistical differences in arteriole density were observed between groups.

DISCUSSION

Microvascular surgery is becoming more prevalent in the field yet alternatives to the use of autologous submillimeter grafts have not yet fully developed. There is a dearth of clinically efficacious artificial submillimeter diameter vascular grafts. The primary causes of failure of vascular grafts at this size scale are thrombogenicity and material mismatch (particularly, mismatch of diameter and compliance) with the native artery. PVA is commonly used for biomedical applications due to its bioinertness, its ability to imbibe water without compromising mechanical integrity and its tunable mechanical properties. To this end, PVA grafts with submillimeter diameter were mechanically tuned to create a new microvascular graft candidate.

At the microvascular size scale, surgery becomes increasingly difficult and increases risk of blood flow stasis, platelet activation and thrombosis (Sarkar et al., 2006). Nonetheless, the characteristics of PVA grafts were suitable to facilitate anastomosis at this dimension and maintain short-term patency. First, close approximation of the PVA graft mechanical properties, especially the diameter and the compliance, to the rabbit femoral artery likely aided maintenance of normal blood flow and propagation of pulsatile flow. In addition, PVA grafts were easily molded into submillimeter dimensions without loss of mechanical integrity; this contributed to the improved outcome of the anastomosis by minimizing manipulation of the native vessel, which is fragile and susceptible to spasm and thrombosis during clamping (Fujimaki et al., 1977; Siemionow, 1987). Spontaneous luminal opening of PVA graft coupled with its elasticity, suture retention, and overall ease of handling likewise aided the anastomosis, which invariably contributed to graft patency (Siemionow, 1987; Chen et al., 2001). In contrast, the use of the relatively stiff vascular graft made of ePTFE with 1 mm ID showed a dismal 8% patency rate after 2 weeks in the rabbit femoral artery despite a good caliber match (Lidman et al., 1980). Ganske et al. (1982)reported even more drastic outcomes of thrombosis within 48 h postimplantation of ePTFE grafts implanted in the same location. The group further reported that the only patent ePTFE graft showed good tissue attachment but without any indication of endothelialization.

Second, improved resistance to thrombosis and patency can also be attributed to the low thrombogenic potential *in vitro* and endothelialization *in vivo* of the submillimeter PVA vascular grafts. Flat PVA films were previously demonstrated by Ino et al. (2013) to induce similar platelet adherence and thrombin generation with the classic vascular graft material ePTFE. Recently, PVA graft thrombogenicity was tested using a baboon *ex vivo* assay, a more physiologically relevant system that mimics the hydrostatics, hemodynamics and blood chemistry found in small diameter vascular grafts after implantation (Cutiongco et al., 2015a). The authors have reported that PVA grafts with diameter of ~3.75 mm have a lower platelet accumulation profile and total fibrin deposition compared with ePTFE. Thus, tuning the mechanical properties of submillimeter diameter PVA grafts did not deteriorate its low thrombogenic potential.

After 2 weeks of implantation, we observed the patency of 67% of PVA grafts. In at least one of the grafts, an endothelial layer was observed on the luminal surface. The observations are made more remarkable by the fact that the animal subjects did not receive any anticoagulant or antithrombotic regimen. Overall, the mechanical and surface properties of submillimeter diameter PVA graft are strongly advantageous for clinical application in microvascular surgery.

However, PVA vascular grafts are far from universal in its application in microvascular surgery. Natural tapering compounded with variation in blood vessel caliber may cause mismatch at the distal anastomosis. The occlusion of PVA2 graft, which showed possible intimal hyperplastic tissue toward the distal end, supported this notion. It may be necessary to create PVA grafts with gradual tapering to accommodate natural changes in vessel diameter.

In addition to accommodating caliber, changes in compliance, tensile strength, and other mechanical properties should be accommodated. PVA can theoretically be adapted to accommodate multiple types of arteries from different anatomical location. Here, cross-linking degree of PVA was modified by manipulating the cross-linking temperature. PVA cross-linking is speculated to depend on the local concentration of alkaline, which is highly dependent on water evaporation rate. The myriad types of PVA available, with different acetylation degrees and molecular weight, present flexibility in the characteristics of the hydrogel obtained. For instance, this study and that of Ino et al. (2013) cross-linked PVA with different acetylation degrees, resulting in PVA with different material properties. The crosslinker STMP and the alkaline content contributed by sodium hydroxide can also be easily modified to control the rate and extent of cross-linking between the PVA chains and STMP. By increasing STMP and sodium hydroxide content, Chaouat et al. (2008) PVA graft (2 mm ID) matched mechanical properties of the rat abdominal aorta. The flexibility of the material and the cross-linking conditions make PVA an outstanding material that can potentially be used as an off-the-shelf vascular graft for various vascular applications.

It should be noted that Chaouat et al. has previously shown patency of PVA grafts with millimeter dimensions in the rat abdominal aorta. While both rat abdominal aorta and rabbit femoral artery share similar diameters (Byrom et al., 2010) different hemodynamics and hematology of the animal species may contribute to dissimilar graft performance. The high blood flow and shear stress in the aorta, combined with the decreased blood coagulation profile, possibly led to better patency in the rat model. In contrast, rabbits have coagulation profile more closely resembling those of humans (Byrom et al., 2010). Furthermore, the rabbit femoral artery has reduced blood flow from the multilevel arterial occlusion. It is known that increasing severity of distal arterial occlusion is correlated with lower graft patency and limb salvage in humans (O'Mara et al., 1981; Toursarkissian et al., 2002). Though the etiology is not well understood, the main suspect for graft failure in presence of poor blood outflow is the hemodynamic changes caused by distal vessel occlusion. The patency of the submillimeter PVA graft observed in this stringent rabbit model further exemplifies the usefulness of this graft for vascular applications.

AUTHOR CONTRIBUTIONS

EY, JH, CLV and JP were responsible for conception and design of the study. MC, MK, JP, MY, JY, AR, and EY performed data collection. MC, MK, CLV, AR, JH, and EY were responsible for data analysis and interpretation. MC and EY were mainly responsible for writing the manuscript. All authors approve this final version of the article.

CONFLICT OF INTEREST STATEMENT

The authors declare that the research was conducted in the absence of any commercial or financial relationships that could be construed as a potential conflict of interest.

ACKNOWLEDGMENTS

This research is funded by the Singapore Ministry of Health's National Medical Research Council Exploratory/Developmental Grant Scheme (NMRC/EDG/0068/2009). The work was also partially funded by Singapore A*STAR-ANR (1122703037) and the National Research Foundation, Prime Minister's Office, Singapore under its Research Center of Excellence programme administered by the Mechanobiology Institute.

The authors are grateful to Prof. Kofidis from the NUS Department of Surgery for generously lending the Doppler ultrasound machine. The authors would like to thank Prof. PT Wong at the NUS Department of Pharmacology for generously providing the laser Doppler flowmeter. The authors would like to acknowledge Mr. Bryan Chua for the mechanical testing; Dr. Mie Yamamoto, Mr. AAK Moe and Ms. Ervi Sju for setting up the animal surgery; and Mr. Brian Teo, Mr. James Low, and Ms. Mafe Villejo for assisting in the surgeries. KM, JP, and MY contributed equally to this work. MC thanks the support of the NMRC fund.

REFERENCES

1. Barnes, R. W. (1980). Hemodynamics for the vascular surgeon. *Arch. Surg.* 115, 216–223. doi:10.1001/archsurg.1980.01380020082021
2. Barzin, J., and Madaeni, S. S. (2007). Hemodialysis membranes prepared from poly(vinyl alcohol): effects of the preparation conditions on the morphology and performance. *J. Appl. Polym. Sci.* 104, 2490–2497. doi:10.1002/app.25627
3. Byrom, M. J., Bannon, P. G., White, G. H., and Ng, M. K. C. (2010). Animal models for the assessment of novel vascular conduits. *J. Vasc. Surg.* 52, 176–195. doi:10.1016/j.jvs.2009.10.080
4. Chaouat, M., Le Visage, C., Baille, W. E., Escoubet, B., Chaubet, F., Mateescu, M. A., et al. (2008). A novel cross-linked poly(vinyl alcohol) (PVA) for vascular grafts. *Adv. Func. Mater.* 15, 2855–2861. doi:10.1002/adfm.200701261
5. Chen, Y. X., Chen, L. E., Seaber, A. V., and Urbaniak, J. R. (2001). Comparison of continuous and interrupted suture techniques in microvascular anastomosis. *J. Hand. Surg.* 26, 530–539. doi:10.1053/jhsu.2001.22933
6. Cutiongco, M. F. A., Anderson, D. E. J., Hinds, M. T., and Yim, E. K. F. (2015a). In vitro and ex vivo hemocompatibility of off-the-shelf modified poly(vinyl alcohol) vascular grafts. *Acta Biomater.* 25, 97–108. doi:10.1016/j.actbio.2015.07.039
7. Cutiongco, M. F. A., Choo, R. K. T., Shen, N. J. X., Chua, B. M. X., Sju, E., Choo, A. W. L., et al. (2015b). Composite scaffold of poly(vinyl alcohol) and interfacial polyelectrolyte complexation fibers for controlled biomolecule delivery. *Front. Bioeng. Biotechnol.* 3:3. doi:10.3389/fbioe.2015.00003
8. Cutiongco, M. F. A., Goh, S.-H., Aid-Launais, R., Le Visage, C., Yee, L. H., and Yim, E. K. F. (2016). Planar and tubular patterning of micro and nano-topographies on poly(vinyl alcohol) hydrogel for improved endothelial cell responses. *Biomaterials* 84, 184–195. doi:10.1016/j.biomaterials.2016.01.036
9. Doi, K., Tominaga, S., and Shibata, T. (1977). Bone grafts with microvascular anastomoses of vascular pedicles: an experimental study in dogs. *J. Bone Joint Surg. Am.* 59, 809–815.
10. Fathi, E., Nassiri, S. M., Atyabi, N., Ahmadi, S. H., Imani, M., Farahzadi, R., et al. (2013). Induction of angiogenesis via topical delivery of basic-fibroblast growth factor from polyvinyl alcohol-dextran blend hydrogel in an ovine model of acute myocardial infarction. *J. Tissue Eng. Regen. Med.* 7, 697–707. doi:10.1002/

term.1460

11. Feng, S., Chen, H., Liu, Y., Huang, Z., Sun, X., Zhou, L., et al. (2013). A novel vitreous substitute of using a foldable capsular vitreous body injected with polyvinylalcohol hydrogel. *Sci. Rep* 3, 1838. doi:10.1038/srep01838
12. Fujimaki, A., O'Brien, B., Kurata, T., and Threlfall, G. (1977). Experimental micro-anastomosis of 0.4-0.5 mm vessels. *Br. J. Plast. Surg.*30, 269–272. doi:10.1016/0007-1226(77)90115-1
13. Ganske, J. G., Demuth, R. J., Miller, S. H., Buck, D. C., and Dolph, J. L. (1982). Comparison of expanded polytetrafluoroethylene microvascular grafts to autogenous vein grafts. *Plast. Reconstr. Surg.* 70, 193–201. doi:10.1097/00006534-198208000-00013
14. Gemmell, C. H., Yeo, E. L., and Sefton, M. V. (1997). Flow cytometric analysis of material-induced platelet activation in a canine model: elevated microparticle levels and reduced platelet life span. *J. Biomed. Mater. Res.* 37, 176–181. doi:10.1002/(SICI)1097-4636(199711)37:2<176:AID-JBM5>3.0.CO;2-O
15. Griffin, J. R., and Thornton, J. F. (2005). Microsurgery: free tissue transfer and replantation. *Selected Readings Plast. Surg.* 10, 1–41.
16. Harris, J. R., and Seikaly, H. (2002). Evaluation of polytetrafluoroethylene micrografts in microvascular surgery. *J. Otolaryngol.* 31, 89–92. doi:10.2310/7070.2002.18928
17. Iglarz, M., Silvestre, J. S., Duriez, M., Henrion, D., and Levy, B. I. (2001). Chronic blockade of endothelin receptors improves ischemia-induced angiogenesis in rat hindlimbs through activation of vascular endothelial growth factor-no pathway. *Arterioscler. Thromb. Vasc. Biol.* 21, 1598–1603. doi:10.1161/hq1001.097065
18. Ino, J. M., Sju, E., Ollivier, V., Yim, E. K. F., Letourneur, D., and Le Visage, C. (2013). Evaluation of hemocompatibility and endothelialization of hybrid poly(vinyl alcohol) (PVA)/gelatin polymer films. *J. Biomed. Mater. Res.* 101, 1549–1559. doi:10.1002/jbm.b.32977
19. Judet, H., Judet, J., and Gilbert, A. (1981). Vascular microsurgery in orthopaedics. *Int. Orthop* 5, 1–9. doi:10.1007/s00586-016-4494-4
20. Kobayashi, M., Chang, Y.-S., and Oka, M. (2005). A two year in vivo study of polyvinyl alcohol-hydrogel (PVA-H) artificial meniscus.*Biomaterials* 26, 3243–3248. doi:10.1016/j.biomaterials.2004.08.028
21. Lamponi, S., Leone, G., Consumi, M., Greco, G., and Magnani, A. (2012). In vitro biocompatibility of new PVA-based hydrogels as vitreous body substitutes. *J. Biomater. Sci. Polym. Ed.* 23, 555–575. doi:10.1163/092050611X554499
22. Lanzetta, M. (1995). Clinical use of microvascular PTFE grafts. *Microsurgery* 16, 412–415. doi:10.1016/j.jacc.2015.11.066
23. Lidman, D. H., Faibisoff, B., and Daniel, R. K. (1980). Expanded polytetrafluoroethylene as a microvascular graft: an experimental study. *Microsurgery* 1, 447–456. doi:10.1002/micr.1920010607

24. O'Mara, C. S., Flinn, W. R., Neiman, H. L., Bergan, J. J., and Yao, J. S. (1981). Correlation of foot arterial anatomy with early tibial bypass patency. *Surgery* 89, 743–752.

25. Sarkar, S., Salacinski, H. J., GG, H., and Seifalian, A. M. (2006). The mechanical properties of infrainguinal vascular bypass grafts: their role in influencing patency. *Eur. J. Vasc. Endovasc. Surg.* 31, 627–636. doi:10.1016/j.ejvs.2006.01.006

26. Sarkar, S., Schmitz-Rixen, T., Hamilton, G., and Seifalian, A. M. (2007). Achieving the ideal properties for vascular bypass grafts using a tissue engineered approach: a review. *Med. Biol. Eng. Comput.* 45, 327–336. doi:10.1007/s11517-007-0176-z

27. Shen, T., Mitchell, G., Morrison, W., and O'Brien, B. (1988). The use of long synthetic microvascular grafts to vascularise free flaps in rabbits. *Br. J. Plast. Surg.* 41, 305–312. doi:10.1016/0007-1226(88)90116-6

28. Siemionow, M. (1987). Evaluation of long-term patency rates of different techniques of arterial anastomosis in rabbits. *Microsurgery* 8, 25–29. doi:10.1002/micr.1920080108

29. Silvestre, J. S., Mallat, Z., Duriez, M., Tamarat, R., Bureau, M. F., Scherman, D., et al. (2000). Antiangiogenic effect of interleukin-10 in ischemia-induced angiogenesis in mice hindlimb. *Circ. Res.* 87, 448–452. doi:10.1161/01.RES.87.6.448

30. So, T. Y. (1998). Freeze-dried vessels as interpositional grafts in microsurgery. *Microsurgery* 18, 248–255. doi:10.1002/(SICI)1098-2752(1998)18:4<248::AID-MICR7>3.0.CO;2-F

31. Toursarkissian, B., D'Ayala, M., Stefanidis, D., Shireman, P. K., Harrison, A., Schoolfield, J., et al. (2002). Angiographic scoring of vascular occlusive disease in the diabetic foot: relevance to bypass graft patency and limb salvage. *J. Vasc. Surg.* 35, 494–500. doi:10.1067/mva.2002.120046

32. Uchida, N., Emoto, H., Kambic, H., Harasaki, H., Chen, J. F., Hsu, S. H., et al. (1989). Compliance effect on patency of small diameter vascular grafts. *ASAIO Trans.* 35, 556–558. doi:10.1097/00002480-198907000-00124

33. Wan, W. K., Campbell, G., Zhang, Z. F., Hui, A. J., and Boughner, D. R. (2002). Optimizing the tensile properties of polyvinyl alcohol hydrogel for the construction of a bioprosthetic heart valve stent. *J. Biomed. Mater. Res.* 63, 854–861. doi:10.1002/jbm.10333

34. Yim, E. K. F., Liao, I. C., and Leong, K. W. (2007). Tissue compatibility of interfacial polyelectrolyte complexation fibrous scaffold: evaluation of blood compatibility and biocompatibility. *Tissue Eng.* 13, 423–433. doi:10.1089/ten.2006.0113

13
CHAPTER

ANALYTICAL SIDE-TO-SIDE RELATED ANASTOMOTIC STRATEGIES AND ARTERY PATCHING

P.C Roussis, A.E Giannakopoulos, H.P Charalambous

Keywords: Artery patching, elastic mismatch, end-to-side anastomosis, side-to-side anastomosis, suture line intimal thickening, suture line stress concentration

INTRODUCTION

In the field of cardiovascular surgery, there are several studies driven by the need to assess and prevent post-surgery complications. In the case of end-to-side and side-to-side anastomosis, long-term complications primarily involve the development of intimal hyperplasia that results in stenosis of the blood vessel. From the literature, among the factors considered to induce intimal hyperplasia are the arterial wall mechanics, hemodynamics, biological activities and compliance between the host artery and the graft. Yet, it is not completely clear which are the factors that influence most the development of intimal hyperplasia and in what specific way.

Special attention has been given to the effect of elastic (compliance) mismatch between the graft and the host artery. Recent end-to-side anastomosis techniques that use "compliant" patches or cuffs, are the Taylor-patch anastomosis and Miller-cuff anastomosis. Studies suggest that these techniques may reduce the stress concentrations at the suture line and therefore the generation of intimal hyperplasia [1, 2].

An end-to-side anastomosis develops intimal hyperplasia at two regions of the anastomosis: the suture line and the artery floor opposite of the distal anastomosis [3, 4]. Bassiouny *et al.* [3] found that the development of intimal hyperplasia at the suture line of conventional end-to-side anastomosis is promoted by healing mechanisms,

Citation: P.C Roussis, A.E Giannakopoulos, H.P Charalambous, Analytical Side-to-Side Related Anastomotic Strategies and Artery Patching, DOI: 10.2174/97816809436271150901.

compliance mismatch and triangulation of the anastomotic junction that may result in complex hemodynamic patterns. They also suggested that intimal hyperplasia on the artery floor is developed due to low wall shear stresses and hemodynamic factors that generate stagnation points at that region. Noberto *et al.* [5] experimentally investigated the effect of the expansibility of vein cuffs by jacketing the cuff with an artificial material. They concluded that the good patency rates of Miller-cuff technique are not correlated to the mechanical properties of the cuffs. Moreover, Noori *et al.* [6] studied the flow patterns of different end-to-side techniques and found that only the Miller-cuff technique appears to have better flow patterns due to its wider anastomotic cavity. Furthermore, clinical studies on side-to-side anastomosis showed that this technique has larger patency rates and better fluid dynamics [7,8]. Our study does not deal with the hemodynamic analysis and flow patterns of side-to-side related anastomosis. It focuses primarily on the suture line behavior in terms of displacements, strains, and stress concentration.

To identify the problem of side-to-side related anastomosis by means of stress concentration, it must be noted that the local stress concentration of an arterial branch (referring to a branch that was not surgically formed) is primarily affected by the geometry of the junction [9]. In the case of anastomosis, the junction is additionally stressed due to the suture-arterial tissue contact at the stitching holes. The present study aims to investigate if the elastic mismatch constitutes a third factor for further stress concentration at the suture line, thereby influencing the development of intimal hyperplasia. Results of this study suggest that elevated elastic mismatch between the artery and the graft/patch does not affect the internal forces of the blood vessels and the system is dominated by almost uniform axial hoop stress. Furthermore, elevated elastic mismatch decreases the radial displacements of the graft, the graft strains and the radial displacement at the junction. The far-field stresses of the artery and the graft are of the same magnitude regardless of the stiffness of the materials. The incompatible angle of the junction appears to be an important response parameter that is affected by the artery/graft compliance mismatch, whereas there is no correlation between elastic mismatch and elevated stress concentration at the suture line.

METHODS

This section presents the mathematical formulation governing the static response of the side-to-side related arterial anastomosis. The system response is described in terms of the internal forces, the radial and tangential displacements, the strains of the blood vessels, and the rotation angle of their cross section. In addition, the dynamic behavior of the model is evaluated in order to examine its significance.

Anastomosis Model and Response to Static Loading

Fig. (1) shows the three end-to-side anastomoses and the side-to-side anastomosis techniques that can be analyzed by the proposed method. End-to-side anastomosis techniques include the conventional anastomosis, Taylor-patch anastomosis and Miller-cuff anastomosis [1-6, 10].

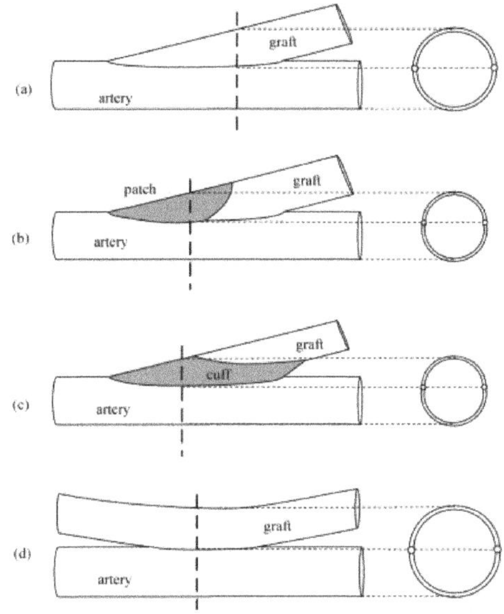

Figure 1: Sections that can be modeled as two hinged circular systems: (a) conventional end-to-side anastomosis; (b) Taylor-patch anastomosis; (c) Miller-cuff anastomosis; (d) side-to-side anastomosis.

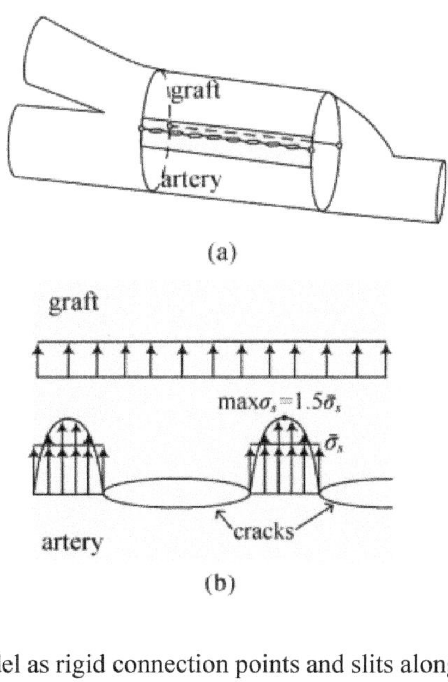

Figure 2: (a) Stitching model as rigid connection points and slits along the suture line, (b) Stress concentration at the suture line.

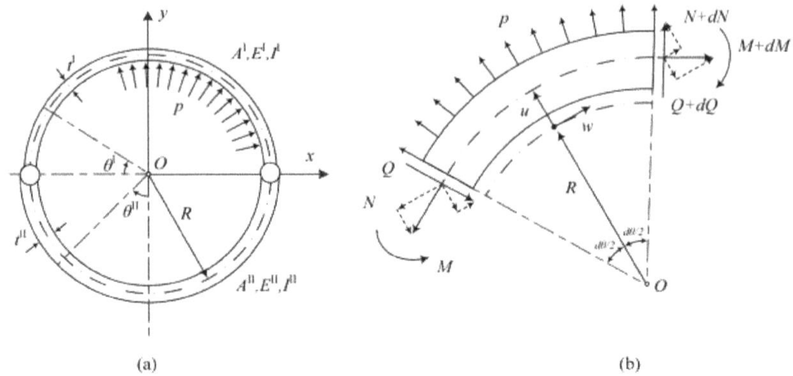

Figure 3: (a) Two-hinged anastomosis model, (b) Typical element of circular sector under static loading.

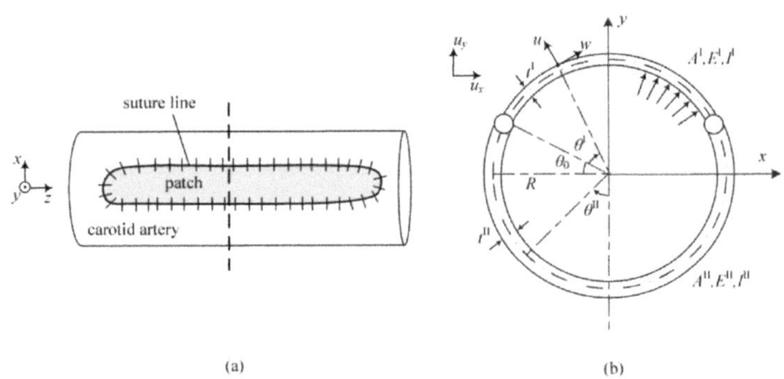

Figure 4: (a) Carotid endrarterectomy with longitudinal patch, (b) Two hinged anastomosis model with the hinges placed at the ends of any chord of the centerline. (I: patch, II: artery).

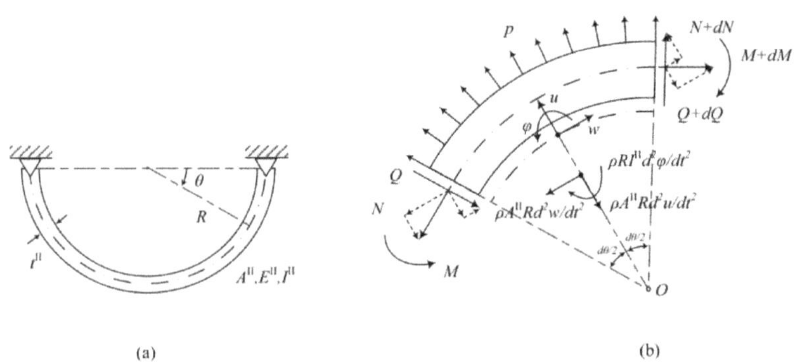

Figure 5: (a) Two-hinged artery segment under the assumption of rigid graft, (b) Typical element of arterial circular sector under dynamic loading.

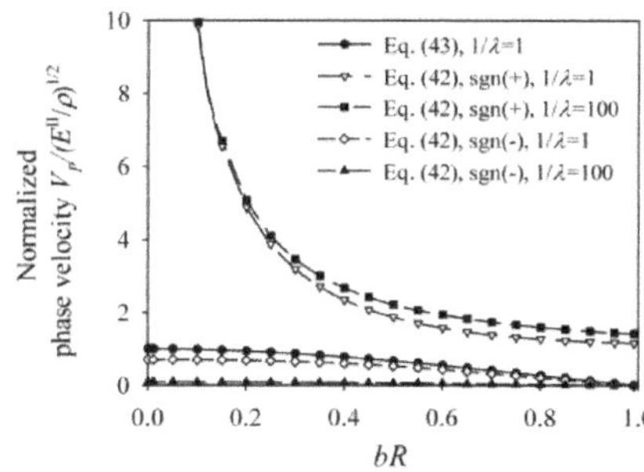

Figure 6: Dispersion curves.

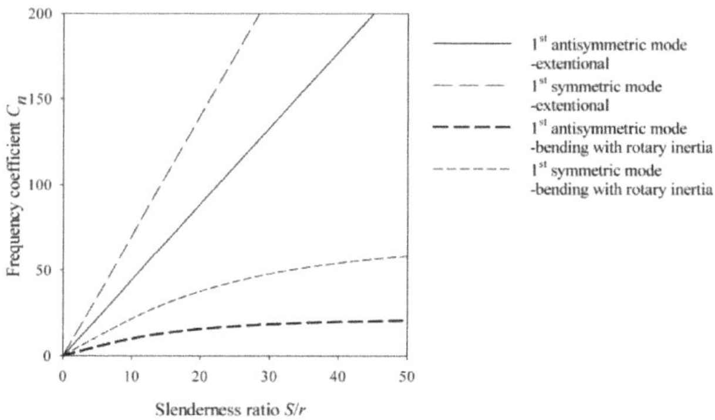

Figure 7: Frequency curves of first antisymmetric and symmetric modes.

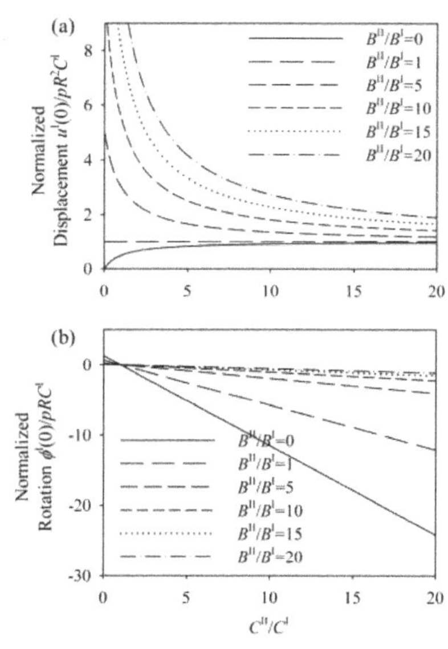

Figure 8: (a) Normalized displacement at the junction, (b) Normalized rotation of the cross section at the junction.

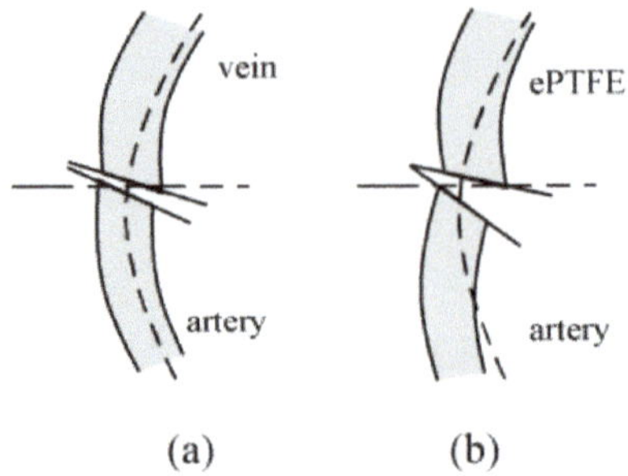

Figure 9: Rotation of the cross sections at the junction of (a) artery/vein anastomosis, (b) artery/ ePTFE anastomosis.

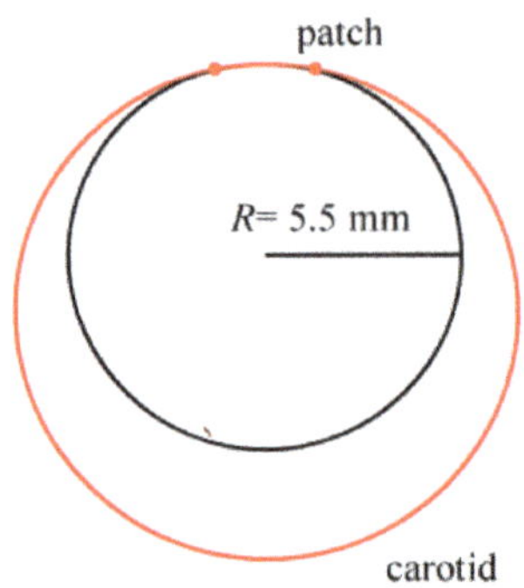

Figure 10: Scheme of global deformation of patched carotid model. The scales of the undeformed and deformed configurations are equal.

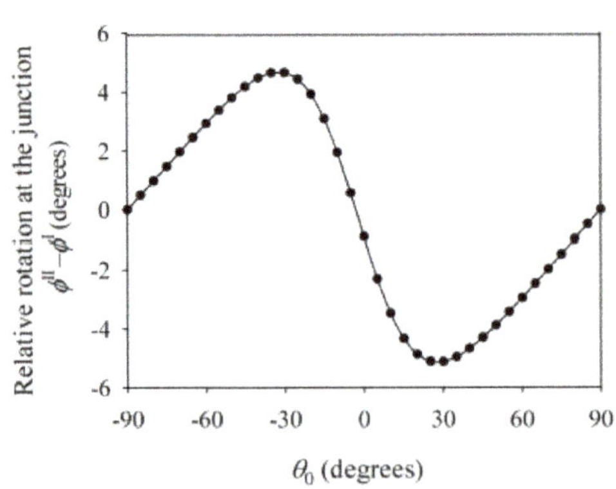

Figure 11: Relative rotation of the cross section of the PTFE patch and the carotid artery at the junction as a function of angle θ0. Large values of θ0 correspond to thinner patches.

The detailed stitching at the suture line can be modeled as a solid surface with cracks (microslits) as shown in Fig. (2a). The cracks are located between the sutures, and the embedding stress σ_s is distributed parabolically along the stitch thickness according to the smooth contact solution of Hertz (Fig. (2b)). Therefore, the maximum embedding stress at the suture line is , where $\sigma_s = 1.5\bar{\sigma}_s$, where $\bar{\sigma}_s$ is the average embedding stress. The average embedding stress increases when the stress concentration or the distance between sequential stitches is increased and/or the suture diameter is decreased.

By considering a vertical plane section in the end-to-side or side-to-side anastomosis of Fig. (1), the resulting system can be approximated by a two hinged circular model, consisting of two semicircles with different elasticity modulus, cross-sectional areas and moments of inertia. The two-hinged circular model consists of element I representing the graft that is connected to the artery side and element II representing the host artery (Fig. (3a)). Element I has thickness t^{I}, cross sectional area A^{I}, Young's modulus E^{I} and moment of inertia I^{I}, whereas element II has thickness t^{II}, cross sectional area A^{II}, Young's modulus E^{II} and moment of inertia I^{II}. The unloaded centerline of the two elements is assumed to form a circle with radius *R*. The sutures are modeled by two hinges that separate the centerline into two semicircles. The varying angles of each element fall in the range $0 \le \theta^{\mathrm{I}} \le \pi$ and $-\pi/2 \le \theta^{\mathrm{II}} \le \pi/2$, respectively, with their origins indicated in Fig. (3a). When subjected to uniform internal pressure p, the system is deformed in the radial direction by $u(\theta)$ and in the tangential direction by $w(\theta)$.

The problem is solved as a boundary value problem of continuous curved beams [11,12]. The static differential equations governing the response of the system can be derived by considering the equilibrium of forces acting on an infinitesimal element of the circular ring shown in Fig. (3b), where $N(\theta)$ is the tangential tensile force, $Q(\theta)$ is the shearing force, and $M(\theta)$ is the in-plane bending moment. By using the radial, tangential and moment equilibrium of the infinitesimal element the resulting equations are, respectively

$$\frac{dQ^i(\theta)}{d\theta} - N^i(\theta) = -pR \tag{1}$$

$$\frac{dN^i(\theta)}{d\theta} + Q^i(\theta) = 0 \tag{2}$$

$$\frac{dM^i(\theta)}{d\theta} - RQ^i(\theta) = 0 \tag{3}$$

Notation i takes the forms I, II when referring to elements I and II respectively. By assuming extensibility of the centerline, the tangential force $N^i(\theta)$ and moment $M^i(\theta)$ can be expressed in terms of displacements as

$$M^{i}(\theta)=\frac{E^{i}I^{i}}{R^{2}}\left(\frac{dw^{i}(\theta)}{d\theta}-\frac{d^{2}u^{i}(\theta)}{d\theta^{2}}\right) \tag{4}$$

$$N^{i}(\theta)=\frac{E^{i}A^{i}}{R}\left(u^{i}(\theta)+\frac{dw^{i}(\theta)}{d\theta}\right) \tag{5}$$

The symmetric boundary conditions of elements I and II are respectively

$$M^{\mathrm{I}}(0)=0,\ w^{\mathrm{I}}(0)=0,\ w^{\mathrm{I}}\left(\frac{\pi}{2}\right)=0,\ \frac{du^{\mathrm{I}}}{d\theta}\left(\frac{\pi}{2}\right)=0,\ Q^{\mathrm{I}}\left(\frac{\pi}{2}\right)=0 \tag{6}$$

$$M^{\mathrm{II}}\left(\frac{\pi}{2}\right)=0,\ w^{\mathrm{II}}\left(\frac{\pi}{2}\right)=0,\ w^{\mathrm{II}}(0)=0,\ \frac{du^{\mathrm{II}}}{d\theta}(0)=0,\ Q^{\mathrm{II}}(0)=0 \tag{7}$$

and the continuity equations between the two elements are

$$N^{\mathrm{I}}(0)=N^{\mathrm{II}}\left(\frac{\pi}{2}\right),\ Q^{\mathrm{I}}(0)=Q^{\mathrm{II}}\left(\frac{\pi}{2}\right),\ u^{\mathrm{I}}(0)=u^{\mathrm{II}}\left(\frac{\pi}{2}\right) \tag{8}$$

By combining Eqs. (1) through (8), the response of the two elements in terms of axial forces, shear forces, moments, radial and tangential displacements can be derived. For element I ($0\le\theta^{\mathrm{I}}\le\pi$) the normalized response is given by

$$\frac{N^{\mathrm{I}}(\theta)}{pR}=A\sin\theta+1 \tag{9}$$

$$\frac{Q^{\mathrm{I}}(\theta)}{pR}=-A\cos\theta \tag{10}$$

$$\frac{M^{\mathrm{I}}(\theta)}{pR^{2}}=-A\sin\theta \tag{11}$$

$$\frac{u^{\mathrm{I}}(\theta)}{R}=B^{\mathrm{I}}ApR\cos\theta+\left(\frac{1}{2A^{\mathrm{I}}E^{\mathrm{I}}}-\frac{R^{2}}{2E^{\mathrm{I}}I^{\mathrm{I}}}\right)ApR\sin\theta-\frac{2B^{\mathrm{I}}}{\pi}ApR\theta\cos\theta+C^{\mathrm{I}}pR \tag{12}$$

$$\frac{w^{\mathrm{I}}(\theta)}{R}=-B^{\mathrm{I}}ApR\sin\theta+\frac{2B^{\mathrm{I}}}{\pi}ApR\theta\sin\theta \tag{13}$$

In which

$$A=\frac{C^{\mathrm{II}}-C^{\mathrm{I}}}{B^{\mathrm{II}}+B^{\mathrm{I}}} \tag{14}$$

$$B^{\mathrm{I}} = \frac{\pi}{4}\left(\frac{1}{A^{\mathrm{I}}E^{\mathrm{I}}} + \frac{R^2}{E^{\mathrm{I}}I^{\mathrm{I}}}\right) \tag{15}$$

$$B^{\mathrm{II}} = \frac{\pi}{4}\left(\frac{1}{A^{\mathrm{II}}E^{\mathrm{II}}} + \frac{R^2}{E^{\mathrm{II}}I^{\mathrm{II}}}\right) \tag{16}$$

$$C^{\mathrm{I}} = \frac{1}{A^{\mathrm{I}}E^{\mathrm{I}}} \tag{17}$$

$$C^{\mathrm{II}} = \frac{1}{A^{\mathrm{II}}E^{\mathrm{II}}} \tag{18}$$

Furthermore, the strain of the middle-wall surface and the rotation of the cross section at any point along the circular arch are respectively

$$\varepsilon^{\mathrm{I}}(\theta) = \frac{u^{\mathrm{I}}(\theta)}{R} + \frac{1}{R}\frac{dw^{\mathrm{I}}(\theta)}{d\theta} = pRC^{\mathrm{I}}\left(A\sin\theta + 1\right) \tag{19}$$

$$\varphi^{\mathrm{I}}(\theta) = \frac{1}{R}\left(\frac{du^{\mathrm{I}}(\theta)}{d\theta} - w^{\mathrm{I}}(\theta)\right) \tag{20}$$

Parameter A indicates the elastic and geometric mismatch between the host artery and the graft. The response of the artery (element II) can be easily obtained from equations (9) through (18) by assuming that the artery represents element I and the graft represents element II.

The Case of Patched Carotid Artery

The problem of patching with longitudinal graft materials can be solved by developing a similar model in which the graft occupies a smaller part of the model. Longitudinal patches are frequently used for carotid endarterectomies [13]. The main post-surgery complications of this technique are the development of intimal hyperplasia, suture line bleeding and patch infection.

Fig. (4a) shows a patched carotid artery and the vertical plane section that can be approximated by two circular parts connected by two hinges (Fig. (4b)). The hinge locations correspond to the suturing position. To appropriately model this system we solved the general problem in which the hinges can be placed at the edges of any chord of the centerline. The origins of the varying angles of each part are shown in Fig. (4b) and have range $0 \le \theta^{\mathrm{I}} \le \pi - 2\theta_0$ (patch) and $-\pi/2 - \theta_0 \le \theta^{\mathrm{II}} \le \pi/2 + \theta_0$ (artery), respectively.

The static differential equations governing the response of the system are expressed by Eqs. (1) through (5) and the symmetric boundary conditions of parts I and II are respectively

$$M^{I}(0)=0,\ u_y^{I}(0)=0,\ u_x^{I}\left(\frac{\pi}{2}-\theta_0\right)=0,\ \frac{du_y^{I}}{d\theta}\left(\frac{\pi}{2}-\theta_0\right)=0,\ Q^{I}\left(\frac{\pi}{2}-\theta_0\right)=0 \tag{21}$$

$$M^{II}\left(\frac{\pi}{2}+\theta_0\right)=0,\ u_y^{II}\left(\frac{\pi}{2}+\theta_0\right)=0,\ u_x^{II}(0)=0,\ \frac{du_y^{II}}{d\theta}(0)=0,\ Q^{II}(0)=0 \tag{22}$$

where u_x^i and u_y^i are the global horizontal and vertical displacements respectively (i = I for patch and i = II for artery). The continuity equations between the two parts are

$$N^{I}(0)=N^{II}\left(\frac{\pi}{2}+\theta_0\right),\ Q^{I}(0)=Q^{II}\left(\frac{\pi}{2}+\theta_0\right),\ u_x^{I}(0)=u_x^{II}\left(\frac{\pi}{2}+\theta_0\right) \tag{23}$$

After calculations the response of the system is solved, providing the axial forces, shear forces, moments, radial and tangential displacements, strains of the middle wall surface and the relative rotation at the hinges. The complete expressions of the solution are presented in the Appendix.

Effect of Dynamic Excitation

To answer the question if the dynamic vibration of the artery is significant and must be taken into consideration, the long-term dynamic response of element II has to be evaluated. The evaluation is performed in terms of dispersion graphs and the frequency coefficient. In particular, the graft is assumed to be rigid and the artery is modeled as a pinned circular arch (Fig. (5a)). This model constitutes the most unfavorable case of elevated elastic mismatch.

The analysis includes an extensibility of the centerline of the arch and rotary inertia, whereas shear deformations are ignored. By considering the equilibrium of forces acting on the infinitesimal element of Fig. (5b) the in-plane dynamic response is described by the following equations of motion:

$$\frac{\partial Q^{II}(\theta,t)}{\partial\theta}-N^{II}(\theta,t)=\rho A^{II}R\frac{\partial^2 u^{II}(\theta,t)}{\partial t^2}-p(\theta,t)R \tag{24}$$

$$\frac{\partial N^{II}(\theta,t)}{\partial\theta}+Q^{II}(\theta,t)=\rho A^{II}R\frac{\partial^2 w^{II}(\theta,t)}{\partial t^2} \tag{25}$$

$$\frac{\partial M^{II}(\theta,t)}{\partial\theta}-RQ^{II}(\theta,t)=\rho RI^{II}\frac{\partial^2 \varphi^{II}(\theta,t)}{\partial t^2} \tag{26}$$

where ρ is the artery density and $\varphi^{II}(\theta,t)$ is the rotation of the artery cross section. The rotation is expressed in terms of displacements as

$$\varphi^{II}(\theta,t)=\frac{1}{R}\left(\frac{\partial u^{II}(\theta,t)}{\partial\theta}-w^{II}(\theta,t)\right) \tag{27}$$

The tangential force $N^{\mathrm{II}}(\theta,t)$ and moment $M^{\mathrm{II}}(\theta,t)$ are expressed in terms of displacements as

$$M^{\mathrm{II}}(\theta,t)=\frac{E^{\mathrm{II}}I^{\mathrm{II}}}{R^2}\left(\frac{\partial w^{\mathrm{II}}(\theta,t)}{\partial\theta}-\frac{\partial^2 u^{\mathrm{II}}(\theta,t)}{\partial\theta^2}\right) \tag{28}$$

$$N^{\mathrm{II}}(\theta,t)=\frac{E^{\mathrm{II}}A^{\mathrm{II}}}{R}\left(u^{\mathrm{II}}(\theta,t)+\frac{\partial w^{\mathrm{II}}(\theta,t)}{\partial\theta}\right) \tag{29}$$

By solving Eq. (26) for $Q^{\mathrm{II}}(\theta,t)$ and using Eqs. (27) and (28), the shear force is

$$Q^{II}(\theta,t)=\frac{E^{II}I^{II}}{R^3}\left(\frac{\partial^2 w^{II}(\theta,t)}{\partial\theta^2}-\frac{\partial^3 u^{II}(\theta,t)}{\partial\theta^3}\right)+\frac{\rho I^{II}}{R}\frac{\partial^2}{\partial t^2}\left(\frac{\partial u^{II}(\theta,t)}{\partial\theta}-w^{II}(\theta,t)\right) \tag{30}$$

By substituting Eqs. (28) through (30) into Eqs. (24) and (25), and by assuming free-vibration conditions $(p(\theta,t)=0)$, we obtain two equations that include terms of displacements only:

$$\frac{E^{II}I^{II}}{R^3}\left(\frac{\partial^3 w^{II}(\theta,t)}{\partial\theta^3}-\frac{\partial^4 u^{II}(\theta,t)}{\partial\theta^4}\right)+\frac{\rho I^{II}}{R}\frac{\partial^2}{\partial t^2}\left(\frac{\partial^2 u^{II}(\theta,t)}{\partial\theta^2}-\frac{\partial w^{II}(\theta,t)}{\partial\theta}\right)-\frac{E^{II}A^{II}}{R}\left(u^{II}(\theta,t)+\frac{\partial w^{II}(\theta,t)}{\partial\theta}\right) \tag{31}$$

$$\frac{E^{II}A^{II}}{R}\left(\frac{\partial u^{II}(\theta,t)}{\partial\theta}+\frac{\partial^2 w^{II}(\theta,t)}{\partial\theta^2}\right)+\frac{E^{II}I^{II}}{R^3}\left(\frac{\partial^2 w^{II}(\theta,t)}{\partial\theta^2}-\frac{\partial^3 u^{II}(\theta,t)}{\partial\theta^3}\right)+\frac{\rho I^{II}}{R}\frac{\partial^2}{\partial t^2}\left(\frac{\partial u^{II}(\theta,t)}{\partial\theta}-w^{II}(\theta,t)\right) \tag{32}$$

These partial differential equations are coupled through the radial and tangential displacement. By assuming a harmonic solution (with frequency ω) of the form

$$u^{\mathrm{II}}(\theta,t)=U(\theta)e^{i\omega t} \tag{33}$$

$$w^{\mathrm{II}}(\theta,t)=W(\theta)e^{i\omega t} \tag{34}$$

Eqs. (31) and (32) become

$$\left(-\frac{\partial^4}{\partial\theta^4}-\frac{\partial^2}{\partial\theta^2}k\lambda+k-\frac{1}{\lambda}\right)U-\left[-\frac{\partial^3}{\partial\theta^3}+\frac{\partial}{\partial\theta}\left(\frac{1}{\lambda}-k\lambda\right)\right]W\equiv L_1U-L_2W=0 \tag{35}$$

$$\left[-\frac{\partial^3}{\partial\theta^3}+\frac{\partial}{\partial\theta}\left(\frac{1}{\lambda}-k\lambda\right)\right]U-\left[\frac{\partial^2}{\partial\theta^2}\left(-1-\frac{1}{\lambda}\right)-k\lambda-k\right]W\equiv L_3U-L_4W=0 \tag{36}$$

in which $k=\rho A^{\mathrm{II}}R^4\omega^2/(E^{\mathrm{II}}I^{\mathrm{II}})$, $\lambda=I^{\mathrm{II}}/(A^{\mathrm{II}}R^2)$ and U and W are the normal functions of u^{II} and w^{II}. The system of equations is then decoupled as

$$\left(L_1L_4 - L_2L_3\right)U = 0 \tag{37}$$

$$\left(L_1L_4 - L_2L_3\right)W = 0 \tag{38}$$

Therefore, the decoupled differential equations of the radial and tangential displacements are identical and are expressed respectively as

$$U^{(6)} + U^{(4)}\left(2 + 2k\lambda\right) + U^{(2)}\left(1 - k + k\lambda + k^2\lambda^2\right) + U\left(k + k\lambda - k^2\lambda - k^2\lambda^2\right) = 0 \tag{39}$$

$$W^{(6)} + W^{(4)}\left(2 + 2k\lambda\right) + W^{(2)}\left(1 - k + k\lambda + k^2\lambda^2\right) + W\left(k + k\lambda - k^2\lambda - k^2\lambda^2\right) = 0 \tag{40}$$

in which $U^{(n)}$, $W^{(n)}$ denote the nth partial derivative of U and W with respect to θ .

To the authors' best knowledge, this is the first time that the decoupled equations of free vibration of an extensible circular arch with rotary inertia (by ignoring shear deformation) are correctly derived. The usual practice is to either include or ignore both rotary inertia and shear deformation. In this study, we deal with the problem of thin rings in which the effect of shear deformation is insignificant.

Dispersion Curves

By using the wave propagation theory, the dynamic response of the system can be evaluated through the dynamic dispersion curves [14]. We assume that the radial and tangential displacements are expressed by the waves of type

$$u^{\mathrm{II}}(\theta,t) = Ue^{i(b\theta R - \omega t)} \tag{41}$$

$$w^{\mathrm{II}}(\theta,t) = We^{i(b\theta R - \omega t)} \tag{42}$$

where b denotes the wave number. The wave equations along the circular ring are:

$$U(\theta) = Ue^{ib\theta R} \tag{43}$$

$$W(\theta) = We^{ib\theta R} \tag{44}$$

The expression $V_P = \omega / b$ denotes the phase velocity of the system. The differential equations of the radial and tangential displacement are identical, therefore by substituting Eq. (43) in Eq. (39) and solving for the normalized phase velocity $V_p / (\sqrt{E^{\mathrm{II}} / \rho})$, one can obtain the dispersion relations of the circular ring as

$$\frac{V_p}{\sqrt{\frac{E^{II}}{\rho}}}=\sqrt{\frac{\left(2b^4R^4+\frac{b^2R^2}{\lambda}-b^2R^2+\frac{1}{\lambda}+1\right)\pm\sqrt{\left(2b^4R^4+\frac{b^2R^2}{\lambda}-b^2R^2+\frac{1}{\lambda}+1\right)^2-4b^2R^2\left(b^2R^2-1\right)^2\left(b^2R^2+\frac{1}{\lambda}+1\right)}}{b^2R^2\left(b^2R^2+\frac{1}{\lambda}+1\right)}}$$

(45)

In the case where the centerline of the ring is inextensible, the dispersion relation is given by

$$\frac{V_p}{\sqrt{\frac{E^{II}}{\rho}}}=\sqrt{\lambda}\,\frac{1-b^2R^2}{\sqrt{1+b^2R^2}}$$

(46)

Fig. (6) presents the dispersion curves of the system. All the curves decrease with increased wave number, indicating that the system is dispersive and its energy attenuates. Therefore, there is no concern of exhibiting abnormal increase of amplitude under dynamic loading.

Frequency Curves

The free vibration of circular arches has been studied thoroughly by many researchers [15-20]. Veletsos *et al.* [17] and Austin and Veletsos [18] suggested approximate formulas to calculate the frequency coefficient spectrum of pinned circular arches. These formulas have proven to have adequate accuracy and are suitable for calculating the natural frequencies of such systems easily.

The final frequency curves are a combination of the bending and extensional frequency coefficient curves, with the mathematical correlation of the natural frequency ω to the frequency coefficient C_n being $\omega = C_n/\left(R^2\pi^2\right)\sqrt{E^{II}I^{II}/\left(\rho A^{II}\right)}$. The bending (including rotary inertia) antisymmetric and symmetric frequency coefficients are expressed respectively as

$$C_n=m^4\pi^4\frac{\left[1-\left(\frac{1}{m}\right)^2\right]^2}{1+3\left(\frac{1}{m}\right)^2}\frac{\frac{S}{m\pi r}}{\sqrt{\left(\frac{S}{m\pi r}\right)^2+\Omega+\left[1+\Omega\left(\frac{m\pi r}{S}\right)^2\right]^{-1}}},\quad m=2n$$

(47)

$$C_n=m^4\pi^4\frac{\left[1-\left(\frac{1}{m}\right)^2\right]^2}{1+\frac{1}{m^2}+2\left(\frac{1}{m}\right)^2}\frac{\frac{S}{m\pi r}}{\sqrt{\left(\frac{S}{m\pi r}\right)^2+\Omega+\left[1+\Omega\left(\frac{m\pi r}{S}\right)^2\right]^{-1}}},\quad m=2n+1$$

(48)

where n is the number of mode, S is equal to π R , and r is the radius of gyration $\sqrt{I^{II} / A^{II}}$. In order to neglect shear deformation, the shear flexibility factor Ω is set equal to 10.

$$C_m = m\pi \frac{S}{r}\sqrt{1+\left(\frac{1}{m}\right)^2} \tag{49}$$

Odd values of m represent antisymmetric modes, whereas even values of *m* represent symmetric modes of vibration.

As shown in Fig. (7) the resultant frequency curve and subsequently the free-vibration characteristics of the system are dominated by the first antisymmetric bending mode. It is clear that the natural frequency of a two-hinged artery is much larger than the frequency of the applied force (the frequency of a typical cardiac pulse is about 7 rad/sec). Therefore, the dynamic response of the system can be adequately approximated by the static response.

RESULTS

The dynamic investigation of the anastomosis response, suggests that the dynamic effect is not significant for the long-term behavior of the two hinged model. The first natural frequency of the two-hinged circular arch appears to be large compared to the frequency of vibration (at least ten times larger). Additionally, the system is dispersive. Therefore, the static analysis constitutes an adequate approach for evaluating the anastomosis response.

We are particularly interested in calculating the response of the suture line in means of suture force f_s, displacements, strains and rotation of the cross section at the junction. The suture force is the resultant force of the tangential and radial forces at the junction ($\theta^I = 0$). The normalized suture tensile force f_s / pR constitutes a stress concentration factor due to the artery/graft compliance mismatch and is calculated as

$$\frac{f_s}{pR} = \sqrt{\left(\frac{N^I(0)}{pR}\right)^2 + \left(\frac{Q^I(0)}{pR}\right)^2} = \sqrt{1+A^2} \tag{50}$$

The normalized radial displacement at the junction ($\theta^I = 0$), is obtained from Eq. (12) and expressed as

$$\frac{u^I(0)}{pR^2C^I} = \frac{\left(B^{II}/B^I\right)+\left(C^{II}/C^I\right)}{1+B^{II}/B^I} \tag{51}$$

Furthermore, the normalized rotation of the cross section at the junction, for $C^I \ll B^I$, can be derived from Eq. (20) as

$$\frac{\varphi^I(0)}{pRC^I} \approx \frac{4}{\pi}\frac{1-C^{II}/C^I}{1+B^{II}/B^I} \tag{52}$$

For typical values of geometric and mechanical properties of the two blood vessels, parameter A ranges from 0 to ±0.01. Thus, the stress concentration at the suture is insignificant. Furthermore, as can be seen from Eqs. (9) through (11), for low values of parameter A , the solution is dominated by almost uniform axial hoop stress N = pR , and the moments and shear forces acting along the blood vessel wall are almost zero. Based upon the situation, the strain of a blood vessel can be approximated by $\varepsilon'(\theta) \approx pRC'$ and it depends on the elastic modulus of that blood vessel.

Fig. (8) plots the normalized radial displacement and approximate normalized rotation at the junction for a range of the ratios B^{II} / B^{I} and C^{II} / C^{I} . From Eq. (51) and Fig. (8a), the radial displacement at the junction is minimized for values B^{II} / B^{I} lower than 1. The radial displacement will never be equal to zero, due to the fact that B^{II} / B^{I} will always have nonzero positive values. Equation (52) and Fig. (8b) indicate that the rotation of the cross section is minimized for large values of the ratio BII / BI and is equal to zero when C^{II} / C^{I} is equal to unity, meaning that the term $A^{I} E^{I}$ is equal to $A^{II}E^{II}$.

The maximum rotation of the artery is developed when the graft is rigid (applies when $A^{II}E^{II} \rightarrow \infty$ and $E^{II} I^{II} \rightarrow \infty$). In this case, the cross section of the graft will not rotate, whereas the cross section of the artery will undergo large rotation approximated as

$$\varphi^{II}(\pi/2) \approx \frac{4pR}{\pi A^{II} E^{I}} \tag{53}$$

For typical values of anastomosis properties, the resultant maximum value of Eq. (53) is about 10°.

Numerical Example of End-to-Side Anastomosis

The proposed analytical model is applied to an end-to-side anastomosis problem and the elastic parameters and response quantities are calculated in order to illustrate the applicability of the proposed relations. The geometric and mechanical properties of the models of Perktold *et al.* [1] are adopted, and the far-field stress values of this paper are verified against the finite element calculations of Perktold *et al.* Table 1 lists the problem parameters and response values of a conventional anastomosis (artery-ePTFE graft) and a Taylor-patch anastomosis (artery-vein patch-ePTFE graft).

Table 1: Parameters of end-to-side anastomosis of Perktold et al. and response values as proposed by this study

	Artery(II) /*vein*(I)	*Artery*(II) /*ePTFE graft*(I)
	$p = 13.33$ kPa, $R = 2$ mm, $E^{II} = 410$ kPa, $t^{II} = 0.5$ mm	
E^{I} (kPa)	820	7500
t^{I} (mm)	0.5	0.35
B^{I}	0.3678	0.1175
B^{II}	0.7356	0.7356
C^{I}	2.439e-3	3.809e-4
C^{II}	4.878e-3	4.878e-3
A	0.00221	0.005271
$\varepsilon^{I}(0)/\varepsilon^{I}(\pi/2)$	0.0650/0.0652	0.0101/0.0102
$\varepsilon^{II}(\pi/2)$	0.13	0.13
$u^{I}(0)/u^{I}(\pi/2)$ (mm)	0.173/0.092	0.053/-0.0006
σ^{I} (kPa)	53.33	75.00
σ^{II} (kPa)	53.32	53.32

Table 2: Rotation angles at the anastomosis junction as proposed by this study

	Artery(II) /vein(I)	*Artery(II) /ePTFE graft(I)*
$\varphi^{I}(0)$ (degrees)	-1.58	-1.20
$\varphi^{II}(\pi/2)$ (degrees)	-3.16	-7.52

Table 3: Parameters and response values of the patched carotid

Parameters	
p (kPa)	17.332
R (mm)	5.5
t^{I} (mm)	0.3
t^{II} (mm)	0.6
E^{I} (kPa)	8000
E^{II} (kPa)	845
θ_0 (degrees)	76
Response values	
D_1^{II} (N)	-0.00398
D_2^{II}	0.000993
$f_s/(pR)$	1
$\varepsilon^{I}(0)$	0.0397
$\varepsilon^{II}(\pi/2+\theta_0)$	0.188
$\sigma^{I}(0)$ (kPa)	317.76
$\sigma^{II}(\pi/2+\theta_0)$ (kPa)	158.88
$u_x^{I}(0)$ (mm)	-0.0529
$\lvert u^{I}_{max} \rvert$ (mm)	0.0128
$\lvert u^{II}_{max} \rvert$ (mm)	1.985
$\lvert w^{I}_{max} \rvert$ (mm)	0.0513
$\lvert w^{II}_{max} \rvert$ (mm)	0.908
$\varphi^{I}(0)$ (degrees)	-0.00185
$\varphi^{II}(\pi/2+\theta_0)$ (degrees)	-1.386
$\varphi^{III}-\varphi$ (degrees)	-1.384

Table 4: Comparison between results of Kamenskiy et al. and this study

	Kamenskiy *et al.* calculations	This study
Patch maximum cyclic strain	0.02	0.0214
Carotid maximum cyclic strain	0.1	0.1012
Patch far field stress $\log_{10}(\sigma_{eff})$ (Pa)	5.5	5.502
Carotid far field stress $\log_{10}(\sigma_{eff})$ (Pa)	5.4	5.201

The radial displacement of the junction appears to be larger in the case of artery/vein anastomosis than in the case of artery/ePTFE anastomosis, whereas the stiffer the blood vessel or graft the lower is the developed strain. The far-field stresses are approximated according to Hooke's law ($\sigma = E\varepsilon$). We can observe that the stresses are not affected by the mechanical properties of the blood vessels, due to the fact that a stiffer graft (large elasticity modulus) will develop lower strains than a soft blood vessel (low elasticity modulus). The far-field stress of the graft would be exactly equal to the far-field stress of the artery if they had the same thicknesses. For the artery and vein the far-field stress as calculated by this study is 53 kPa and for the ePTFE graft the far-field stress is 75 kPa. The finite element results of Perktold *et al.* are 50 kPa and 60 kPa respectively, which they compare well with our results.

The rotation of each cross section at the junction, as calculated by Eq. (20), is listed in Table 2. In both cases, element I is stiffer than the host artery, causing larger rotations angles for the host artery than the graft or vein. When the ePTFE graft is used, instead of the vein, the rotation angle of the artery is increased, creating larger incompatible angles that may cause injury of the arterial tissue and may promote the development of intimal hyperplasia. Fig. (9) shows the incompatible angles at the junction of the artery/vein anastomosis and the artery/ePTFE graft anastomosis.

Numerical Example of a Patched Carotid Artery

Kamenskiy *et al.* [13] studied a finite element model of a patched carotid artery. They used an exponential hyperelastic material law and modeled the stitches as fixed rigid contacts.

Table 3. lists the properties used in the analysis and the corresponding response values derived from our analysis. The geometric data of the model of Kamenskiy *et al.* were not given explicitly, therefore we used their figures and typical values for carotid arteries from the literature [21, 22]. The patch width was taken from Kamenskiy *et al.* to be about 2.7 mm. The elastic modulus for our calculations was taken at a pre-stretch of 1.08.

Fig. (10) plots the total displacements along the PTFE patch and the artery. We can observe that the artery response is much larger than the patch response and that the most significant response value appear to be the relative rotation between the artery and the patch at the junction $\varphi^{III}(\pi/2+\theta_0)-\varphi(0)$ (Table 3). Note that, the forces and strains are found to be almost uniform along the patch and the carotid. Kamenskiy et al. particularly calculated the cyclic strain (the difference of Von Misses strain between systole and diastole) and the Misses effective stress σ_{eff} values. Table 4. list the maximum cyclic strain and the far field stresses as calculated by Kamenskiy et al. and by this study. Our calculations compare well with the finite element calculations of Kamenskiy et al. Note that the far-field stresses strongly depend on the thickness of the blood vessel and that Kamenskiy et al. modeled the stitches as rigid contacts resulted to stress concentration at the suture line. On the other hand, the model proposed in this study has hinges that result in relative rotations of the connected parts.

If the size of the patch is increased, i.e the angle θ_0 is decreased, the relative rotation of the carotid and the patch at the junction will be increased (Fig. (11)). The largest relative rotation at the stitched junction is developed when $\theta_0 \approx 30°$. Therefore, thinner strips of patches seem to be more appropriate in order to prevent post-surgery complications.

DISCUSSION

The present study examined the correlation of elastic (compliance) mismatch against the suture stress concentration and development of intimal hyperplasia at the suture line of side-to-side related anastomosis. The static analysis of the system under internal pressure appears to give an adequate estimation of the long-term response, compared to the dynamic analysis, and is utilized to calculate the displacement at the junction (Eq. (51)), the strains developed at each blood vessel (Eq. (19)), and the incompatible angles at the junction (Eq. (20)).

The analysis considers an idealized two-hinged circular model, consisting of two semicircles. Therefore, the applicability of this study is limited to the analysis of anastomosis regions that can be approximated by the idealized model of Fig. (3).

Results of this study suggest that elevated elastic mismatch between the artery and the graft does not affect the internal forces of the blood vessels and the system is dominated by almost uniform axial hoop stress $N = pR$. Furthermore, elevated elastic mismatch reduces the radial displacements and strains of the graft, reduces the radial displacement at the junction, whereas the far-field stresses are of the same magnitude regardless of the material used. For typical geometrical and mechanical properties of the artery, parameter A has very low values. This favors the suture response by indicating insignificant stress concentration at the suture line in the presence of elastic mismatch (Eq. (50)).

From Fig. (8b) and Fig. (9) the incompatible angle of the junction appears to be affected by the difference between the mechanical properties of the two blood vessels. Whenever blood flow creates almost zero shear stresses at the artery wall (e.g. stagnation points, low fluid velocities, reverse flows etc.), conditions for hyperplasia set in. At such cases, the compliance mismatch between the prosthetic graft and the host artery plays an important role in the development of intimal hyperplasia in the following sense. The higher the compliance mismatch, the higher will be the incompatible angle at the junction between the graft and the artery and the blood flow at the suture line is disturbed even more. In order to minimize the rotation of the arterial cross section and avoid elevated intimal thickening, the term $A^I E^I$ must be equal to $A^{II} E^{II}$. Frequently, the graft is stiffer than the host artery. Therefore, in order to obtain zero rotation the graft thickness has to be decreased to satisfy the equality $A^I E^I = A^{II} E^{II}$. In the case of geometric mismatch (when the thicknesses of the two blood vessels differ), the far-field stresses and therefore the embedding stresses of the host artery and the graft are not equal. Their values are of the same magnitude as long as thicknesses are also of the same magnitude. Additionally, when the graft thickness is increased the compliance parameter A is also increased.

For the case that the hinges are placed at the edges of any chord of the full circle, the response value that is significantly affected is the rotation at the junction. By increasing the absolute value of angle θ_0 the relative rotation at the junction is decreased (Fig. (11)). In the case of the patched carotid, the arterial part exhibits large displacements that may lead to softening of the tissue and development of aneurysm after a long time period. Additionally, it is likely that the large rotation angle at the junction promotes (along with other parameters) the development of intimal hyperplasia, injury of the arterial tissue, and infection of the patched region.

In conclusion, the primary contribution of this study is that through the proposed model and analysis the optimal graft characteristics can be obtained in order to minimize the incompatible angle at the anastomosis junction and the development of intimal hyperplasia. The proposed model is analytical and is characterized by generality. In order to minimize the post-surgery complications of end-to-side anastomosis, side-to-side anastomosis or artery patching the following techniques are proposed for surgical application: (a) Ideally, the graft and the host artery should have the same elasticity modulus and same thickness; (b) If the graft is stiffer than the host artery, the graft thickness should be smaller than the artery thickness (aiming to satisfy the equality $A^I E^I = A^{II} E^{II}$); and (c) In the case of artery patching, given that the patch is stiffer than the artery, the patch width should be as small as possible.

CONFLICT OF INTEREST

Authors P.C. Roussis and H.P. Charalambous declare that they have no competing interests. Author A.E. Giannakopoulos has received research grant under the "ARISTEIA II" Action of the "OPERATIONAL PROGRAMME EDUCATION AND LIFELONG LEARNING", co-founded by the European Social Fund (ESF) and National Resources.

ACKNOWLEDGEMENTS

A.E. Giannakopoulos acknowledges that part of this project was implemented under the "ARISTEIA II" Action of the "OPERATIONAL PROGRAMME EDUCATION AND LIFELONG LEARNING" and is co-founded by the European Social Fund (ESF) and National Resources.

APPENDIX

The problem of patching with longitudinal graft materials can be solved by the general model that has two hinges placed at the edges of any chord of the full circle scheme (Fig. (4b)). By combining Eqs. (1) through (5) and Eqs. (21) through (23) the response of the two elements in terms of axial forces, shear forces, moments, radial and tangential displacements of the artery/element II $(-\pi/2-\theta_0 \le \theta^{II} \le \pi/2+\theta_0)$ are respectively

$$N^{II}(\theta) = D_1^{II}\cos\theta + pR \quad (54)$$

$$Q^{II}(\theta) = D_1^{II}\sin\theta \quad (55)$$

$$M^{II}(\theta) = -RD_1^{II}(\sin\theta_0 + \cos\theta) \quad (56)$$

Furthermore, the strain of the middle wall surface and the rotation of the cross section at any point along the circular arch are respectively

$$u^{II}(\theta) = D_2^{II}\cos\theta + D_1^{II}\left[\frac{\theta}{2}\sin\theta\left(\frac{R}{A^{II}E^{II}} + \frac{R^3}{E^{II}I^{II}}\right) + \frac{R^3}{E^{II}I^{II}}\sin\theta_0\right] + \frac{pR^2}{A^{II}E^{II}} \quad (57)$$

$$w^{II}(\theta) = -D_2^{II}\sin\theta + D_1^{II}\left[\left(\frac{R}{2A^{II}E^{II}} - \frac{R^3}{2E^{II}I^{II}}\right)\sin\theta + \frac{\theta}{2}\cos\theta\left(\frac{R}{A^{II}E^{II}} + \frac{R^3}{E^{II}I^{II}}\right) - \frac{R^3}{E^{II}I^{II}}\theta\sin\theta_0\right] \quad (58)$$

In which

$$D_1^{II} = \frac{pR^2\cos\theta_0\left(\frac{1}{A^IE^I} - \frac{1}{A^{II}E^{II}}\right)}{\frac{\sin\theta_0\cos\theta_0}{2}\left(\frac{R}{A^IE^I} - \frac{R^3}{E^II^I} - \frac{R}{A^{II}E^{II}} + \frac{R^3}{E^{II}I^{II}}\right) + \left(\frac{\pi}{4} - \frac{\theta_0}{2}\right)\left(\frac{R}{A^IE^I} + \frac{R^3}{E^II^I}\right) + \left(\frac{\pi}{4} + \frac{\theta_0}{2}\right)\left(\frac{R}{A^{II}E^{II}} + \frac{R^3}{E^{II}I^{II}}\right) + \sin\theta_0\left\{\frac{R^3}{E^II^I}\left[\sin\theta_0\left(\frac{\pi}{2} - \theta_0\right) - \cos\theta_0\right] + \frac{R^3}{E^{II}I^{II}}\left[\sin\theta_0\left(\frac{\pi}{2} + \theta_0\right) + \cos\theta_0\right]\right\}} \quad (59)$$

And

$$D_2^{II} = \frac{pR^2\sin\theta_0}{A^{II}E^{II}} + D_1^{II}\left\{\cos^2\theta_0\left[\frac{R}{2A^{II}E^{II}} - \frac{R^3}{2E^{II}I^{II}}\right] + \sin\theta_0\frac{R^3}{E^{II}I^{II}}\left[\sin\theta_0 - \cos\theta_0\left(\frac{\pi}{2} + \theta_0\right)\right]\right\} \quad (60)$$

$$\varepsilon^{II}(\theta) = \frac{u^{II}(\theta)}{R} + \frac{1}{R}\frac{dw^{II}(\theta)}{d\theta} = \frac{pR}{A^{II}E^{II}} + \frac{D_1^{II}\cos\theta}{A^{II}E^{II}} \quad (61)$$

$$\varphi^{II}(\theta) = \frac{D_1^{II}R^2}{E^{II}I^{II}}(\sin\theta + \theta\sin\theta_0) \quad (62)$$

The strain and rotation at the junction ($\theta = \pi/2 + \theta_0$) are

$$\varepsilon^{II}\left(\frac{\pi}{2}+\theta_0\right)=\frac{pR}{A^{II}E^{II}}-\frac{D_1^{II}\sin\theta_0}{A^{II}E^{II}} \tag{63}$$

$$\varphi^{II}\left(\frac{\pi}{2}+\theta_0\right)=\frac{D_1^{II}R^2}{E^{II}I^{II}}\left[\cos\theta_0+\sin\theta_0\left(\frac{\pi}{2}+\theta_0\right)\right] \tag{64}$$

The response of the graft (element I) can be easily obtained by using equations (54) through (64) and by assuming that element II represents the graft and element I represents the artery.

The normalized suture tensile force f_s / pR constitutes a stress concentration factor due to the artery/graft compliance mismatch and can be calculated as

$$\frac{f_s}{pR}=\sqrt{\left(\frac{N^{II}(\frac{\pi}{2}+\theta_0)}{pR}\right)^2+\left(\frac{Q^{II}(\frac{\pi}{2}+\theta_0)}{pR}\right)^2}=\sqrt{\left(D_1^{II}\right)^2-2D_1^{II}pR\sin\theta_0+(pR)^2} \tag{65}$$

REFERENCES

1. K. Perktold, A. Leuprecht, M. Prosi, T. Berk, M. Czerny, W. Trubel, and H. Schima, "Fluid dynamics, wall mechanics, and oxygen transfer in peripheral bypass anastomoses", Ann. Biomed. Eng., vol. 30, no. 4, pp. 447-460, 2002.
2. A. Leuprecht, K. Perktold, M. Prosi, T. Berk, W. Trubel, and H. Schima, "Numerical study of hemodynamics and wall mechanics in distal end-to-side anastomoses of bypass grafts", J. Biomech., vol. 35, no. 2, pp. 225-236, 2002.
3. H. S. Bassiouny, S. White, S. Glagov, E. Choi, D. P. Giddens, and C. K. Zarins, "Anastomotic intimal hyperplasia: mechanical injury or flow induced", J. Vasc. Surg., vol. 15, no. 4, pp. 708-716; discussion 716-717, 1992.
4. P. D. Ballyk, C. Walsh, J. Butany, and M. Ojha, "Compliance mismatch may promote graft-artery intimal hyperplasia by altering suture-line stresses", J. Biomech., vol. 31, no. 3, pp. 229-237, 1998.
5. J. J. Norberto, A. N. Sidawy, K. S. Trad, B. A. Jones, R. F. Neville, S. F. Najjar, M. K. Sidawy, and R. G. DePalma, "The protective effect of vein cuffed anastomoses is not mechanical in origin", J. Vasc. Surg., vol. 21, no. 4, pp. 558-566, 1995.
6. N. Noori, R. Scherer, K. Perktold, M. Czerny, G. Karner, M. Trubel, P. Polterauer, and H. Schima, "Blood flow in distal end-toside anastomoses with PTFE and a venous patch: results of an in vitro flow visualisation study", Eur. J. Vasc. Endovasc. Surg., vol. 18, no. 3, pp. 191-200, 1999.
7. K. M. Vural, E. Sener, and O. Taşdemir, "Long-term patency of sequential and individual saphenous vein coronary bypass grafts", Eur. J. Cardiothorac. Surg., vol. 19, no. 2, pp. 140-144, 2001.
8. Song Min-Ho, Tokuda Yoshiyuki, and Ito Toshiaki, "Revival of the side-to-side

approach for distal coronary anastomosis", J. Cardiothorac. Surg., vol. 2, no. 1, p. 2, 2007. Available from: http://www.cardiothoracicsurgery.org/content/2/1/2

9. M. J. Thubrikar, S. K. Roskelley, and R. T. Eppink, "Study of stress concentration in the walls of the bovine coronary arterial branch", J. Biomech., vol. 23, no. 1, p. 15-26, 1990.
10. X.-M. Li and S. E. Rittgers, "Computational simulation of biomechanics in e-PTFE and venous Miller's cuffs: implications for intimal hyperplasia", J. Med. Eng. Technol., vol. 29, no. 4, pp. 187-196, 2005.
11. A. E. H. Love, A Treatise on the mathematical theory of elasticity. Dover: New York 1944.
12. S. S. Rao, "Vibration of Continuous Systems", John Wiley & Sons, USA, 2007.
13. A. V. Kamenskiy, I. I. Pipinos, A. S. Desyatova, Y. E. Salkovskiy, L. Yu Kossovich, I. V. Kirillova, L. A. Bockeria, K. M. Morozov, V. O. Polyaev, T. G. Lynch, and Y. A. Dzenis, "Finite element model of the patched human carotid", Vasc. Endovasc. Surg., vol. 43, no. 6, pp. 533-541, 2009.
14. K. F. Graff, "Wave Motion in Elastic Solids", Courier Dover Publications: USA, 1975.
15. L. L. Philipson, "On the role of extension in the flexural vibrations of rings", J. Appl. Mech., vol. 23, pp. 364-366, 1956.
16. D. G. Ashwell, A. B. Sabir, and T. M. Roberts, "Further studies in the application of curved finite elements to circular arches", Int. J. Mech. Sci., vol. 13, no. 6, pp. 507-517, 1971.
17. A. S. Veletsos, W. J. Austin, L. Pereia, C. A, and S.-J. Wung, "Free In-Plane Vibration of Circular Arches", J. Eng. Mech. Div., vol. 98, no. 2, pp. 311-329, 1972.
18. W. J. Austin and A. S. Veletsos, "Free vibration of arches flexible in shear", J. Eng. Mech. Div., vol. 99, no. 4, pp. 735-753, 1973.
19. J. Kirkhope, "In-plane vibration of a thick circular ring", J. Sound Vib., vol. 50, no. 2, pp. 219-227, 1977.
20. M. S. Issa, T. M. Wang, and B. T. Hsiao, "Extensional vibrations of continuous circular curved beams with rotary inertia and shear deformation, I: Free vibration", J. Sound Vib., vol. 114, no. 2, pp. 297-308, 1987.
21. A. Delfino, N. Stergiopulos, J. E. Moore Jr, and J.-J. Meister, "Residual strain effects on the stress field in a thick wall finite element model of the human carotid bifurcation", J. Biomech., vol. 30, no. 8, pp. 777-786, 1997.
22. A. V. Kamenskiy, J. N. MacTaggart, I. I. Pipinos, J. Bikhchandani, and Y. A. Dzenis, "Three-Dimensional Geometry of the Human Carotid Artery", J. Biomech. Eng., vol. 134, no. 6, pp. 064502.1- 064502.7, 2012.

14
CHAPTER

RELATIONSHIP OF SHORT-TERM BLOOD PRESSURE VARIABILITY WITH CAROTID INTIMA-MEDIA THICKNESS IN HYPERTENSIVE PATIENTS

Yujie Chen, Huahua Xiong, Dan Wu, Sandeep Pirbhulal, Xiaohong Tian3, Ruiqin Zhang, Minhua Lu, Wanqing Wu and Wenhua Huang

Keywords: Blood pressure variability, Intima-media, Hypertension

BACKGROUND

High blood pressure (BP) is the most important risk factor for stroke [1, 2, 3] and other vascular events, accounting for approximately 54% of stroke and 47% of ischemic heart disease worldwide [4]. Physiologically, BP undergoes continuous fluctuations over time as a result of a complex interaction among cardiovascular control mechanisms. Recently, the study suggests that blood pressure variability (BPV) has been proved to be promising in providing potential regulatory mechanisms of the cardiovascular system [5]. Frattola et al. also constitute the first longitudinal evidence that cardiovascular complications of hypertension may depend on the degree of 24-h BPV [6]. Moreover, the population-based prospective studies [7, 8] have shown that ambulatory blood pressure (ABP) better predicts than clinic BP measurements the risk of subsequent cardiovascular events. So in our study the assessment of short-term BPV in the clinical setting is made possible by the growing use of ambulatory BP monitoring (ABPM) [7, 9]. From these recordings, it is possible to examine the prognostic of ABPM and its BPV evaluated with standard deviation (SD), coefficient of variation (CV), and average real variability (ARV) over the hypertensive people in the southern area of China.

In previous studies, in both longitudinal [6, 10, 11, 12] and cross-sectional studies [13, 14, 15, 16], has clearly shown that useful information may arise from analysis of BPV, and variation in blood pressure has also been reported to be associated with

Citation: Yujie Chen, Huahua Xiong, Dan Wu, Sandeep Pirbhulal, Xiaohong Tian, Ruiqin Zhang, Minhua Lu, Wanqing Wu and Wenhua Huang, Relationship of short-term blood pressure variability with carotid intima-media thickness in hypertensive patients, DOI: 10.1186/s12938-015-0059-8.

cerebrovascular diseases. One cause link for this association was the development of atherosclerosis [11, 17]. And the widely use of B-mode ultrasound offers the opportunity to assess the intima-media thickness (IMT) of carotid artery as a reliable market for the extent of atherosclerosis [18, 19]. Date from previous investigations indicated that the carotid IMT was positively correlated to ambulatory blood pressure measurement (ABPM) [13, 14]. For example, in the study of Sander et al. [14], they found that the SD of diurnal systolic BPV as the strongest predictor for IMT. The previous research [15] also showed that both the daytime, and 24 h systolic BPV evaluated by SD, CV, and ARV are positively associated with IMT. Mena et al. [20] found that ARV added prognostic value to the ABPM [15] and could prompt the use of therapeutic measures to control BPV. Therefore the question that has arisen from the above findings is obviously which pressure has the greater clinical significance and can thus be taken as the best predictor of the patient's cerebrovascular risk.

This paper will address this issue on the basis of the relationship between BPV and IMT to demonstrate the major impact of circadian blood pressure patterns on the development of early carotid atherosclerosis. In our study, we calculate SD, CV, and ARV of average systolic (SBP), diastolic (DBP), and mean BP values over the 24 h, with the daytime and the nighttime periods separately considered. We designed this study to prospectively analyze the relationship between changes in circadian blood pressure patterns and the progression of early carotid atherosclerosis. The aim is to found the greater association between IMT and BPV evaluated by three indices in hypertension, in the hope of promoting the application of 24-h BPV for the assessment of preclinical atherosclerosis.

METHODS

Study population

The study was conducted in the Second People's Hospital of Shenzhen, Guangdong Province, China. 78 individuals aged 28–79 years (57.7% male gender) were enrolled in this study. They fulfilled the following inclusion criteria: (1) patients with a clinical diagnosis of essential hypertension; (2) no history or clinical evidence of diabetes mellitus (fasting serum glucose <7.0 mmol/L; non fasting serum glucose <11.1 mmol/L); (3) both 24 h BP monitoring and carotid artery ultrasound measurement were performed; (4) the valid BP measurements within 24 h $>90\%$. The Institutional Ethics Committee of the Second People's Hospital of Shenzhen (China) approved this study, and the informed consent was obtained from every subject.

Ambulatory BP measurement

All of the subjects underwent 24 h ABPM on a day of daily activity. A proper cuff was selected according to the size of subject's arm and placed on the non-dominant arm. The subjects were asked to keep their arms still at the time of measurements. The ambulatory BP was recorded automatically using a commercial device (MobilGraph 24 h ABP-Control). The daytime BP monitoring was from 7:00 to 22:59, measured automatically every 30 min, and during the nighttime, from 23:00 to 6:59, the BP was measured once an hour. According to the recorded 24 h BP measurements, BPV was evaluated through the calculations of SD, CV, and ARV of the SBP and diastolic BP (DBP) during daytime, nighttime, and over 24 h. For the short-term (with 24 h) BPV analysis, SD, CV, and ARV are the common indices of BPV in time domain.

Carotid artery ultrasound examination

The carotid artery ultrasound was examined using a high-resolution ultrasound Doppler system (iU22, Philips Ultrasound, Bothell, WA, USA), with a 7.5 MHz liner array transducer. During the examination, the subjects were supine in the bed, with the head turned 45° away from the examined side. The left and right common carotid arteries, carotid bulbs, and internal carotid arteries were scanned in three angles (lateral, anterior, and posterior). Thus, we can assess the mean IMT in each position from the three measurements in different angles. The specific places we measured in the carotid artery were defined as follows: the IMT at the common carotid artery was measured on the far wall of blood vessel, 10–20 mm proximal to the carotid bifurcation. The carotid bulb we measured was in the carotid bifurcation, and the IMT at the internal carotid artery was measured over a distance of 10–20 mm from the bifurcation. In our study, the correlation analysis will focus on the common carotid artery, and thus carotid IMT in this paper represents the IMT at the common carotid artery, which is an average of right and left IMT. Besides, the abnormal IMT is defined that the IMT at the common carotid artery is more than 1.0 mm.

Statistical analysis

All statistical analyses were performed using SPSS statistical package (SPSS Inc., Chicago, IL, USA). Simple regression analyses for BPV and IMT/number of plaques were determined. Quintile analysis was applied to determine the relation between BPV and IMT, in which subjects were divided into five groups according to the distribution of the variability. Multiple regression analyses were also performed to evaluate the relation between BPV and IMT. We defined the carotid IMT/number of plaques as the dependent factor and the BPV estimated with SD, CV, and ARV as the independent factors, respectively. When the correlation coefficient r was close to 1, it indicated that the BPV had highly positive correlation with IMT. On the contrary, when r was close to −1, the relativity about BPV and IMT was negative. A P value of <0.05 was considered significant. Data are reported as mean ± SD.

RESULTS

Among all of the hypertensive participants, we excluded the cases that had the incomplete or invalid measurements. Finally, a total of 78 patients aged 28–79 (male 57.7%) were successfully obtained in the study. Of those, 43 subjects had the normal carotid IMT, and 35 subjects had a carotid IMT more than 1.0 mm, which is defined as the abnormal IMT. Table 1 summarized the clinical characteristics of all the subjects and two subgroups: the subjects with the normal IMT and the subjects with the abnormal IMT. The data of clinical characteristics were expressed as means ± SDs or percentages. In this table, mean SBP and DBP in different periods of time, mean PP in daytime and nighttime, BP decreasing percent from day to night, IMTs at different carotid arteries and the plaque status were reported. No significant differences were documented between the normal IMT group and abnormal IMT group regarding the BP values. However, for the baseline characteristics, the subjects in the abnormal IMT group were significantly older than the subjects in the normal IMT group ($P < 0.05$). And smoking rates in the abnormal IMT group was higher (34.3%), which is statistical significance ($P < 0.05$). Besides, in the abnormal IMT group, 77.1% of subjects had the plaques, which is higher than that in the normal IMT group ($P < 0.001$). Moreover, the abnormal IMT group had a significantly greater IMT both at bulb and internal carotid artery than the normal IMT group ($P < 0.001$), and most of them tended to suffer from the prevalence of the atherosclerotic plaques ($P < 0.001$). We evaluated the BPV using SD, CV, and ARV, and the average BPV values quantified with three indices in 24 h were reported in Table 2. We compared the correlations of these BPV values in each group of the two using Pearson's test. Except the DBPV in nighttime between CV and SD, ARV respectively. ($P > 0.05$), no significant differences were found among the three indices of BPV, they had strongly positive correlation ($P < 0.01$). Moreover, we found that all of the systolic blood pressure variability (SBPV) values were greater than those of DBPV when evaluated using SD and ARV. In contrast, the DBPV values were found to be greater than SBPV when using CV as a measure.

Table 1: Clinical characteristics of all the subjects and the two subgroups: normal IMT group and abnormal IMT group

Characteristics	All subjects (N = 78)	IMT <1.0 mm (N = 43)	IMT ≥1.0 (N = 35)	T(x^2)值	P value
Age (years)	55.9 ± 13.0	51.7 ± 12.9	61.1 ± 11.4	−3.374	0.001**
Male gender (%)	57.7	55.8	60	−0.368	0.714
Smoking (%)	23.1	14	34.3	−2.088	0.041*
IMT ≥1.0 mm	44.9	0	100	−9.950	0.000**
Presence of plaque (%)	51.3	30.2	77.1	−4.601	0.000**
CCA IMT (mm)	1.0 ± 0.2	0.78 ± 0.12	1.16 ± 0.11	−14.474	0.000**
Bulb IMT (mm)	0.8 ± 0.3	0.67 ± 0.14	1.00 ± 0.26	−6.754	0.000**
ICA IMT (mm)	0.6 ± 0.1	0.52 ± 0.08	0.66 ± 0.13	−5.630	0.000**
24 h SBP (mmHg)	125.1 ± 15.4	124.5 ± 13.4	125.9 ± 17.7	−0.394	0.695
24 h DBP (mmHg)	81.5 ± 12.8	82.7 ± 11.8	80.0 ± 14.0	0.928	0.356
24 h PP (mmHg)	43.6 ± 8.6	41.8 ± 6.4	45.9 ± 10.5	−2.030	0.047*
Daytime SBP (mmHg)	126.2 ± 15.3	125.5 ± 13.2	127.0 ± 17.7	−0.430	0.669
Daytime DBP (mmHg)	84.3 ± 15.8	84.8 ± 12.9	83.7 ± 18.9	0.284	0.777
Daytime PP (mmHg)	41.9 ± 11.3	40.7 ± 8.4	43.4 ± 14.1	−0.973	0.335
Nighttime SBP (mmHg)	121.0 ± 17.6	120.4 ± 16.0	121.6 ± 19.6	−0.298	0.767

Nighttime DBP (mmHg)	77.6 ± 13.7	78.3 ± 12.8	76.8 ± 14.9	0.484	0.630
Nighttime PP (mmHg)	43.3 ± 10.0	42.1 ± 7.8	44.8 ± 12.2	−1.109	0.272
SBP decrease (%)	2.3 ± 6.8	2.7 ± 5.2	1.9 ± 8.2	0.371	0.713
DBP decrease (%)	4.1 ± 7.2	4.2 ± 5.4	4.0 ± 8.6	0.102	0.919

Table 2: The blood pressure variabilities evaluated with SD, CV, and ARV for all subjects (N = 78)

Variables	**SD (mmHg)**		**CV (%)**		**ARV (mmHg)**	
	Mean ± SD	**$r(P)^1$**	**Mean ± SD**	**$r(P)^2$**	**Mean ± SD**	**$r(P)^3$**
Daytime SBPV	11.2 ± 3.5	0.865** (0.000)	9.2 ± 2.5	0.687** (0.000)	9.1 ± 2.7	0.801** (0.000)
Daytime DBPV	9.1 ± 2.7	0.286* (0.011)	13.4 ± 4.1	0.497** (0.000)	9.1 ± 2.9	0.623** (0.000)
Nighttime SBPV	9.5 ± 3.6	0.377** (0.001)	9.3 ± 3.0	0.377** (0.001)	10.1 ± 4.6	0.861** (0.000)
Nighttime DBPV	8.0 ± 2.6	0.164 (0.152)	14.4 ± 4.6	0.093 (0.420)	8.9 ± 2.9	0.768** (0.000)
24 h SBPV	11.6 ± 3.2	0.891** (0.000)	9.3 ± 2.6	0.731** (0.000)	9.1 ± 2.7	0.823** (0.000)
24 h DBPV	9.2 ± 2.0	0.453** (0.000)	13.9 ± 4.0	0.439** (0.000)	8.0 ± 1.9	0.662** (0.000)

Table 3 depicted the correlation coefficients between different indices of BPV and carotid IMT in all subjects. As the results showed, for all the subjects, there is no significant correlation between the BPV and RCCA-IMT, whereas, the SD, CV, and ARV of daytime SBP showed a positive correlation with LCCA-IMT ($r^1 = 0.312$, $P = 0.005$; $r^1 = 0.255$, $P = 0.024$; $r^1 = 0.284$, $P = 0.012$, resp.). Moreover, 24 h SBPV evaluated by SD and ARV were significantly related to LCCA-IMT ($r^1 = 0.261$, $P = 0.021$; $r^1 = 0.262$, $P = 0.021$, resp.). For the daytime DBPV, ARV indices was significantly related to LCCA-IMT ($r^1 = 0.239$, $P = 0.035$), which differed form BPV evaluated by SD and CV. For the night time, there is no significant correlation between the BPV and IMT. In addition, for the mean CCA-IMT, only daytime SBPV evaluated with SD and ARV indices were significant (for SD, $r^3 = 0.231$, $P = 0.041$; for ARV, $r^3 = 0.266$, $P = 0.019$.). In addition, the correlations between the different indices of BPV and number of plaques also were shown in Table 3. The results indicated that there was no significant correlation between BPV and the number of plaques of RCCA, whereas, the ARV of daytime SBPV, 24 h SBPV and nighttime DBPV showed a positive correlation with the number of plaques of LCCA ($r^1 = 0.356$, $P = 0.008$; $r^1 = 0.297$, $P = 0.027$; $r^1 = 0.278$, $P = 0.040$, resp.). Moreover, for the number of plaques of mean CCA, only daytime SBPV evaluated with ARV was significant ($r^3 = 0.278$, $P = 0.016$).

Table 3: The correlation between the blood pressure variability (evaluated with SD, CV, and ARV) and carotid intima-media thickness/number of plaques in all the subjects

Variables	IMT			Number of plaques		
	r(P)[1]	**r(P)[2]**	**r(P)[3]**	**r(P)[1]**	**r(P)[2]**	**r(P)[3]**
SD						
Daytime SBPV	0.312** (0.005)	0.103 (0.368)	0.231* (0.041)	0.146 (0.286)	0.073 (0.596)	0.065 (0.584)
Daytime DBPV	0.098 (0.391)	0.037 (0.745)	0.076 (0.51)	0.002 (0.989)	−0.105 (0.443)	−0.104 (0.378)
Nighttime SBPV	0.053 (0.646)	0.008 (0.945)	0.033 (0.771)	0.156 (0.255)	0.078 (0.572)	0.014 (0.907)
Nighttime DBPV	0.046 (0.686)	0.136 (0.235)	0.105 (0.359)	0.215 (0.115)	0.149 (0.279)	0.142 (0.227)
24 h SBPV	0.261* (0.021)	0.119 (0.298)	0.213 (0.061)	0.151 (0.272)	0.100 (0.467)	0.065 (0.584)
24 h DBPV	0.098 (0.392)	0.068 (0.555)	0.093 (0.416)	−0.005 (0.970)	−0.058 (0.671)	−0.104 (0.378)
CV						
Daytime SBPV	0.255* (0.024)	0.117 (0.306)	0.208 (0.067)	0.167 (0.223)	0.122 (0.373)	0.105 (0.374)
Daytime DBPV	0.172 (0.132)	0.132 (0.248)	0.172 (0.133)	0.174 (0.203)	0.077 (0.575)	0.097 (0.410)
Nighttime SBPV	0.08 (0.485)	0.146 (0.201)	0.13 (0.258)	0.097 (0.481)	0.080 (0.560)	0.059 (0.616)
Nighttime DBPV	0.007 (0.95)	0.143 (0.212)	0.088 (0.444)	0.172 (0.209)	0.195 (0.153)	0.130 (0.268)
24 h SBPV	0.215 (0.059)	0.146 (0.202)	0.203 (0.075)	0.175 (0.202)	0.142 (0.301)	0.122 (0.301)
24 h DBPV	0.145 (0.206)	0.153 (0.18)	0.169 (0.139)	0.200 (0.142)	0.145 (0.292)	0.118 (0.316)
ARV						
Daytime SBPV	0.284* (0.012)	0.188 (0.099)	0.266* (0.019)	0.356** (0.008)	0.241 (0.077)	0.278* (0.016)
Daytime DBPV	0.239* (0.035)	0.076 (0.511)	0.175 (0.126)	0.150 (0.275)	0.100 (0.467)	0.076 (0.523)
Nighttime SBPV	−0.014 (0.904)	−0.008 (0.941)	−0.013 (0.913)	0.155 (0.259)	0.054 (0.698)	0.025 (0.834)
Nighttime DBPV	0.053 (0.646)	0.16 (0.162)	0.123 (0.285)	0.278* (0.040)	0.137 (0.317)	0.186 (0.113)
24 h SBPV	0.262* (0.021)	0.122 (0.286)	0.215 (0.059)	0.297* (0.027)	0.151 (0.270)	0.188 (0.108)
24 h DBPV	0.202 (0.077)	0.097 (0.398)	0.167 (0.143)	0.241 (0.077)	0.129 (0.348)	0.138 (0.240)

As Fig. 1 showed, the SBPV during daytime and 24 h had greater correlation than DBPV during daytime and 24 h. Moreover, the correlations of the SBPV (evaluated with SD, CV, and AVR) and IMT were almost the same. However, for the DBPV during the daytime and 24 h, the SD and CV indices of BPV had greater correlation with IMT than ARV index.

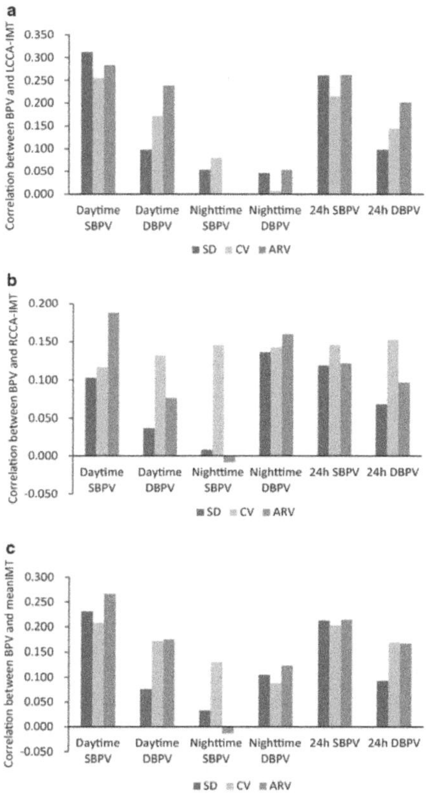

Figure 1: The correlation of the blood pressure variability and carotid intima-media thickness in all subjects. *BPV* blood pressure variability, *IMT* intima-media thickness, *CV* coefficient of variation, *ARV* average real variability, *SBPV*systolic blood pressure variability, *DBPV* diastolic blood pressure variability.

To further compare the results, we described these correlations between variability of SBP and mean CCA-IMT in Fig. 2. It assesses association of increases in mean CCA-IMT with stepwise increases in the variability of 24-h, daytime and nighttime SBP (evaluated with SD, CV, and ARV). The correlation of three indices of SBPV during daytime and mean CCA-IMT were almost the same. Moreover, the mean CCA-IMT of patients who's SD of daytime SBP was 10.5 mmHg and above was significantly higher than that of the patients whose SD of daytime SBP was below 10.5 mmHg.

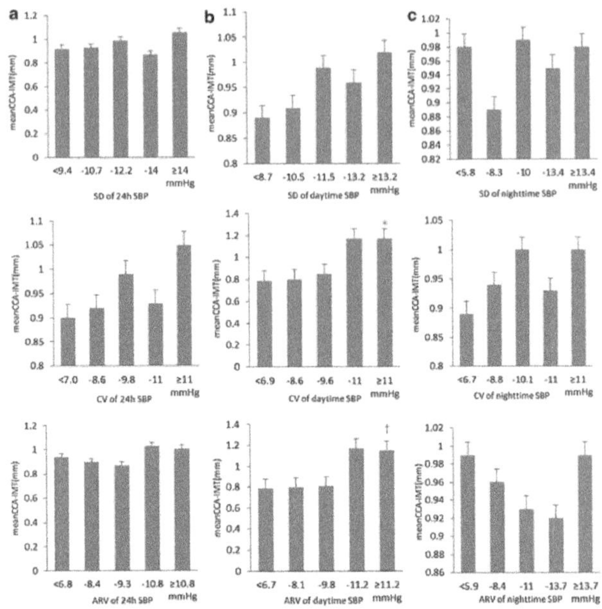

Figure 2: Changes in mean CCA-IMT in association with stepwise increases in SBPV (evaluated with SD, CV, and ARV) in hypertensives. Values are means ± S.E.M. **a** Variability of 24 h SBP. **b** Variability of daytime SBP. *P < 0.05 vs the <6.9 mmHg group. †P < 0.05 vs the <8.1 mmHg group. **c** Variability of nighttime SBP.

The mean CCA-IMT of patients having CV of daytime SBP was 9.6 mmHg and above was significantly higher than that of the patients who are CV of daytime SBP was below 9.6 mmHg. The mean CCA-IMT of patients who's ARV of daytime SBP was 9.8 mmHg and above was significantly higher than that of the patients who are ARV of daytime SBP was below 9.8 mmHg. However, for the increases in 24 h and nighttime SBPV (evaluated with SD, CV, and ARV respectively) showed different mean CCA-IMT values.

The correlations between the average BP values and carotid IMT/number of plaques were analyzed using Pearson's test. The results were shown in Table 4. It indicated that there was no significant correlation between these BP variables and carotid IMT, whereas, 24 h PP, daytime PP, and nighttime PP were positively associated with the number of plaques (for LCCA, $r^1 = 0.485$, $P^1 = 0.000$; $r^1 = 0.465$, $P^1 = 0.000$; $r^1 = 0.510$, $P^1 = 0.000$, resp.; for RCCA, $r^2 = 0.394$, $P^2 = 0.003$; $r^2 = 0.375$, $P^2 = 0.005$; $r^2 = 0.413$, $P^2 = 0.002$, resp.; for mean CCA, $r^3 = 0.358$, $P^3 = 0.002$; $r^3 = 0.353$, $P^3 = 0.002$; $r^3 = 0.374$, $P^3 = 0.001$, resp.). Moreover, a negative correlation was found between the nighttime average DBP and the number of plaques (for LCCA, $r^1 = -0.443$, $P^1 = 0.001$; $r^1 = -0.463$, $P^1 = 0.000$; $r^1 = -0.339$, $P^1 = 0.011$, resp.; for RCCA, $r^2 = -0.412$, $P^2 = 0.002$; $r^2 = -0.416$, $P^2 = 0.002$; $r^2 = -0.369$, $P^2 = 0.006$, resp.; for mean CCA, $r^3 = -0.372$, $P^3 = 0.001$; $r^3 = -0.391$, $P^3 = 0.001$; $r^3 = -0.308$, $P^3 = 0.008$, resp.). In addition, the number of plaques in LCCA had higher correlation with PP and DBP than that in RCCA.

Table 4: The correlation between mean blood pressure values and carotid intima-media thickness/number of plaques in all the subjects

Variables	IMTc			Number of plaques		
	r(P)[1]	r(P)[2]	r(P)[3]	r(P)[1]	r(P)[2]	r(P)[3]
24 h SBP	0.073 (0.525)	−0.048 (0.673)	0.011 (0.921)	−0.083 (0.548)	−0.111 (0.420)	−0.109 (0.356)
24 h DBP	−0.033 (0.776)	−0.190 (0.096)	−0.129 (0.259)	−0.443** (0.001)	−0.412** (0.002)	−0.372** (0.001)
24 h PP	0.177 (0.120)	0.194 (0.089)	0.211 (0.064)	0.485** (0.000)	0.394** (0.003)	0.358** (0.002)
Daytime SBP	0.059 (0.606)	−0.040 (0.725)	0.009 (0.940)	−0.122 (0.373)	−0.132 (0.338)	−0.135 (0.251)
Daytime DBP	−0.059 (0.610)	−0.167 (0.145)	−0.130 (0.257)	−0.463** (0.000)	−0.416** (0.002)	−0.391** (0.001)
Daytime PP	0.161 (0.159)	0.176 (0.123)	0.191 (0.093)	0.465** (0.000)	0.375** (0.005)	0.353** (0.002)
Nighttime SBP	0.100 (0.382)	−0.059 (0.605)	0.020 (0.086)	0.036 (0.795)	−0.046 (0.738)	−0.025 (0.833)
Nighttime DBP	0.045 (0.699)	−0.160 (0.161)	−0.170 (0.544)	−0.339* (0.011)	−0.369** (0.006)	−0.308** (0.008)
Nighttime PP	0.113 (0.324)	0.118 (0.303)	0.131 (0.252)	0.510** (0.000)	0.413** (0.002)	0.374** (0.001)
SBP decrease (%)	−0.062 (0.702)	−0.087 (0.590)	−0.087 (0.588)	−0.200 (0.216)	−0.127 (0.434)	−0.169 (0.299)
DBP decrease (%)	−0.064 (0.690)	0.029 (0.856)	−0.021 (0.895)	−0.129 (0.428)	0.024 (0.882)	−0.031 (0.849)

To further compare the effects of different indices of BPV on LCCA-IMT, Multiple regression analysis for 4 independent factors indicated significant correlations between LCCA-IMT and age and smoking in Table 5. Thus, LCCA-IMT may not only be influenced by age or smoking but also by the SD index of daytime SBPV. However, LCCA-IMT was not correlated with any other ambulatory BPVs.

Table 5: Multiple regression analysis of left carotid intima-media thickness and blood pressure variabilities

Factors	β (95% CI)	P value	R^2
Age	0.006 (0.002 to 0.011)	0.005	0.296
Smoking	0.220 (0.104 to 0.336)	0.000	
Hypertension duration	0.002 (−0.004 to 0.008)	0.440	
24 h SBPV (SD)	0.008 (−0.008 to 0.024)	0.324	

Age	0.006 (0.002 to 0.010)	0.007	0.330
Smoking	0.222 (0.110 to 0.029)	0.000	
Hypertension duration	0.002 (−0.003 to 0.008)	0.400	
daytime SBPV (SD)	0.015 (0.001 to 0.029)	0.035	
Age	0.006 (0.002 to 0.010)	0.007	0.307
Smoking	0.229 (0.116 to 0.342)	0.000	
Hypertension duration	0.003 (−0.003 to 0.008)	0.399	
Daytime SBPV (CV)	0.014 (−0.006 to 0.034)	0.154	
Age	0.006 (0.002 to 0.011)	0.007	0.292
Smoking	0.222 (0.105 to 0.338)	0.000	
Hypertension duration	0.002 (−0.004 to 0.008)	0.426	
24 h SBPV (ARV)	0.007 (−0.012 to 0.026)	0.457	
Age	0.006 (0.002 to 0.010)	0.006	0.298
Smoking	0.218 (0.102 to 0.334)	0.000	
Hypertension duration	0.002 (−0.004 to 0.008)	0.457	
Daytime SBPV (ARV)	0.009 (−0.008 to 0.027)	0.283	
Age	0.007 (0.002 to 0.011)	0.002	0.291
Smoking	0.217 (0.095 to 0.339)	0.001	
Hypertension duration	0.002 (−0.004 to 0.008)	0.452	
Daytime DBPV (ARV)	0.007 (−0.016 to 0.030)	0.522	

DISCUSSION

The results of the present study showed that the SBP fluctuations during daytime and 24 h were significantly associated with the increased carotid IMT. Moreover, for all the subjects, there is no significant correlation between the BPV and right CCA-IMT/number of plaques, whereas, the SD, CV, and ARV of daytime SBP showed a positive correlation with LCCA-IMT. Moreover, the ARV of daytime SBPV, 24 h SBPV and nighttime DBPV showed a positive correlation with the number of plaques of LCCA. In addition, quintile stepwise analyses showed that the correlation of three indices of SBPV during daytime and mean CCA-IMT were almost the same, and the carotid IMT showed a progressively greater value from the quintile with the lowest to the quintile with the highest daytime SBPVs. But it did not show any noticeable or consistent variation from the quintile with the lowest to the quartile with the highest 24 h or nighttime SBPVs. For further multiple regression analysis, we found that the daytime SBPV evaluated with SD was significantly associated with carotid IMT.

In earlier studies, BP fluctuations being the result of a complex interaction between environmental stimuli and the response of cardiovascular control mechanisms [21, 22, 23]. BPV is characterized by marked short-term BPV occurring within a 24-h period (beat-to-beat, minute-to-minute, hour-to-hour, and day-to-night changes) and also by long-term BPV occurring over more-prolonged periods of time (days, weeks, months, seasons, and even years) [24]. Compared with long-term BPV, short-term BPV indicators were easier to measure and collect. Previous studies also demonstrated that good control of ambulatory BP has a more beneficial effect on cardiovascular organ damage in hypertensive patients than good control of clinic BP [25], and reported that the association between short-term BPV derived from 24-h ABPM and carotid IMT [11, 13, 15, 26, 27, 28, 29]. Thus, tight BP control throughout the 24-h period structurally and functionally improves the stiffened arterial walls of hypertensive patients.

Our results corroborate previous findings. Firstly, in the earlier study [15], it was reports that the relationship between the 24 h BPV and carotid IMT. They found that both the daytime, and 24 h systolic BPV evaluated by SD, CV, and ARV are positively associated with IMT (for daytime SBPV, $r = 0.408$, $P = 0.001$; $r = 0.381$, $P = 0.003$; $r = 0.396$, $P = 0.002$, resp.; for 24 h SBPV, $r = 0.339$, $P = 0.002$; $r = 0.376$, $P = 0.003$; $r = 0.339$, $P = 0.008$, resp.). They also found the relationship between carotid IMT and DBPV during the daytime and 24 h, the SD and CV indices of BPV had greater correlation than ARV index (for daytime DBPV, $r = 0.293$, $P = 0.023$; $r = 0.302$, $P = 0.019$, resp.; for 24 h DBPV, $r = 0.328$, $P = 0.010$; $r = 0.323$, $P = 0.012$, resp.). The similar conclusions were proposed from the study of Sander et al. [11]. They indicated that the progression of IMT was significantly greater in the patients with increased SBPV, multivariate regression analysis also revealed the daytime SBPV to be the best predictor for the progression of IMT. Our study presents new evidence because the previous demonstrations of its significant conclusion have been derived mainly from population-based study [15] rather than hypertensive patients. We also suggested that the results of correlation analysis for the relationship between SBPV and IMT in hypertensive patient were consistent with their studies.

Secondly, previous studies mostly focused on exploring the association between 24 h ambulatory BP variability and mean carotid IMT [11, 15], and comparing the effects on the carotid artery structure for different indices of BPV [20, 30]. In the earlier study [15], they found that daytime systolic BPV evaluated with ARV is the best variable to represent the increasing of carotid IMT. The similar conclusions have been show in the study of Mena et al. [20] and Hansen et al. [30]. Mena et al. found that the commonly used SD index may be more sensitive to the sampling frequency of the ABPM devices, and ARV index ($RR = 1.611$, $P = 0.004$) is a more reliable representation of time series variability than SD ($RR = 1.103$, $P = 0.571$) for the prognostic significant BPV. Hansen et al. also suggested that BPV was a significant and independent predictor of mortality and of cardiovascular and stroke events, ARV24 was a better predictor than SD24 and SDdn. Thus, ARV24 might be a more specific measure of BPV than SD. In our present study, we not only found that for the daytime DBPV evaluated with ARV was significantly related to LCCA-IMT ($r^1 = 0.239$, $P = 0.035$), which differed form BPV evaluated by SD and CV, but also there is no significant correlation between the BPV and RCCA-IMT, whereas, the SD, CV, and ARV of daytime SBP showed a positive correlation with LCCA-IMT. Moreover, the present study indicated that there was no significant correlation between these BP variables and carotid IMT, whereas, the ARV of daytime SBPV, 24 h SBPV and nighttime DBPV showed a positive correlation with the number of plaques of LCCA. So the results also show that ABP better predicts than clinic BP measurements the risk of subsequent cardiovascular events as before studies [7, 8]. Moreover, 24 h PP, daytime PP, and nighttime PP were positively associated with the number of plaques in hypertensive patients. And a negative correlation was found between the nighttime average DBP and the number of plaques. The similar conclusions were proposed from the earlier study [15]. In addition, the number of plaques in LCCA had higher correlation with PP, DBP, SBPV and DBPV than that in RCCA. Despite this, more evidence is still required to assess whether the correlation between BPV and LCCA-IMT/number of plaques is stronger than the right.

Thirdly, we found that the correlation of three indices of SBPV during daytime and mean CCA-IMT were almost the same. Moreover, the maximum IMT increased progressively from the quintile with the lowest to the quintile with the highest daytime BPV evaluated with CV. However, for the increases in 24 h and nighttime SBPV (evaluated with SD, CV, and ARV respectively) showed different growing trends with mean CCA-IMT values, especially for the nighttime SBPV. In the earlier study, Mancia et al. showed that the end-of-treatment carotid CBM_{max} increased progressively and significantly from the quartile with the lowest to the quartile with the highest on-treatment 24-h SBP mean. But carotid CBM_{max} showed no significant difference between quartiles of on-treatment 24-h SBP CV or SD [31]. In our present study, we also did not find any significant difference between quintiles of SDs, CVs or ARVs in hypertensive patients. This study demonstrated growing trends between mean CCA-IMT and BPV evaluated with SD, CV and ARV.

Besides, other findings of our study also deserve to be discussed. The earlier study [15] suggested that no significant differences were found among the three indices of BPV when compared the correlations of these BPV values in each group of two using Pearson's test, they had strongly positive correlation ($P < 0.01$). In our study, we did not find that the DBPV in nighttime showed positive correlation between CV and SD, ARV in hypertensive patients ($P > 0.05$). Moreover, in our multiple regression analysis, it showed that the correlation between daytime SBP evaluated with SD and the increased carotid IMT independent of the well-known confounding factors, such as age, smoking. Although the previous outcome-based studies which showed the superiority of night-time over daytime ambulatory BP averages for prediction of a composite pool of cardiovascular events [32, 33]. Kikuya et al. also demonstrated that an excessive BP variability, evaluated by an increased SD of night-time SBP, adds prognostic information to that provided by a wide ambulatory PP [34]. Our finding was consistent with the study of Sander et al. [14], they found that the SD of diurnal SBPV as the strongest predictor for IMT. The previous research [15] also showed that both the daytime, and 24 h systolic BPV evaluated by SD, CV, and ARV are positively associated with IMT.

Finally, certain limitations of the present study should be acknowledged. First, in our study, the BPV during the night time was not associated with IMT. Because in the present study, BP variability was measured as the SD, CV, and ARV of BP measurements every 30 min during the daytime and every 60 min during the night time. Time frequency of BP measurements is important at the time to estimate variability from non-invasive ABPM techniques. Therefore, the results of the present study should be confirmed by ambulatory BP measurements at a shorter interval. Second, both the relatively small size of the subjects and the cross-sectional survey are the important limitations in our present study. So the link between ambulatory BP variability and carotid atherosclerosis is unable to deduce a causal sequential conclusion. Third, the correlation between mean CCA-IMT and DBP variability evaluated with SD, CV and ARV were not demonstrated in present study. This issue remains to be addressed in future studies. In conclusion, though the limitations exist in our study, we also obtained the suggestive and significant conclusions. All important abbreviation used in this research paper are mentioned above.

CONCLUSIONS

Our study provides the evidence that the SBPV during daytime and 24 h had significant correlation with IMT, for the hypertensive subjects from the southern area of China. Moreover, we also found the daytime SBPV to be the best predictor for the progression of IMT in multivariate regression analysis. In addition, the present study suggests that the correlation between BPV and LCCA-IMT/number of plaques is stronger than the right. However, more evidence is still required to assess whether the correlation between BPV and LCCA-IMT/number of plaques is stronger than the right in future studies. We also will conduct the large-scale trials and perform more analysis to investigate how to predict the risks of cardiovascular disease and mortality from the alteration of carotid structure and function.

DECLARATIONS

Authors' contributions

WH and WW helped in coordination, defined the research theme, conducted the literature re and provided technical supports. YC, HX and DW participated in data analyzing and design of the study, YC was in charge of thesis writing, and SP helped in English correction and formatting. HX and ML carried out the clinical examination and participated in collecting the carotid artery ultrasound measurement. WW and ML performed ultrasound data processing and analyzing. XT and RZ carried out the clinical examination and provided clinical supports and guidance. All authors read and approved the final manuscript.

Acknowledgements

This work was supported in part by the National Basic Research Program 863 (no.

2012AA02A603), the Guangzhou Science and Technology Planning Project (no. 2014J4100153), the Key Lab for Health Informatics of the Chinese Academy of Sciences, the Enhancing Program of Key Laboratories of Shenzhen City (ZDSY20120617113021359), Shenzhen Development and Reform Commission's Stroke Screening and Prevention Public Service Platform, Shenzhen Innovation Funding (JCYJ20140414170821190), and the National Natural Science Foundation of China (no. 81101120), the science technology and innovation committee of Shenzhen for research projects (Grant CXZZ20140909004122087, JYJC20130327093948937, JCYJ20140414170821285 and JCYJ20130401164750005).

REFERENCES

1. Collaborative ESCHD. Blood pressure, cholesterol, and stroke in eastern Asia. Lancet. 1998;352(9143):1801–7.
2. Kannel WB. Role of blood pressure in cardiovascular morbidity and mortality. Prog Cardiovasc Dis. 1974;17(1):5–24.
3. Lawes CM, Bennett DA, Feigin VL, Rodgers A. Blood pressure and stroke an over of published res. Stroke. 2004;35(3):776–85.
4. Lawes CM, Vander Hoorn S, Rodgers A. Global burden of blood-pressure-related disease, 2001. Lancet. 2008;371(9623):1513–8.
5. Mancia G, Grassi G. Mechanisms and clinical implications of blood pressure variability. J Cardiovasc Pharmacol. 2000;35:S15–9.
6. Frattola A, Parati G, Cuspidi C, Albini F, Mancia G. Prognostic value of 24-h blood pressure variability. J Hypertens. 1993;11(10):1133–7.
7. Verdecchia P, Porcellati C, Schillaci G, Borgioni C, Ciucci A, Battistelli M, et al. Ambulatory blood pressure. An independent predictor of prognosis in essential hypertension. Hypertension. 1994;24(6):793–801.
8. Clement DL, De Buyzere ML, De Bacquer DA, de Leeuw PW, Duprez DA, Fagard RH, et al. Prognostic value of ambulatory blood-pressure recordings in patients with treated hypertension. N Engl J Med. 2003;348(24):2407–15.
9. Mancia G, Di Rienzo M, Parati G. Ambulatory blood pressure monitoring use in hypertension research and clinical practice. Hypertension. 1993;21(4):510–24.
10. Mancia G, Bombelli M, Facchetti R, Madotto F, Corrao G, Trevano FQ, et al. Long-term prognostic value of blood pressure variability in the general population results of the Pressioni Arteriose Monitorate e Loro Associazioni Study. Hypertension. 2007;49(6):1265–70.
11. Sander D, Kukla C, Klingelhöfer J, Winbeck K, Conrad B. Relationship between circadian blood pressure patterns and progression of early carotid atherosclerosis A 3-year follow-up study. Circulation. 2000;102(13):1536–41.
12. Pickering TG, James GD. Ambulatory blood pressure and prognosis. J Hypertens Suppl Off J Int Soc Hypertens. 1994;12(8):S29–33.
13. Mancia G, Parati G, Hennig M, Flatau B, Omboni S, Glavina F, et al. Relation between blood pressure variability and carotid artery damage in hypertension:

baseline data from the European Lacidipine Study on Atherosclerosis (ELSA). J Hypertens. 2001;19(11):1981–9.

14. Sander D, Klingelhofer J. Diurnal systolic blood pressure variability is the strongest predictor of early carotid atherosclerosis. Neurology. 1996;47(2):500–7.
15. Xiong H, Wu D, Tian X, Lin W-H, Li C, Zhang H et al. The relationship between the 24 h blood pressure variability and carotid intima-media thickness: a compared study. Comput Math Methods Med. 2014;2014:1–9.
16. Goldstein IB, Bartzokis G, Hance DB, Shapiro D. Relationship between blood pressure and subcortical lesions in healthy elderly people. Stroke. 1998;29(4):765–72.
17. Crouse JR, Goldbourt U, Evans G, Pinsky J, Sharrett AR, Sorlie P, et al. Risk factors and segment-specific carotid arterial enlargement in the Atherosclerosis Risk in Communities (ARIC) cohort. Stroke. 1996;27(1):69–75.
18. Pignoli P, Tremoli E, Poli A, Oreste P, Paoletti R. Intimal plus medial thickness of the arterial wall: a direct measurement with ultrasound imaging. Circulation. 1986;74(6):1399–406.
19. Hodis HN, Mack WJ, LaBree L, Selzer RH, Liu C-R, Liu C-H, et al. The role of carotid arterial intima-media thickness in predicting clinical coronary events. Ann Intern Med. 1998;128(4):262–9.
20. Mena L, Pintos S, Queipo NV, Aizpurua JA, Maestre G, Sulbaran T. A reliable index for the prognostic significance of blood pressure variability. J Hypertens. 2005;23(3):505–11.
21. Parati G, Ochoa JE, Salvi P, Lombardi C, Bilo G. Prognostic value of blood pressure variability and average blood pressure levels in patients with hypertension and diabetes. Diabetes Care. 2013;36(Supplement 2):S312–24.
22. Mancia G. Short-term and long-term blood pressure variability. Special Issues in Hypertension. Springer; 2012. p. 91–102.
23. Franklin SS, Larson MG, Khan SA, Wong ND, Leip EP, Kannel WB, et al. Does the relation of blood pressure to coronary heart disease risk change with aging? The Framingham Heart Study. Circulation. 2001;103(9):1245–9.
24. Parati G, Ochoa JE, Lombardi C, Bilo G. Assessment and management of blood-pressure variability. Nat Rev Cardiol. 2013;10(3):143–55.
25. Cuspidi C, Meani S, Fusi V, Valerio C, Catini E, Magrini F, et al. Isolated ambulatory hypertension and changes in target organ damage in treated hypertensive patients. J Hum Hypertens. 2005;19(6):471–7.
26. Zanchetti A, Bond MG, Hennig M, Neiss A, Mancia G, Dal Palù C, et al. Risk factors associated with alterations in carotid intima—media thickness in hypertension: baseline data from the European Lacidipine Study on Atherosclerosis. J Hypertens. 1998;16(7):949–61.
27. Shintani Y, Kikuya M, Hara A, Ohkubo T, Metoki H, Asayama K, et al. Ambulatory blood pressure, blood pressure variability and the prevalence of carotid artery alteration: the Ohasama study. J Hypertens. 2007;25(8):1704–10.

28. Skalidi SJ, Manios ED, Stamatelopoulos KS, Barlas G, Michas F, Toumanidis ST, et al. Brain edema formation is associated with the time rate of blood pressure variation in acute stroke patients. Blood Press Monit. 2013;18(4):203–7.

29. García-García Á, García-Ortiz L, Recio-Rodríguez JI, Patino-Alonso MC, Agudo-Conde C, Rodriguez-Sanchez E, et al. Relationship of 24-h blood pressure variability with vascular structure and function in hypertensive patients. Blood Press Monit. 2013;18(2):101–6.

30. Hansen TW, Thijs L, Li Y, Boggia J, Kikuya M, Björklund-Bodegård K, et al. Prognostic value of reading-to-reading blood pressure variability over 24 h in 8938 subjects from 11 populations. Hypertension. 2010;55(4):1049–57.

31. Mancia G, Facchetti R, Parati G, Zanchetti A. Visit-to-visit blood pressure variability, carotid atherosclerosis and cardiovascular events in the European Lacidipine Study on Atherosclerosis. Circulation. 2012:CIRCULATIONAHA. 112.107565.

32. Dolan E, Stanton A, Thijs L, Hinedi K, Atkins N, McClory S, et al. Superiority of ambulatory over clinic blood pressure measurement in predicting mortality the Dublin outcome study. Hypertension. 2005;46(1):156–61.

33. Hansen TW, Jeppesen J, Rasmussen S, Ibsen H, Torp-Pedersen C. Ambulatory blood pressure and mortality a population-based study. Hypertension. 2005;45(4):499–504.

34. Kikuya M, Hozawa A, Ohokubo T, Tsuji I, Michimata M, Matsubara M, et al. Prognostic significance of blood pressure and heart rate variabilities the Ohasama study. Hypertension. 2000;36(5):901–6.

15
CHAPTER

LONGITUDINAL FOLLOW UP OF COILED INTRACRANIAL ANEURYSMS: THE IMPACT OF CONTRAST ENHANCED MRA IN COMPARISON TO 3DTOF MRA AT 3T

Nicoletta Anzalone, C. De Filippis, F. Scomazzoni, G. Calori, A. Iadanza, F. Simionato and C. Righi

BACKGROUND

The role of Magnetic Resonance Angiography (MRA) in the follow up of coiled cerebral aneurysms is well recognized. Many papers have reported the high accuracy of 3DTOF MRA in depicting aneurysms recanalization when compared to DSA (Digital Subtraction Angiography) [1]. Moreover the use of higher field has shown to improve accuracy [2, 5].

Contrast enhanced MRA (CEMRA) has been proposed in the follow up of coiled aneurysms with the aim to reduce the impact of coils artifacts on the evaluation of aneurysm recanalization. Data from the literature are partly incoherent in showing the advantage of CEMRA in aneurysms patency depiction, partly due to the small sample size in the series [3, 4, 6, 7, 9, 10, 12]; nevertheless there is a general agreement in recognizing the advantage of contrast acquisitions in the better depiction of aneurysm remnant either small or large.

A higher sensitivity of CEMRA has been particularly proved in the evaluation of small type 1 patencies (NR), often not evident at 3DTOF where the aneurysm is judged occluded [5, 12]. Nevertheless a clear advantage of this finding, relative to patient treatment is not known; generally such remnants are not considered to be worth a retreatment by most endovascular therapists and we do not know if they will grow to become treatable. Consequentely a clear advantage of CEMRA on a clinical perspective

Citation: Nicoletta Anzalone, C. De Filippis, F. Scomazzoni, G. Calori, A. Iadanza, F. Simionato and C. Righi, Longitudinal follow up of coiled intracranial aneurysms: the impact of contrast enhanced MRA in comparison to 3DTOF MRA at 3T, DOI 10.1186/s40809-015-0008-8.

is unknown. No real data on the longitudinal follow up of coiled aneurysms with the aim to compare unenhanced with enhanced acquisitions are available. Pierot L et al. [8] have reported a series of cases with coiled cerebral aneurysms followed up with 3DTOF and CEMRA with a mean interval time from treatment of 22.7 months. They came to the conclusion that 3DTOF MRA was equivalent to CEMRA in the detection of occlusion and better in showing coils. Nevertheless, their data do not cover the span of a longitudinal FU monitoring and therefore no predictiveness test is available of previous to subsequent stages of FU monitoring data. Our aim was to compare 3DTOF MRA and CEMRA in the longitudinal follow up of a series of coiled cerebral aneurysms and verify wether or not a higher depiction of neck remnants at CEMRA at earlier stages of FU is predictive of subsequent growth and if it played a significant impact on management decisions.

METHODS

According to internal procedure all patients with ruptured or unruptured cerebral aneurysms treated with coils are followed up with MRA at 3T within one year from the procedure and then once a year for at least 5 years. DSA is performed when retreatment is considered in the presence of aneurysm recanalization.

From June 2004 to December 2010 all coiled aneurysms that were regularly followed up with 3DTOF and 3DCEMRA at 3T for at least 4 years were included in this retrospective evaluation.

MRA

Magnetic resonance angiography exams were performed on 3T Philips equipment (Intera from 2004 upgraded to Achieva in December 2012, Philips, Best, The Netherlands); the parameters are shown in Table 1. 3DTOF acquisition was acquired first, followed by 3DCEMRA after bolus injection of 0.2-0.1 ml/kg of gadolinium (GDBOPTA, Bracco - Gadobutrol, Bayer Healthcare) at 2 ml/sec followed by 20 ml of saline with a bolus track technique.

Table 1: Parameters of 3DTOF and 3DCEMRA at 3T

	3D-TOF	**CEMRA**
TE (ms)	3.5	1.8
TR (MS)	23	5.9
FOV	250	220
Matrix	1024 x 1024	304 (ric. 512)
SENSE factor	2.5	3
Slices	180	180
Voxel size	0.5x0.5x1 mm	0.72x0.72x0.80 mm
		(ric 0.4x0.4x0.4)

Time acquisition	7 min	24 sec

Data collection

Clinical data regarding patients (age and gender), aneurysm size, location and history (ruptured and unruptured) were collected.

Aneurysm location was classified in four groups: anterior communicating artery (AcoA), middle cerebral artery (MCA), internal carotid artery (ICA), vertebro-basilar system (VB).

Aneurysm size was classified into: small< 10 mm (separated in smaller and larger than 5 mm), large between 10 mm and 25 mm, giant>25 mm.

During follow up retreated cases were registered; moreover cases judged suitable for retreatment on the MRA results, but not retreated due to clinical-technical unfavourable conditions were also registered as "intention to treat" group.

Data analysis

MRA datasets included source images, MIP reconstructions and volume rendering reconstructions from both acquisitions for all the four years follow up.

All images were evaluated by a senior neuroradiologist dedicated to MRA. 3DTOF and 3DCEMRA were evaluated blindly and separately in a random order. In all the cases the pre-treatment and end of procedure DSA exams were also evaluated to have notion of aneurysm location, shape, end procedure results and coil position. This is of particular importance in the evaluation of neck remnants.

Aneurysm status was evaluated using the three grade score on the Montreal scale [14, 15]: 0 (Total Occlusion:TO), 1 (Neck Remnant:NR), 2 (Aneurysm Remnant:AR).

Then, Montreal score was assigned to each aneurysm both by 3DTOF and CEMRA acquisitions for each year of follow up.

Statistical analysis

Kappa statistics were used to obtain intertechnique agreement at year 1 and year 4 for each investigation. The interpretation of K was as follow, according to Landis and Koch: $k<0$ indicated no agreement; $k=0\text{-}0.19$ poor agreement; $k=0.20\text{-}0.39$ fair agreement, $k=0.40\text{-}0.59$ moderate agreement; $K=0.60\text{-}0.79$ substantial agreement; and $k=0.80\text{-}1.00$ almost perfect agreement [16].

McNemar –Bowker test was calculated for each MRA technique to investigate score modifications during the entire length of follow up.

Area under receiver –operating characteristics (ROC) curves were calculated in order to compare the predictive role of 3DTOF and 3DCEMRA at 1 year on the judgement of suitableness to retreatment.

Analysis were performed with SPSS 18 version.

RESULTS

A total of 64 cases satisfied the inclusion criteria and were included in the retrospective evaluation. The population consisted of 14 males and 50 women, age: 33–74 years, mean 56,2+− 11,1 years, median 55 years.

Thirthy aneurysms were ruptured (46,8 %) and 34 (53,12 %) unruptured. Aneurysms location was ACA/AcomA in 35, ICA in 15,VB in 14. According to pre-treatment aneurysms size, 50 aneurysms measured <5 mm, 12 between 5 and 10 mm, and 2>10 mm. Montreal scale score at the end of procedure was: 33 aneurysms TO, 28 NR, 3 AR.

A total of 512 MRA datasets were evaluated.

Aneurysm occlusion/patency

AT 1 year FU, TO to NR to AR Montreal scale scores ratios were 31/23/10 (48/36/16 %) and 22/31/11 (34/49/17 %) at 3DTOF and CEMRA respectively, whereas at 4 years FU they evolved to 28/22/14 (44/34/22 %) and 19/28/17 (30/44/26 %) respectively.

Among 22 cases scored TO in both techniques at 1 year FU, only 3 evolved to NR only at CEMRA. Among the 22 cases scored NR in both techniques at 1 year FU, 3 evolved to AR at 4 year FU in both techniques and 3 additional cases evolved to AR only at CEMRA. In 9 cases scored NR only at CEMRA, none evolved further and 3DTOF ended up scoring NR as well at 4 years FU in 3 of them (Fig. 1).

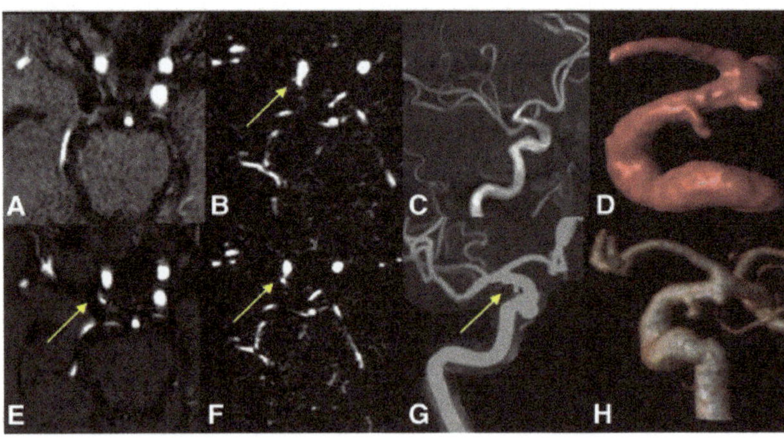

Figure 1: Internal carotid artery treated aneurysm at 1 year (above) and 4 years (below) FU. At early follow up the remnant is not evident at 3DTOF MRA (a and c) while it is evident at 3D CEMRA (b and d, arrow)). At late follow-up the neck remnant is evident at both 3DTOF (e, g, arrows) and 3DCEMRA (f, h, arrow), stable.

Fifteen patencies (all AR) out of 64 aneurysms (23 %) were judged suitable of retreatment evaluation during FU and 8 (12,5 %) retreatments were effectively performed after overall benefit/risk ratio considerations. All 15 reopenings were equally depicted by both techniques (Fig. 2) except one that was depicted earlier on CEMRA (Fig. 3).

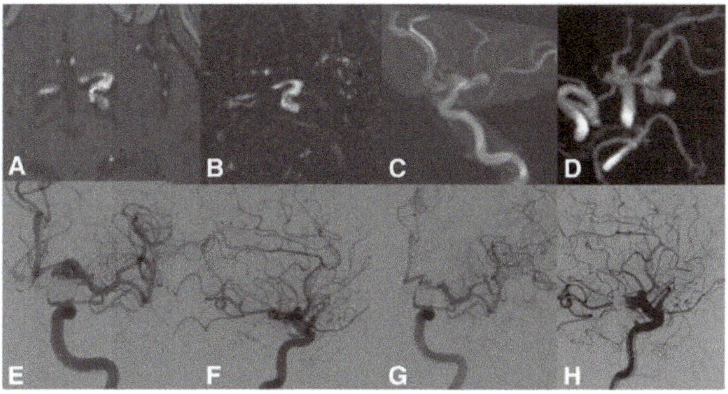

Figure 2: Internal carotid artery retreated aneurysm. The AR was equally demonstrated at early and late follow up by both 3DTOF (a, c) and 3DCEMRA (b, d). DSA confirmed the entity of the patency (e, f) and the aneurysm was retreated with subtotal occlusion at post procedural DSA (g, h).

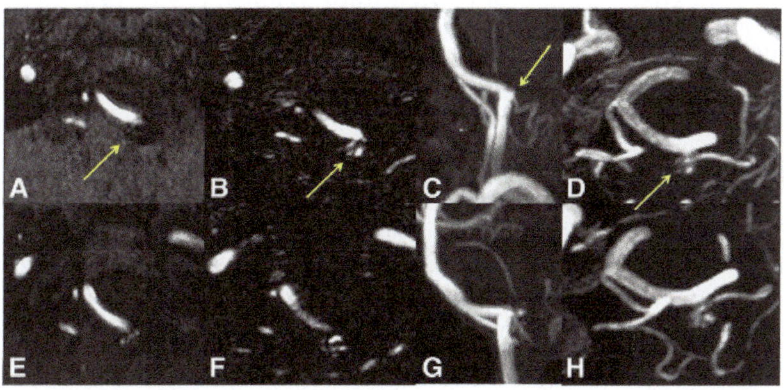

Figure 3: Left vertebral artery treated aneurysm at 1 year (above) and 4 year (below) FU. At early follow up 3DTOF MRA (a, c, arrows) scored the aneurysm as NR, while 3DCEMRA (b, d, arrows) as AR. At late FU the larger remnant was evident also at 3DTOF (e, g) equally to 3DCEMRA (f, h).

Intermodality agreement and aneurysms grade modification during follow up according to MRA technique

3DTOF/CEMRA intertechnique agreement in Montreal scale scoring was 0.75 (E.S.: 0,07) at 1 year and 0.72 (E.S.: 0,07) at 4 years FU, showing a substantial agreement for both exams.

Both 3DTOF score (p=0.030) and 3DCEMRA score (p=0.011) significantly changed at 4 years compared to 1 year; three out of 31 and 3 out of 22 cases rated TO at 1 year FU in 3DTOF and CEMRA respectively evolved to NR at 4 years FU, while 4 out of 23 and 6 out of 31 cases rated NR at 1 year FU in 3DTOF and CEMRA respectively evolved to AR at 4 years FU (Fig. 4).

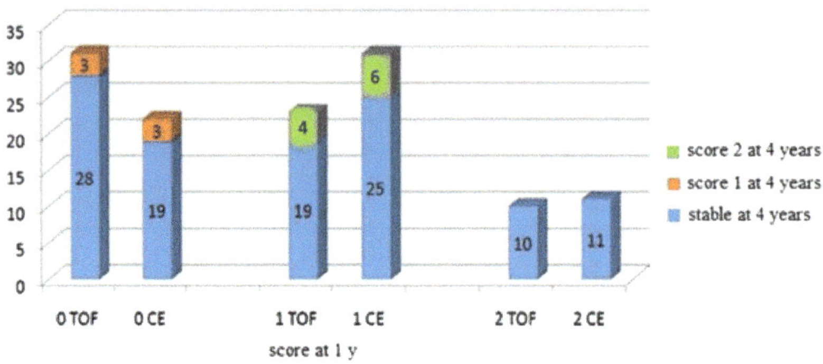

Figure 4: Treated aneurysms status modifications at 4 years FU compared to 1 year FU.

Aneurysm recanalization and retreatment according to MRA techniques

Area under ROC curves indicated that the performance of 3DTOF and 3DCEMRA in predicting retreatment was very good and very similar, being 0.94 (95 % CI: 0.88; 1) and 0.93 (95 % CI: 0.84; 1) respectively.

DISCUSSION

Our data confirm the higher prevalence of aneurysm recanalization together with better depiction of residual patency in favour of 3DCEMRA that has been already reported in previous studies [5, 12, 13]. Though most of the recanalizations, as known, occur within the first year from treatment, score changes according to Montreal scale are also evident in longer follow up [15]. Longitudinal evaluation of unenhanced and enhanced MRA available from our data clearly shows that this change is concordant for both techniques and, despite the higher detection of patency with 3DCEMRA, their concordance is good. Most important the data on aneurysms recanalization (AR) showed that all the retreated cases (15,6 %) were equally depicted both temporally and in score assignment by both techniques. Moreover most of AR (14 out of 17) were equally depicted at both techniques, while only 3 cases out of 17 were underscored as NR at 3DTOF; none of these 3 patencies with differential 3DTOF/CEMRA NR to AR scores was considered suitable for retreatment. Among the 15 patencies considered suitable for retreatment evaluation, only in one case 3DCEMRA anticipated the presence of aneurysm remnant that was nevertheless disclosed at 3DTOF as well, only later in time. As a consequence a clear influence on patient management of CEMRA better depiction of aneurysms patencies over 3DTOF does not emerge from our data, even if endovascular therapists may feel sometime more confident in the evaluation of aneurysm recanalization on the basis of CEMRA images. The higher detection by CEMRA of aneurysms patencies can be a sum of less sensitivity to slow flow and to susceptibility artifacts related to coils presence, artifacts known to affect 3DTOF evaluation [11]. Due to the higher sensitivity to slow flow of 3DTOF MRA, it is possible that residual flow at the neck of the treated aneurysm is not evident with this technique, as in the presence of a residual aneurysm with slow or turbolent flow where 3DTOF can underestimate the entity of the patency.

Another important result that came out from our study was the stability in time of most cases rated as NR by CEMRA, rated as TO by 3DTOF. The higher sensitivity of 3DCEMRA in showing small remnants has been already reported but no data were previously available about the predictive role for further aneurysm recanalization. Our data showed that most of the cases scored as small patencies remained stable and no one enlarged to a higher score.

Another relevant data regard TO rate at one year that in most of the cases (22/28) was equally depicted at both techniques and remained stable (19/22) at following FU. This observation confirms data reported in the literature on large series of treated aneurysms [15].

Sprengers et al. [7] and Pierot et al. [8] had already reported the similar performance of 3DTOF and 3DCEMRA at 3T in the evaluation of aneurysm occlusion, both concluding that the latter is unnecessary in this condition. Our data show that in the presence of aneurysm occlusion at 3DTOF, 3DCEMRA can either show TO or NR, either one avoid of any tendency to further relevant growth in following FU. In this context it seems therefore possible to avoid CEMRA.

Pierot et al. [8] underlie the advantage of 3DTOF in showing coils; indeed the lesser sensitivity to susceptibility artifacts of 3DCEMRA, that allows better evidence of aneurysm enhancing remnant, obscures the images of the aneurysm shape filled of coils that can help in understanding the relationship between the coils and the remnant. On the other hand, if appropriately acquired and timed to the arterial phase, 3DCEMRA acquisitions are less disturbed by movements related artifacts than unenhanced acquisitions.

In our institution we do not regularly perform DSA to follow up coiled aneurysm and arteriography is planned only when a possible aneurysm retreatment is considered. We have a long experience in MRA follow up of coiled aneurysms and from previous published data we have reported a high diagnostic accuracy of both MRA techniques at either 1,5 T and 3T [5, 12]. Moreover as well known, DSA may not always be the ideal technique to disclose aneurysm remnant, due to the frequent possible superimposition of vessels and the consequent "helmet effect" due to the presence of coils that obscure aneurysm or neck patency. We strongly support the utilization of MRA for coiled aneurysms FU evaluation considering it mature enough to substitute DSA even as gold standard for large series data reporting.

A limitation of this study is the relative small number of cases that does not allow to draw definite conclusions on the possible beneficial impact on outcome of the superiority of CEMRA in the higher demonstration of residual patency in the treated aneurysms.

Nevertheless the data of this first longitudinal follow up evaluation of 3DTOF and 3DCEMRA at 3T in coiled aneurysms show that, despite a higher prevalence of aneurysm and neck remnants demonstrated at 3DCEMRA, no modification in patients management emerged. In front of 3DTOF MRA test negative for residual patency in early FU stages, eventual patencies disclosed by CEMRA proved to be stable at later FU stages.

As opposite, in case of patencies detected at 3DTOF MRA, CEMRA may allow better depiction of the remnant and possibly disclose a larger patency.

CONCLUSIONS

Even if from our data CEMRA superiority in the depiction of intracranial aneurysms recanalization is confirmed, a clear impact in patient management is apparently not evident. As a consequence the adjunct of CEMRA to 3DTOF MRA in front of aneurysm patency may be planned on a case to case rather than on a routinary basis, following diagnostic or interventional neuroradiologists judgement. However awareness about a possible underestimation of patencies should be bared in mind.

Evidence of occlusion at 3DTOF FU may not need the addition of a CEMRA study.

AUTHORS' CONTRIBUTIONS

NANA: project and protocol development, data management, manuscript editing. CDF: data collection and management. FS: data collection, manuscript writing. CG: Statistical analysis. AI: data collection and management. FS: data collection. CR: data collection, protocol design. All authors read and approved the final manuscript.

REFERENCES

1. Kwee TC, Kwee RM. MR angiography in the follow-up of intracranial aneurysms treated with Guglielmi detachable coils: systematic re and meta-analysis. Neuroradiology. 2007;49:703–13.
2. Urbach H, Dorenbeck U, von Falken hausen M, Wilhelm K, Willinek W, Schaller C, et al. Three dimensional time-of-flight MR angiography at 3T compared to digital subtraction angiography in the follow-up of ruptured and coiled aneurysms. Neuroradiology. 2008;50:383–9.
3. Kaufmann TJ, Huston J, Cloft HJ, Mandrekar J, Gray L, Bernstein MA, et al. A prospective trial of 3T and 1.5T time-of-flight and contrast-enhanced MR angiography in the follow-up of coiled intracranial aneurysms. AJNR Am J Neuroradiol. 2010;31:912–8.
4. Pierot L, Delcourt C, Bouquigny F, Breidt D, Feuillet B, Lanoix O, et al. Follow-up of intracranial aneurysms selectively treated with coils: prospective evaluation of contrast-enhanced MR angiography. AJNR Am J Neuroradiol. 2006;27:744–9.
5. Anzalone N, Scomazzoni F, Cirillo M, Righi C, Simionato F, Cadioli M, et al. Follow-up of coiled aneurysms at 3T: comparison of 3D time-of-flight MR angiography and contrast-enhanced MR angiography. AJNR Am J Neuroradiol. 2008;29:1530–6.

6. Ramgren B, Siemund R, Cronqvist M, Undrén P, Nilsson OG, Holtås S, et al. Follow-up of intracranial aneurysms treated with detachable coils: comparison of 3D inflow MRA at 3T and 1.5T and contrast-enhanced MRA at 3 T with DSA. Neuroradiology. 2008;50:947–54.
7. Sprengers ME, Schaafsma JD, van Rooij WJ, van den Berg R, Rinkel GJ, Akkerman EM, et al. Evaluations of the occlusion status of coiled aneurysms with MR angiography at 3T: is contrast enhancement necessary? AJNR Am J Neuroradiol. 2009;30:1665–71.
8. Pierot L, Portefaix C, Boulin A, Gauvrit JY. Follow-up of coiled intracranial aneurysms: comparison of 3D time-of-flight and contrast-enhanced magnetic resonance angiography at 3T in a large, prospective series. Eur Radiol. 2012;22:2255–63.
9. Gauvrit JY, Leclerc X, Pernodet M, Lubicz B, Lejeune JP, et al. Intracranial aneurysms treated with Guglielmi detachable coils: usefulness of 6-month imaging follow-up with contrast-enhanced MR angiography. AJNR Am J Neuroradiol. 2005 Mar;26(3):515-21.
10. Cirillo M, Scomazzoni F, Cirillo L, Cadioli M, Simionato F, Iadanza A, et al. Comparison of 3D TOF-MRA and 3D CE-MRA at 3T for imaging of intracranial aneurysms. Eur J Radiol. 2013 Dec;82(12):e853-9.
11. Anzalone N, Scomazzoni F, Cirillo M, Cadioli M, Iadanza A, Kirchin MA, et al. Follow-up of coiled cerebral aneurysms: comparison of three-dimensional time-of-flight magnetic resonance angiography at 3 tesla with three-dimensional time-of-flight magnetic resonance angiography and contrast-enhanced magnetic resonance angiography at 1.5 Tesla. Invest Radiol. 2008 Aug;43(8):559-67.
12. Agid R, Willinsky RA, Lee SK, Terbrugge KG, Farb RI. Characterization of aneurysm remnants after endovascular treatment: contrast-enhanced MRA versus catheter digital subtraction angiography. AJNR Am J Neuroradiol. 2008 Sep;29(8):1570-4.
13. Raymond J, Guilbert F, Weill A, Georganos SA, Juravsky L, Lambert A, et al. Long-term angiographic recurrences after selective endovascular treatment of aneurysms with detachable coils. Stroke 2003; 34: 1398-403.
14. Raymond J, Guilbert F, Weill A, Georganos SA, Juravsky L, Lambert A, et al. Long-term angiographic recurrences after selective endovascular treatment of aneurysms with detachable coils. Stroke. 2003;34:1398–403.
15. Roy D, Milot G, Raymond J. Endovascular treatment of unruptured aneurysms. Stroke. 2001;32:1998–2004.
16. Landis JR, Koch GG. The measurement of observer agreement for categorical data. Biometrics. 1977;33:159–74.

16
CHAPTER

COMPUTATIONAL FLUID DYNAMICS OF COMPUTED TOMOGRAPHY ANGIOGRAPHY TO DETECT THE HEMODYNAMIC IMPACT OF INTRACRANIAL ATHEROSCLEROTIC STENOSIS

Xinyi Leng, Fabien Scalzo, Albert K Fong, Mark Johnson, Hing Lung Ip, Yannie Soo, Thomas Leung, Liping Liu, Edward Feldmann, Ka Sing Wong and David S Liebeskind

Keywords: Cerebral hemodynamics, Cerebrovascular disease, Stroke, Computational flow dynamics, Computed tomography angiography

BACKGROUND

As the most common cause of ischemic stroke and transient ischemic attack in Asian populations and an important cause of stroke as well in other populations, intracranial atherosclerotic stenosis (ICAS) has attracted attention both in clinical practice and relevant research fields in recent decades [1-3]. The degree of anatomic stenosis was noted as an independent predictor for recurrent ischemic *s*troke *i*n the *t*erritory of the index artery (SIT), for instance, in the Warfarin-Aspirin Symptomatic Intracranial Disease (WASID) trial [4]. However, the fact also existed that nearly half of the SIT occurred in patients with 50-69% ICAS in the WASID trial [4]. According to the Chinese IntraCranial AtheroSclerosis Study, recurrent stroke also occurred in a considerable percentage of patients with <50% ICAS [5]. On the other hand, factors affecting hemodynamics of ICAS, for instance, collateralization, have been found to dramatically alter subsequent stroke risks in the WASID and the Stenting and Aggressive Medical Management for Preventing Recurrent stroke in Intracranial Stenosis (SAMMPRIS) trial [6,7]. Therefore, hemodynamics plays an important role in the case of ICAS,

Citation: Xinyi Leng, Fabien Scalzo, Albert K Fong, Mark Johnson, Hing Lung Ip, Yannie Soo, Thomas Leung, Liping Liu, Edward Feldmann, Ka Sing Wong and David S Liebeskind, Computational fluid dynamics of computed tomography angiography to detect the hemodynamic impact of intracranial atherosclerotic stenosis, DOI: 10.1186/s40809-014-0001-7.

concerning subsequent risk of SIT. Evaluation of hemodynamic impact of ICAS will probably facilitate in the risk stratification of patients with symptomatic ICAS.

Computational fluid dynamic (CFD) techniques, when applied in simulation of blood flow, can quantitatively reveal hemodynamic characteristics of arterial stenosis. Noninvasive fractional flow reserve (FFR), which is the distal to proximal pressure ratio (PR) across a stenosis, measured through CFD reconstruction of coronary computed tomography angiography (CTA), has been identified of high diagnostic accuracy for the hemodynamic significance of stenosed coronary arteries as compared with FFR obtained invasively, and this is promising in guiding patient selection for percutaneous coronary intervention [8,9]. More recently, virtual FFR obtained from CFD models based on coronary angiograms by assigning averaged generic downstream boundary conditions without simulating hyperemic conditions, was also found to be substantially accurate to define hemodynamically significant coronary lesions (accuracy of 97%), as compared with invasively measured FFR under induced hyperemia [10]. In addition, CFD could also be used to reveal the hemodynamic effects of ICAS [11,12]. In the present pilot study, we evaluated the feasibility to discern hemodynamic impact of ICAS using CFD models reconstructed from routinely obtained CTA images with a small sample size, to pave the way for generalized application of this technique in larger clinical studies in the near future.

METHODS

Subjects

This was a retrospective observational study. Ten patients, each with a symptomatic ICAS lesion (50-99% luminal stenosis, WASID criteria [13]) of a major intracranial artery [intracranial portion of internal carotid artery (ICA); M1 segment of middle cerebral artery (MCA-M1); or basilar artery (BA)] identified on CTA, were retrospectively selected from a prospective clinical study at Prince of Wales Hospital in Hong Kong. All patients had given written informed consent for the previously approved prospective clinical study, and the current retrospective study was also approved by the Joint Chinese University of Hong Kong-New Territories East Cluster Clinical Research Ethics Committee (the Joint CUHK-NTEC CREC). Patients' characteristics were collected from clinical records. CTA source images were retrieved and anonymized from the picture archiving and communication system and transferred to University of California, Los Angeles for reconstruction of CFD models.

CT protocol

All CT examinations were performed on a 64-slice CT scanner (Lightspeed VCT, GE Healthcare, US), including non-contrast CT scan of the whole brain and CTA of intracranial arteries. The non-contrast CT scan was performed in axial mode, covering the skull base to vertex region, and obtained at 120 kV 320 mA and 1.0 sec rotation. CTA was performed in helical mode with no tilting, covering the skull base to the level of lateral ventricles, and obtained at 120 kV 550 mA and 0.4 sec rotation. Intravenous contrast (70 ml Omnipaque 300, 3–3.5 ml/s) was injected via the antecubital vein using a power injector. Axial CTA images were reconstructed at 0.625 mm intervals and stored as source images for further image analysis.

CFD simulations of hemodynamics

The scientific basis of evaluating hemodynamics of ICAS lesions, such as the trans-stenotic pressure gradient, using simulated models constructed out of standard CTA source images, was that the hemodynamic features of such lesions could be calculated via the CFD technique by applying several assumptions on the three-dimensional (3D) vessel geometry obtained from CTA source images. CFD simulations of hemodynamics were performed through the following procedures. Firstly, the location of the target arterial segment was visually identified and delineated with a region-of-interest on CTA images. The region-of-interest was then segmented using a gradient-driven level set method [14] to extract the vascular volume. Centerlines were then computed from selected inlet and outlet points placed at the extreme points of the vessel. The diameter of the vessel along the centerline was derived using the Voronoi method which allowed a 3D geometry of the vessel to be constructed.

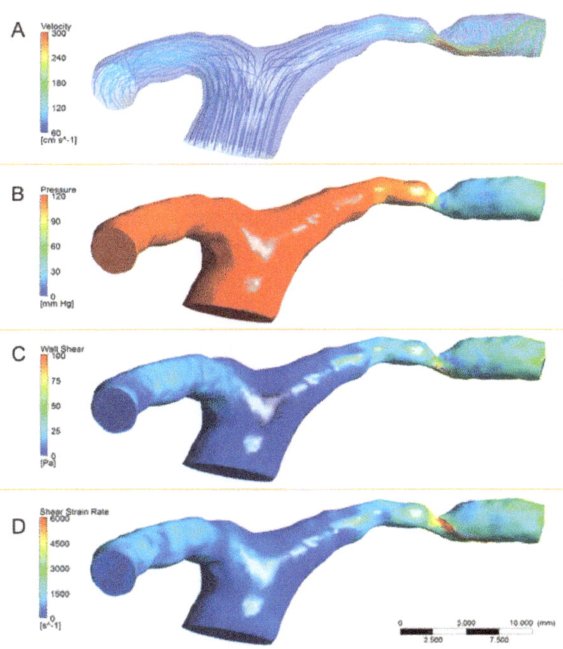

Figure 1: The CFD model showing hemodynamic characteristics of a 70% MCA-M1 stenosis (Case #4). Blood flow velocity(A), wall shear stress (C) and shear rates (D) dramatically increased and pressure (B) greatly decreased in situ and downstream to the lesion. Besides, turbulence and a recirculating flow was noted immediately distal to the ICAS lesion (panel A). CFD indicates computational fluid dynamics; MCA-M1, M1 segment of middle cerebral artery.

A mesh of the 3D surface was then created using ANSYS ICEM-CFD (ANSYS,

Inc.), composed of approximately 500,000 tetrahedral cells. Blood flow simulation was then performed on this mesh using ANSYS CFX software. It was assumed that blood was an incompressible Newtonian fluid with a constant viscosity of 0.004 $kg{\cdot}m^{-1}{\cdot}s^{-1}$ and could be governed by the Navier–Stokes equations [15]. It was also assumed that blood has a density of 1060 kg/m^3. The boundary conditions placed on this simulation was one that assumed rigid, non-compliant walls with no-slip flow conditions. The inlet boundary condition was set to be 120 mmHg while the outlet velocity was prescribed as 60 cm/s. As it has been assumed that the vessel is non-compliant, the velocity downstream can be assumed to also follow ideal pipe-flow and thus physiological velocities. The simulation results were post-processed in ANSYS CFX-post (ANSYS, Inc.), for extraction of flow parameters, for instance, velocity, pressure, wall shear and shear strain rates (Figure 1). Generation of mesh, simulation of blood flow and post-processing of simulation results were run on a Cray CX1 cluster (Cray Inc.).

Measurement of anatomic characteristics of ICAS

Proximal normal vessel diameter, anatomic severity, and length of the stenoses were measured on reconstructed 3D models. Anatomic severity of ICAS was measured according to the WASID criteria [13]. Length of a lesion was defined as the distance between the first normal diameters distal and proximal to the stenosis.

Evaluation of hemodynamic impact of ICAS

Evaluation of the CFD models was also performed in ANSYS CFX-post (ANSYS, Inc.). Hemodynamic impact of ICAS was evaluated by using 2 indices in the present study, which were PR and pressure gradient (PG) across the lesion. Pressures were measured at the 1st normal diameters distal and proximal to the lesion, for which spherical volumes-of-interest with the same radius of the vessel were selected within the vessel domain to get the mean pressure value. PR was defined as the distal to proximal pressure ratio, and PG (mmHg/cm) was defined as pressure drop across the ICAS divided by length of the lesion. Since this was a preliminary study, and that there had been no data about the cut-point value of PR to define a hemodynamically significant ICAS, we used the same cut-point of PR (0.80) as is used in the cardiac field for FFR [16], with a PR less than or equal to 0.80 considered hemodynamically significant in the present study.

Statistical analysis

Descriptive statistics were used in the current study to describe demographics of patients recruited and imaging characteristics of the symptomatic ICAS lesions.

RESULTS

Among the 10 patients recruited in this study, the CTA source images of 9 subjects (median age was 62, and 7 were males) were successfully processed to CFD models. In the other one case, vessel geometry of the arterial segment containing the ICAS lesion failed to be extracted from the CTA source images due to poor image quality.

Table 1: Patient demographics and ICAS characteristics*

Patient #	Gender	Age	ICAS			Proximal vessel diameter (mm)	Proximal pressure (mmHg)	Distal pressure (mmHg)	Pressure ratio	Pressure gradient (mmHg/cm)
			Location	Anatomic severity (%)	**Length (mm)**					
1	M	44	MCA-M1	50	20	3.5	118	104	0.88	7
2	M	68	MCA-M1	51	11	2.7	118	107	0.91	10
3	M	51	MCA-M1	53	13	2.9	119	102	0.86	13
4	M	61	MCA-M1	70	10	2.7	120	29	0.24	93
5	F	74	MCA-M1	78	14	3.0	119	−184	−1.55	223
6	F	65	MCA-M1	79	9	2.5	120	−156	−1.30	300
7	M	62	MCA-M1	80	17	3.5	117	−8,847	−75.70	5,382
8	M	69	ICA distal	50	10	4.2	120	118	0.98	2
9	M	50	BA	62	5	3.4	116	67	0.58	98

*Patients are listed in the table by the lesion location and sequentially arranged according to the degree of luminal stenosis (%) of the lesions.

ICAS indicates intracranial atherosclerotic stenosis; MCA-M1, M1 segment of middle cerebral artery; ICA, internal carotid artery; BA, basilar artery.

The reconstructed CFD models could quantitatively depict hemodynamic environment at the stenosis. Blood flow velocity, wall shear stress and shear rates increased and pressure decreased in situ and downstream to a stenosis. Figure 1 shows hemodynamic characteristics of a 70% MCA-M1 stenosis (Case #4), revealed by the CFD model.

Among the 9 cases processed, 7 were MCA-M1 lesions, and the other 2 were ICA and BA lesions, respectively. Four cases were 70-99% stenoses. Patient demographics, anatomic characteristics of ICAS, and other parameters and indices measured and calculated from the CFD models are shown in Table 1. The median PR was 0.58 and the median PG was 93 mmHg/cm. Four anatomically severe and 1 anatomically moderate stenoses were considered hemodynamically significant (PR $\leq$0.80) in the current study. Besides, PRs and PGs varied in cases with similar percentages of stenoses (Table 1 and Figure 2). For instance, Case #5, #6 and #7, with similar anatomic severity of stenoses (around 80%) in MCA-M1 but different lesion lengths and proximal vessel diameters, greatly differed in hemodynamic severities as assessed via CFD models (Table 1). The pressure maps of Case #6 and #7 are shown in Figure 2, with PGs of 300 and 5,382 mmHg/cm, respectively.

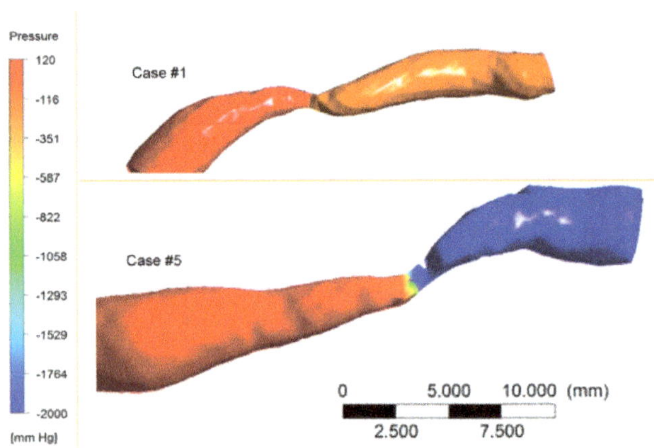

Figure 2: Pressure maps of Case #6 and #7. Both cases were around 80% stenoses of MCA-M1 but with different lengths (double-headed arrows) and proximal vessel diameters. Hemodynamic severities of the two cases differed in terms of PR and PG. The PRs were −1.30 and −75.70, respectively. And PGs were 300 and 5,382 mmHg/cm, respectively. MCA-M1 indicates M1 segment of middle cerebral artery; PR, pressure ratio; PG, pressure gradient.

DISCUSSION

This was a feasibility study. Despite of the small sample size, we demonstrated the feasibility of simulating blood flow across ICAS lesions by CFD modeling based on routinely obtained CTA images, and the feasibility of quantitatively analyzing the hemodynamic characteristics of such lesions on the CFD models. Besides, the study results implied that the severity of luminal stenosis probably was not the only indicator to determine the hemodynamic impact of symptomatic ICAS lesions, which reinforced the urgent need for a more comprehensive paradigm for clinical evaluation of such lesions, to replace, or at least improve, the current unreasonable and misleading method of defining the significance of such lesions only based on the percentage of stenosis.

Patients with symptomatic ICAS are at high risk of recurrent ischemic stroke, despite of medical and/or interventional treatment [17-19]. However, commonly used noninvasive imaging modalities have been found of relatively low positive predictive values for diagnosis of 50-99% intracranial stenosis, compared with digital subtract angiography (DSA) [20,21]. Moreover, the percentage of stenosis itself, even when diagnosed by DSA, was not the only factor that might be able to affect downstream hemodynamics in the case of ICAS. Irregularity and eccentricity of the lesion, which in many cases is influenced by the plaque compositions, as well as the collateral status, may also affect the hemodynamic impact of an ICAS lesion [22]. This may partly explain why patients with ICAS of moderate luminal stenosis would also be at risk of SIT [22,23]. Therefore, we aimed to evaluate hemodynamic impact of ICAS via reconstructed CFD models in the present study, which was found feasible using routinely obtained CTA source images, so that this single noninvasive imaging modality could provide much more information of ICAS beyond the anatomic severity of luminal stenosis.

Although biplane DSA images could also be used to reconstruct CFD models of ICAS [24], and that CTA may not be as accurate as DSA to depict the vessel geometry in ICAS [21], we assumed that CTA images would be a better source for CFD modeling of ICAS lesions from both the technical and clinical points of . On one hand, CTA source images, with its three-dimensional nature, yield a better source for CFD modeling than biplane DSA images, from the technical angle. On the other hand, as a noninvasive imaging modality, CTA is more commonly used and easier to be obtained in clinical practice than DSA, which permits studies with relatively large sample sizes in the future. In addition, although the noninvasive time-of-flight MR angiography can also provide three-dimensional geometry of the cerebral vessels of interest as CTA does, vessel geometry obtained from CTA is more accurate than that from MR angiography, especially in cases with extremely low distal flow beyond the ICAS lesion when MR angiography could overestimate the degree of stenosis.

Hemodynamic impact of ICAS was assessed using PR in our study, paralleled to FFR in the cardiac field, with lower PR indicating more significantly decreased downstream flow. To our knowledge, there had been no data about the cut-point of simulated PR to define a hemodynamically significant ICAS. However, for coronary artery disease, virtual FFR based on CFD models of coronary lesions had been found to be closely correlated with FFR measured under induced hyperemia during percutaneous coronary angiography (correlation coefficient $r = 0.84$), and to be able to accurately identify lesions with FFR <0.80 as mentioned above [10]. Thus for this pilot study, we used the same cut-point of PR (0.80) as is currently used in the cardiac field for invasively measured FFR and virtual FFR [10,16]. But in future studies, we will explore an optimal cut-point of PR to dichotomize ICAS lesions by the hemodynamic impact, for instance, by comparing PR values against brain perfusion results such as quantitative arterial spin labeling MR perfusion imaging. According to the results, distal pressures and PRs of ICAS lesions were in minus values in some cases. This was one of the limitations of CFD modeling in the current study that is further discussed below, and also one of the reasons that we also used another index, PG, to quantify the hemodynamic severity of ICAS.

In the measurement of invasive FFR for coronary artery disease, use of vasodilator could decrease the microcirculatory resistance, magnify the function of existing collaterals, and hence induce hyperemia, under which circumstance the hemodynamic impact of the lesion could be accurately evaluated in most cases [25]. However, it has also been recognized that the invasive FFR might not be reliable in cases with microvascular damage, in which cases maximal hyperemia could not be achieved [10]. In a latest study as mentioned above utilizing the CFD modeling technique to obtain virtual FFR of coronary lesions, generic downstream boundary conditions, including the microvascular resistance and compliance values, were developed and applied to the arterial outlet(s) with a Windkessel model [10,26]. The virtual FFR obtained in this way, not affected by the status of microcirculation and without the need of simulating hyperemic conditions, was proved of substantial consistency with invasively measured FFR, with an average absolute error of ±0.06 [10]. Therefore, virtual fractional flow of arterial stenosis based on vessel geometry and generic boundary conditions is potentially reliable in defining the hemodynamic significance of the lesion. In the current study, we did not take into account the effects of distal microvascular resistance and the collaterals in the CFD models of ICAS lesions, which needs to be addressed in future studies, probably by referring to the method for obtaining virtual FFR for coronary lesions as discussed above.

Fractional flow across ICAS, in terms of PR and PG in our study, was not exclusively determined by percentage of the stenosis. Other morphological characteristics of an ICAS lesion might also impact on the hemodynamic environment in situ and downstream, for instance, length of the lesion as implied by this study, though we did not do any statistical analysis to confirm the speculation concerning the relationships between the lesion length and the hemodynamic impact of an ICAS due to the small sample size, as well as the irregularity and eccentricity of the stenosis that were not yet investigated in the current study. To date, few data existed on relationships between morphology and hemodynamics of ICAS, but length of carotid plaque and patent ICA vessel diameter, besides degree of stenosis, were found to be significantly related to ipsilateral intracranial blood flow in studies of carotid stenosis [27]. Based on vessel geometry and therefore harboring all morphological information of a lesion, simulated CFD blood flow models could comprehensively reflect effects of morphological factors on hemodynamic characteristics of ICAS. Since risk of stroke recurrence could be altered by blood flow hemodynamics in patients with symptomatic ICAS, evaluation of CFD models, instead of using anatomic severity of luminal stenosis as almost the only imaging indicator, might play a role in risk stratification of these patients. In addition, evaluating the hemodynamic parameters embedded within the CFD models of symptomatic ICAS lesions, such as PR, PG, flow velocity, wall shear stress and shear strain rates, may be useful to embrace a better understanding of the effects of hemodynamics on diverse pathomechanisms of ICAS-related ischemic stroke, which are currently understudied. The most important limitation of the present study was that CFD models were simplified and only based on geometry of short vessel segments containing the stenoses, trimming off artery branches and meanwhile ignoring effects of collaterals and other factors that may affect hemodynamics of the lesion. This may be part of the reasons for the minus downstream pressure values as detected in the CFD models of some cases. Besides, the prescribed outflow velocity may also partly contribute to the unrealistic minus pressures in some of the CFD models. In future studies, the following measures could be explored to improve the realistic accuracy of the simulated CFD models: covering longer vessel segments in the CFD models, at least long enough for post-stenotic blood flow to restore laminar flow; and assigning personalized pressures and flow velocities at the inlet and outlet that could be of higher physiological significance, for instance, flow velocities distal to an ICAS lesion at a major intracranial artery detected by transcranial Doppler. Moreover, unlike carotid arteries, intracranial arteries have plenty of braches and perforators, which could alter the hemodynamics of blood flow in a major intracranial artery. Therefore, including main adjacent branches and perforators in the CFD models of ICAS lesions in future studies, as what is currently done for CFD modeling of coronary lesions [9,28], could further optimize the realistic accuracy of the simulating results. Also, it would further enhance the clinical relevance of CFD blood flow simulation of symptomatic ICAS by considering the effects of distal microvascular resistance and collateral status, which might also facilitate better understanding of mechanisms of collateral recruitment in the presence of symptomatic ICAS. In addition, another limitation of the current study lay in that simulated pressure gradients were not validated against direct, invasive measures, or compared with indirect measures with other noninvasive methods, which will also be addressed in future studies.

Apart from the above measures to improve the CFD models of ICAS lesions, meanwhile we also need to balance the complexity and accuracy of the models with its generalizability in clinical studies. Simplified modeling would be less time-consuming for each patient involved and probably more generalizable for large clinical studies in the future, but at the meantime the consequent inaccuracy of simulated hemodynamic environment may compromise its clinical perspective. Thus, achieving an acceptable balance between the realistic accuracy and the generalizability of CFD modeling of symptomatic ICAS lesions is important for this technique to ultimately be of clinical significance and utility in the assessment of such lesions.

CONCLUSIONS

This pilot study demonstrated the feasibility to quantitatively assess hemodynamic impact of ICAS using CFD models reconstructed from routinely obtained CTA. A vast number of studies are required to evaluate the ultimate value of this technique, to seek improvement in the realistic accuracy and the generalizability of CFD modeling of ICAS, and to explore the role of specific hemodynamic characteristics from CFD models in risk stratification of patients with symptomatic ICAS.

AUTHORS' CONTRIBUTIONS

XL contributed to study design, data collection, analysis and interpretation, and manuscript preparation; FS, AKF, MJ and HLI contributed to image processing and computational modeling; YS and TL contributed to data collection and interpretation; LL and EF contributed to study design and manuscript preparation; KSW and DSL contributed to study design, data analysis and interpretation, and manuscript preparation. All authors read and approved the final manuscript.

REFERENCES

1. Wong LKS: Global burden of intracranial atherosclerosis. *Int J Stroke* 2006, 1:158–159.
2. Qureshi AI, Feldmann E, Gomez CR, Johnston SC, Kasner SE, Quick DC, Rasmussen PA, Suri MF, Taylor RA, Zaidat OO:Intracranial atherosclerotic disease: an update. *Ann Neurol* 2009, 66:730–738.
3. Saba L, Anzidei M, Piga M, Ciolina F, Mannelli L, Catalano C, Suri JS, Raz E: Multi-modal CT scanning in the evaluation of cerebrovascular disease patients. *Cardiovasc Diagn Ther* 2014, 4:245–262.
4. Kasner SE, Chimowitz MI, Lynn MJ, Howlett-Smith H, Stern BJ, Hertzberg VS, Frankel MR, Levine SR, Chaturvedi S, Benesch CG, Sila CA, Jovin TG, Romano JG, Cloft HJ, for the Warfarin Aspirin Symptomatic Intracranial Disease (WASID) Trial Investigators: Predictors of ischemic stroke in the territory of a symptomatic intracranial arterial stenosis.*Circulation* 2006, 113:555–563.
5. Wang Y, Liu L, Wang Y, Soo Y, Pu Y, Wong KS: A multicenter study of the prevalence and outcomes of intracranial large artery atherosclerosis among stroke and TIA patients in China [abstract]. *Stroke* 2012, 43:A120.
6. Liebeskind DS, Cotsonis GA, Saver JL, Lynn MJ, Turan TN, Cloft HJ, Chimowitz MI: Collaterals dramatically alter stroke risk in intracranial atherosclerosis. *Ann Neurol* 2011, 69:963–974.
7. Liebeskind DS, Cotsonis GA, Lynn MJ, Cloft HJ, Fiorella DJ, Derdeyn CP, Chimowitz MI, on behalf of the SAMMPRIS Investigators: Collaterals determine risk of early territorial stroke and hemorrhage in the SAMMPRIS trial. *Stroke*2012, 43:A124.
8. Min JK, Koo BK, Erglis A, Doh JH, Daniels DV, Jegere S, Kim HS, Dunning AM, DeFrance T, Lansky A, Leipsic J: Usefulness of noninvasive fractional flow reserve computed from coronary computed tomographic angiograms for intermediate stenoses confirmed by quantitative coronary angiography. *Am J Cardiol* 2012, 110:971–976.
9. Koo BK, Erglis A, Doh JH, Daniels DV, Jegere S, Kim HS, Dunning A, DeFrance T, Lansky A, Leipsic J, Min JK: Diagnosis of ischemia-causing coronary stenoses by noninvasive fractional flow reserve computed from coronary computed tomographic angiograms: results from the prospective multicenter DISCOVER-FLOW (Diagnosis of Ischemia-Causing Stenoses Obtained Via Noninvasive

Fractional Flow Reserve) study. *J Am Coll Cardiol* 2011, 58:1989–1997.

10. Morris PD, Ryan D, Morton AC, Lycett R, Lawford PV, Hose DR, Gunn JP: Virtual fractional flow reserve from coronary angiography: modeling the significance of coronary lesions: results from the VIRTU-1 (VIRTUal Fractional Flow Reserve From Coronary Angiography) study. *JACC Cardiovasc Interv* 2013, 6:149–157.
11. Schirmer CM, Malek AM: Prediction of complex flow patterns in intracranial atherosclerotic disease using computational fluid dynamics. *Neurosurgery* 2007, 61:842–852.
12. Liebeskind DS, Fong A, Scalzo F, Derdeyn CP, Fiorella DJ, Cloft HJ, Chimowitz MI, Feldmann E: SAMMPRIS angiography discloses hemodynamic effects of intracranial stenosis: computational fluid dynamics of fractional flow. *Stroke*2013, 44:A156.
13. Samuels OB, Joseph GJ, Lynn MJ, Smith HA, Chimowitz MZ: A standardized method for measuring intracranial arterial stenosis. *AJNR Am J Neuroradiol* 2000, 21:643–646.
14. Antiga L, Piccinelli M, Botti L, Ene-Iordache B, Remuzzi A, Steinman DA: An image-based modeling framework for patient-specific computational hemodynamics. *Med Biol Eng Comput* 2008, 46:1097–1112.
15. Batchelor GK: *An Introduction to Fluid Dynamics.* Cambridge: Cambridge University Press; 1967.
16. Min JK, Berman DS, Budoff MJ, Jaffer FA, Leipsic J, Leon MB, Mancini GBJ, Mauri L, Schwartz RS, Shaw LJ: Rationale and design of the DeFACTO (Determination of Fractional Flow Reserve by Anatomic Computed Tomographic AngiOgraphy) study. *J Cardiovas Comput Tomogr* 2011, 5:301–309.
17. Chimowitz MI, Lynn MJ, Howlett-Smith H, Stern BJ, Hertzberg VS, Frankel MR, Levine SR, Chaturvedi S, Kasner SE, Benesch CG, Sila CA, Jovin TG, Romano JG: Comparison of warfarin and aspirin for symptomatic intracranial arterial stenosis. *N Engl J Med* 2005, 352:1305–1316.
18. Chimowitz MI, Lynn MJ, Derdeyn CP, Turan TN, Fiorella D, Lane BF, Janis LS, Lutsep HL, Barnwell SL, Waters MF, Hoh BL, Hourihane JM, Levy EI, Alexandrov AV, Harrigan MR, Chiu D, Klucznik RP, Clark JM, McDougall CG, Johnson MD, Pride GL, Jr., Torbey MT, Zaidat OO, Rumboldt Z, Cloft HJ: Stenting versus aggressive medical therapy for intracranial arterial stenosis. *N Engl J Med* 2011, 365:993–1003.
19. Weber R, Kraywinkel K, Diener HC, Weimar C, German Stroke Study C: Symptomatic intracranial atherosclerotic stenoses: prevalence and prognosis in patients with acute cerebral ischemia. *Cerebrovasc Dis* 2010, 30:188–193.
20. Liebeskind DS, Kosinski AS, Saver JL, Feldmann E, for the SONIA Investigators: CT angiography in the Stroke Outcomes and Neuroimaging of Intracranial Atherosclerosis (SONIA) study [abstract]. *Stroke* 2007, 32:477.
21. Feldmann E, Wilterdink JL, Kosinski A, Lynn M, Chimowitz MI, Sarafin J, Smith HH, Nichols F, Rogg J, Cloft HJ, Wechsler L, Saver J, Levine SR,

Tegeler C, Adams R, Sloan M, the SONIA Trial Investigators: The Stroke Outcomes and Neuroimaging of Intracranial Atherosclerosis (SONIA) trial. *Neurology* 2007, 68:2099–2106.

22. Leng X, Wong KS, Liebeskind DS: Evaluating intracranial atherosclerosis rather than intracranial stenosis. *Stroke*2014, 45:645–651.
23. Liebeskind DS, Cotsonis GA, Saver JL, Lynn MJ, Cloft HJ, Chimowitz MI, Warfarin-Aspirin Symptomatic Intracranial Disease Investigators: Collateral circulation in symptomatic intracranial atherosclerosis. *J Cereb Blood Flow Metab* 2011,31:1293–1301.
24. Scalzo F, Hao Q, Walczak AM, Hu X, Hoi Y, Hoffmann KR, Liebeskind DS: Computational hemodynamics in intracranial vessels reconstructed from biplane angiograms. In *Advances in Visual Computing, Part III*, Volume 37. Edited by Bebis G, Boyle R, Parvin B, Koracin D, Chung R, Hammound R, Hussain M, Kar-Han T, Crawfis R, Thalmann D, Kao D, Avila L. Berlin Heidelberg: Springer; 2010:359–367. Lecture Notes in Computer Science.
25. De Bruyne B, Sarma J: Fractional flow reserve: a re. *Heart* 2008, 94:949–959.
26. Westerhof N, Lankhaar JW, Westerhof BE: The arterial Windkessel. *Med Biol Eng Comput* 2009, 47:131–141.
27. Douglas AF, Christopher S, Amankulor N, Din R, Poullis M, Amin-Hanjani S, Ghogawala Z: Extracranial carotid plaque length and parent vessel diameter significantly affect baseline ipsilateral intracranial blood flow. *Neurosurgery*2011, 69:767–773.
28. Min JK, Leipsic J, Pencina MJ, Berman DS, Koo BK, van Mieghem C, Erglis A, Lin FY, Dunning AM, Apruzzese P, Budoff MJ, Cole JH, Jaffer FA, Leon MB, Malpeso J, Mancini GB, Park SJ, Schwartz RS, Shaw LJ, Mauri L: Diagnostic accuracy of fractional flow reserve from anatomic CT angiography. *JAMA* 2012, 308:1237–1245.

17

CHAPTER

CYANOBACTERIA AS A PLATFORM FOR BIOFUEL PRODUCTION

Nicole E. Nozzi, JohnW. K. Oliver and Shota Atsumi

Keywords: Cyanobacteria, biofuel, synthetic biology, metabolic engineering, photosynthesis

INTRODUCTION

On October 31, 2011 world population officially hit seven billion, only 12 years after the six billion mark in 1999. The age of exploration and discovery of untapped land and untouched resources is over, humanity must now learn to cultivate and renew energy sources in the same way that we do for food. The ability of biology to renew and reproduce holds great promise for sustainable fuel production if it can be effectively harnessed. Specifically, photosynthetic life self-replicates the intricate machinery needed for capture and conversion of light energy and waste carbon dioxide. We are already utilizing photosynthesis through the fermentation of farm crops for bioethanol production. However, though this is a renewable source of fuel, it competes with cropland (Witcover et al., 2013). What is needed is biological fuel production that functions orthogonally to food production. The use of plant-derived lignocellulose derived from agricultural waste as a source of fermentable sugars is an option favored by many current start-up companies. However, this material consists mainly of heavily cross-linked polymers responsible for plant structure and strength, thus the process for breaking down such material to a form that can be readily utilized by bacteria for fermentation is a highly energy intensive process (Sanderson, 2011).

Citation: Nozzi NE, Oliver JWK and Atsumi S (2013) Cyanobacteria as a platform for biofuel production. Front. Bioeng. Biotechnol. 1:7. doi: 10.3389/fbioe.2013.00007.

Alternatively, the use of photosynthetic microorganisms as a platform for biological fuel production has gained considerable popularity as an option that could potentially avoid some of the problems aforementioned (Machado and Atsumi, 2012). As photosynthetic microorganisms directly fix carbon dioxide as their primary carbon source, the need for a source of fermentable sugars as a carbon feedstock for biological fuel production could be eliminated. Eukaryotic algae and cyanobacteria have been the primary organisms of interest for this strategy of fuel production. Both can grow much faster than plants and do not need to be grown on arable land (Dismukes et al., 2008). Furthermore, these organisms are grown submerged in water, which allows for the use of CO_2 at higher concentrations than that of ambient air (Sheehan et al., 1998) and could potentially allow for the use of concentrated CO_2 emissions from waste industrial sources. Research on eukaryotic algae has primarily centered on their ability to produce large amounts of lipids for the production of biodiesel (Pate et al., 2011). However despite years of research, eukaryotic algae have yet to realize their industrial potential and synthetic biology techniques for eukaryotic systems remain elusive limiting our ability to improve and diversify these strains (Radakovits et al., 2010). Cyanobacteria, prokarytic organisms, combine of the advantages of both eukaryotic algae, as a photosynthetic microorganism, and *E. coli*, as a tractable and naturally transformable host.

Cyanobacteria have already been engineered to produce a number of different biofuel related compounds (Machado and Atsumi, 2012). In one of the first examples of biofuel production in cyanobacteria,*Synechococcus elongatus* sp. strain PCC 7942 (*S. elongatus*) was successfully engineered to produce ethanol through the addition of a pyruvate decarboxylase and an alcohol dehydrogenase, redirecting carbon from pyruvate (Deng and Coleman, 1999). Cyanobacterial production of ethanol has since been significantly improved (Dexter and Fu, 2009; Gao et al., 2012). Though compatible with current fuel infrastructure as a supplement to gasoline, ethanol serves as a rather poor gasoline substitute due to its hygroscopicity and low energy density. For these reasons efforts have shifted toward longer carbon chain fuels (Table 1). Isobutyraldehyde, an important chemical feedstock for hydrocarbons normally derived from petroleum, was successfully produced in *S. elongatus* by diverting carbon flux from the valine biosynthesis pathway through the addition of a ketoacid decarboxylase, reaching 1.1 g/L in 8 days (Atsumi et al., 2009). Isobutanol, a promising candidate for a gasoline substitute, can easily be obtained from isobutyraldehyde via chemical conversion. Direct biological production of isobutanol from *S. elongatus*was achieved with the addition of an alcohol dehydrogenase reaching 450 mg/L in 6 days (Atsumi et al., 2009). Three heterologous enzymes, acetolactate synthase, 2-acetolactate decarboxylase, and a secondary alcohol dehydrogenase, introduced into *S. elongatus* allowed for the diversion of carbon flux from pyruvate to the production of the chemical feedstock 2,3-butanediol reaching 2.4 g/L in 21 days (Oliver et al., 2013). Other chemicals produced with heterologous biosynthetic pathways from cyanobacteria include 1-butanol (29.9 mg/L) (Lan and Liao, 2012), 2-methyl-1-butanol (200 mg/L) (Shen and Liao, 2012), acetone (36 mg/L) (Zhou et al., 2012), ethylene (~171 mg/L·day) (Takahama et al., 2003; Ungerer et al., 2012), isoprene (0.05 mg/g dry cell·day) (Lindberg et al., 2010), and fatty acids (197 mg/L) (Liu et al., 2011).

Table 1: Titers for various biochemical

Compound	Organism	Titer	Reference
Acetone	*Synechocystis* sp. PCC6803	36 mg/L	Zhou et al. (2012)
2,3-Butanediol	*S. elongatus* sp. PCC7942	2.4 g/L	Oliver et al. (2013)
1-Butanol	*S. elongatus* sp. PCC7942	30 mg/L	Lan and Liao (2012)
Ethanol	*Synechocystis* sp. PCC6803	5.5 g/L	Gao et al. (2012)
Ethylene	*Synechocystis* sp. PCC6803	171 mg/L·day	Ungerer et al. (2012)
Fatty acids	*Synechocystis* sp. PCC6803	197 mg/L	Liu et al. (2011)
Isobutanol	*S. elongatus* sp. PCC7942	450 mg/L	Atsumi et al. (2009)
Isobutyraldehyde	*S. elongatus* sp. PCC7942	1.1 g/L	Atsumi et al. (2009)
Isoprene	*Synechocystis* sp. PCC6803	50 μg/g dry cell·day	Lindberg et al. (2010)
2-Methyl-1-butanol	*S. elongatus* sp. PCC7942	200 mg/L	Shen and Liao (2012)

These successes clearly demonstrate the malleability of cyanobacteria as a chemical production platform. Over the past 15 years we have moved from detection of the first industrial chemicals produced from exogenous genes in cyanobacteria, through a burst of discovery and experimentation with pathways and design in photosynthetic prokaryotes, to our current status of balancing and matching of production to the metabolism of the host (Oliver et al., 2013). In this perspective we seek to highlight the greatest challenges that must be overcome before sustainable biofuel production in cyanobacteria can be fully realized. We will focus mainly on pathway engineering and strain development (Figure 1). Though we will touch on it, the challenges concerning large scale commercialization are largely beyond the scope of this work.

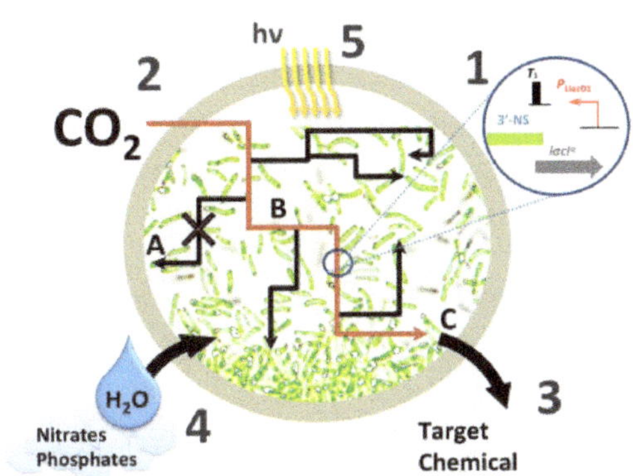

Figure 1: Challenges in cyanobacterial chemical production. (1) Improving available

biological parts at each level of the central dogma for engineering artificial pathways in cyanobacteria; (2) improving carbon fixation; (3), improving metabolic yield with various strategies, A – eliminating competing pathways, B – improving pathway flux, for example via irreversible steps, C – improving tolerance to or continuous removal of the target chemical; (4), management of limited resources that may be stressed upon scale-up; (5), photosynthetic efficiency and bioreactor design.

IMPROVING GENETIC PARTS FOR CYANOBACTERIA

Most engineered pathways in cyanobacteria utilize gene expression systems derived from *E. coli* (Atsumi et al., 2009; Shen and Liao, 2012), however it is known that gene expression in *E. coli* cannot accurately predict gene expression in a photosynthetic host (Huang et al., 2010; Oliver et al., 2013). Many engineered systems have employed endogenous cyanobacterial promoters for constitutive expression (Deng and Coleman, 1999), but few such genetic parts have been specifically characterized for utility in metabolic engineering (Heidorn et al., 2011).

The cyanobacterial RNA polymerase (RNAP) holoenzyme contains different subunits than those found in the RNAPs of most bacteria. Furthermore, though cyanobacteria contain σ factors belonging to the σ^{70}family which are also found in *E. coli*, they do not possess any σ^{54} family σ factors which are found in most bacteria (Imamura and Asayama, 2009). With these differences in mind, the discovery that many promoter sequences commonly employed in *E. coli* engineering, such as the lac inducible expression system, do not function well or at all in cyanobacterial systems may not come as a great surprise (Huang et al., 2010; Oliver et al., 2013). Characterization of endogenous cyanobacterial promoters constitutes a short list including light-inducible and metal-inducible promoters (Heidorn et al., 2011). At the translational level, an analysis of ribosomal binding site (RBS) sequences of all genes in *Synechocystis*6803 revealed that only 26% contained the RBS core sequence compared to 57% in *E. coli* (Ma et al., 2002). Indeed, a comparison of the strength of an RBS sequence modeled after those identified in*Synechocystis* 6803 and three BioBrick sequences further revealed the importance of choosing biological parts adapted specifically for the organism of interest, cyanobacteria in this case (Heidorn et al., 2011). The differences in both transcriptional and translational regulation systems in cyanobacteria must be accounted for if biological parts from *E. coli* are utilized in engineering designs.

Experiments have indicated the operation of anti-sense RNA in regulating gene expression in cyanobacterial systems (Georg and Hess, 2011). Indeed anti-sense suppression has been successfully used in *S. elongatus* to regulate gene expression (Holtman et al., 2005; Cai et al., 2013). Evidence of the CRISPR-Cas system, which has recently become a topic of intense interest, has been identified in most cyanobacterial strains (Cai et al., 2013). The great potential of the CRISPR-Cas system as an engineering tool has already been demonstrated in *E. coli* (Qi et al., 2013).

IMPROVING CO_2 FIXATION

Despite billions of years of evolution, nature's ability to effectively sequester CO_2 would seem on the surface to be strangely inefficient. Ribulose-1,5-bisphosphate carboxylase/oxygenase (RuBisCO), the enzyme responsible for CO_2 fixation, appears to be lacking in the two qualities enzymes are most known for: high catalytic rate and high specificity (Tcherkez et al., 2006). RuBisCO's lack of specificity lies in its inherent tendency to bind O_2 instead of CO_2, which results in a futile use of energy. Attempts to improve this specificity via site-directed mutagenesis have found that improved specificity always comes at the expense of catalytic rate (Tcherkez et al., 2006; Ninomiya et al., 2008). Consequently, RuBisCO may already be perfectly optimized to the best possible compromise between specificity and catalytic efficiency. Among photosynthetic organisms, cyanobacteria have already evolved very efficient carbon concentrating mechanisms (CCM) which allow RuBisCO to operate near V_{max} by lowering the need for high specificity (Savir et al., 2010; Price, 2011).

However, there are large differences between the conditions under which RuBisCO evolved and laboratory or bioreactor conditions which can provide high intensity light and concentrated CO_2. These artificial conditions may allow for some improvement of carbon fixation. For example, expression of heterologous RuBisCO resulted in a twofold increase in isobutyraldehyde production in *S. elongatus*, indicating a possible increase in carbon fixation (Atsumi et al., 2009). However, the localization of heterologous RuBisCO to the cytosol and not the carboxysome (Iwaki et al., 2006) makes it unclear which limitation is alleviated. Even if we evolve organisms to match saturated CO_2 conditions, we will still be limited by photosystem II electron turnover after less than a threefold increase in RuBisCO activity (Iwaki et al., 2006).

IMPROVING METABOLIC YIELD

Titers for cyanobacterial production of bulk products such as chemical feedstocks, remain significantly lower than fermentative systems (Table 1) (Lan and Liao, 2013). Initial studies reported barely detectable production of chemicals from exogenous pathways (Deng and Coleman, 1999; Lindberg et al., 2010; Lan and Liao, 2011). This has improved rapidly along with host specific design techniques (Atsumi et al., 2009; Ungerer et al., 2012; Oliver et al., 2013). Historically the improvement of exogenous chemical production has followed characterization of the organism. In *E. coli*, arguably the most well characterized model organism available, yields increased steadily along with genetic technology and have started approaching theoretical yields only recently (Inokuma et al., 2010; Shen et al., 2011). *E. coli* still finds little application in industrial settings, due to complications in scale-up (Huffer et al., 2012). Cyanobacteria, while often stated as having a wealth of information available compared to eukaryotic algae, are comparatively uncharacterized for metabolic engineering as compared to fermentative systems (see Improving Genetic Parts for Cyanobacteria). Even on the scale of basic metabolism, a missing gene to complete the TCA cycle in cyanobacteria was only recently characterized (Zhang and Bryant, 2011).

General strategies for metabolic optimization can be grouped into three areas: elimination of competing pathways, maximizing pathway flux, and improving tolerance to or separating out toxic products (with gas stripping for example). Specific to photosynthetic organisms, a fourth strategy can be added to this list: improving carbon uptake, which we discuss in Section "Improving CO_2 Fixation." The elimination of competing pathways in cyanobacteria is almost uncharted. Some effort has been put into testing the removal of glycogen pathways (Suzuki et al., 2010), and libraries of knockouts have been constructed (Holtman et al., 2005), however investigations in production optimization similar to those in *E. coli*(Rodriguez and Atsumi, 2012) are hindered by the lack of a strong, standardized chemical production system in cyanobacteria to serve as a benchmark for improvement. In contrast to the strategy of eliminating competing pathways, most work in cyanobacteria has focused on improving pathway flux. For example, production of 2,3-butanediol appears to redirect up to 60% of biomass toward product through the use of irreversible steps, and enzyme screening (Oliver et al., 2013). In the future, computational modeling could be applied to cyanobacteria as it has been to other organisms for the identification of distant pathways that could potentially affect pathway flux, for example in terms of cofactor or ATP availability (Asadollahi et al., 2009; Agren et al., 2013; Misra et al., 2013).

By nature cyanobacteria brings with it an oxygenic atmosphere. This fact automatically limits the list of potential heterologous enzymes available for pathway construction. Many enzymes have displayed lowered activity when transferred into cyanobacteria and have clearly limited production (Lan and Liao, 2012; Ungerer et al., 2012). Changing enzymes in these cases greatly improved yield. Cofactor matching, choosing enzymes that can utilize NADPH versus NADH, is also important when working in a photosynthetic context (Lan and Liao, 2012). Currently pathways exist that appear not to be limited by pathway flux (Oliver et al., 2013), allowing for greater characterization of other limitations in metabolism. Improving tolerance to products should in theory allow for higher titers in culture media (Atsumi et al., 2010), however no investigations into improving cyanobacterial resistance to toxicity have been conducted. Alternatively constant removal of toxic products can increase production (Atsumi et al., 2009;Inokuma et al., 2010; Ungerer et al., 2012), although the feasibility of such processes on an industrial scale remains to be proven.

For continuous production from cyanobacterial strains, culture stability remains a challenge with peak titers occurring after a week in many cases. Loss of production may be due to genetic instability, as carbon diversion creates a selective pressure for spontaneous mutants with an inactive pathway. Production durations have been increased in studies that included codon optimization of key genes to eliminate mutation hotspots, or lowering of end-product toxicity to increase viability of production strains, however more data is needed to clearly define the factors impacting duration (Ungerer et al., 2012; Oliver et al., 2013).

MANAGING INPUTS: NUTRIENT AND WATER REQUIREMENTS

Though cyanobacteria do not compete with food crops in terms of land, there is some concern that competition for nutrients may become an issue. Cyanobacteria require a source of nitrogen and phosphorous just as plants do, and fertilizer production for plant growth is already a huge industry. Large scale culturing of cyanobacteria with similar nutrient requirements could put significant strain on these resources. A study of potential resource impacts for algae scale-up noted that target production greater than 10 billion gallons per year would require nutrient inputs that could double current fertilizer use (Pate et al., 2011). Current production strains could be expected to give similar nutrient requirement projections.

Phosphate for fertilizer use is sourced entirely from the mining of limited resources. While projections conflict on exactly when these mines will be exhausted, the limitation is clear. We must consider nutrient recovery from domestic wastewater and agricultural runoff. Both biological and chemical methods are being considered for phosphate recovery and recycling. Enhanced biological phosphorous removal (EBPR) utilizes polyphosphate accumulating organisms (PAOs), primarily microorganisms belonging to the *Accumulibacter* group (Yuan et al., 2012). Chemical methods include: chemically reactive filters, enhancing natural struvite (magnesium ammonium phosphate) precipitation, nanomaterials, and polymers with high phosphorous affinity (Pratt et al., 2012). While much work is underway concerning the removal of phosphorous from wastewater, the challenge lies in the recovery of the phosphorous in a way that does not carry along heavy metals and pathogens.

Electricity can be used to generate nitrogen in the Haber–Bosch process, however the bioavailable nitrogen generated in this way is not recycled and can end up as nitrous oxide greenhouse gases. To mitigate this problem renewable strategies for algal recycling of nitrogen have been proposed (Huo et al., 2012). Cyanobacteria capable of efficiently fixing nitrogen from air are known, and possibilities for engineering these strains as production systems remain to be explored (Golden et al., 1985; Steinberg and Meeks, 1991). Large scale cyanobacterial production would also require enormous amounts of water. Current metabolic engineering for chemical production has mainly focused on freshwater strains. To avoid competition with drinking water, large scale production must adapt to strains that can grow and produce competitively in wastewater or salt water. Genetic tools for salt-water strains are available (Frigaard et al., 2004), although no specific exogenous chemical production has been investigated. Work is progressing in the application of eukaryotic algae to wastewater treatment (Cabanelas et al., 2013; Hu et al., 2013), similar work should be applied also to engineered cyanobacteria.

PHOTOSYNTHETIC EFFICIENCY AND BIOREACTORS

The simple nutrient requirements of cyanobacteria (mainly light, water, and CO_2) make it an ideal candidate for biofuel production, but the requirement of light exposure makes the design of an industrial bioreactor challenging. To achieve maximum photosynthetic efficiency light must be provided to cells in saturating amounts (Iwaki et al., 2006). Self-shading prevents this from being possible if the culture depth is more than a few inches, and success is highly dependent on the rate of cell mixing (Qiang et al., 1998). Because economy of scale implies longer path lengths (such as raceway ponds) and natural irradiance, industrial outlooks have focused on light as the limiting factor in production calculations. It appears that only 10–15% of sunlight will be available to cells for photosynthesis after non-active radiation, and losses from events such as reflection are subtracted (Robertson et al., 2011). Because of this, maximum production rates measured in high CO_2 and high light conditions, in particular in strains with improved

CO_2 fixation may not be applicable to large scale systems. New bioreactor designs and production strain designs need to find a balance between capturing all of the available sunlight and using the smallest volume possible to reduce the cost of purification.

The large amount of sunlight incident on cells but not available for photosynthesis is capable of creating heat in cultures. Both this and ambient temperatures may impair production in high insolation areas. The engineering of hyperthermophilic bacteria, capable of tolerating up to 70°C, could alleviate this problem (Onai et al., 2004). Another approach is to convert non-photosynthetically active radiation into usable wavelengths (Wondraczek et al., 2013) to prevent heat absorption.

Industrial systems relying on the natural irradiation of sunlight are limited to a diurnal cycle. In 2013 the successful insertion of sugar transporter systems into *S. elongatus* made it possible for this cyanobacterium to grow in the absence of light (McEwen et al., 2013). This development opens the door to the possibility of 24 hour chemical production by mediating the cost that would be required to electrically illuminate large scale cultures. Cyanobacterial strains that are natural photoheterotrophs such as*Synechocystis* sp. PCC 6803 could also be used for this purpose.

FINAL THOUGHTS

Seen as a list together the challenges to be conquered before cyanobacterial biofuel production can be realized on an industrial scale can seem great. However, taking a step back, the benefits such a renewable system could reap far outweigh the investment necessary to achieve its reality. Significant progress has already been made in each challenge area since interest in cyanobacteria was sparked. The greatest potential to be unlocked lies in the characterization of tightly controlled expression systems tailored for cyanobacteria. Until we can engineer cyanobacteria in a predictable manner, all other concerns, such as those related to scale-up, must wait. "Plug-and-play" biological parts must be adapted to the host of interest. Too long have we been trying to run software designed for a different operating system. Once we are speaking the same language, engineering designs for cyanobacterial systems will balloon with possibilities.

CONFLICT OF INTEREST STATEMENT

The authors declare that the research was conducted in the absence of any commercial or financial relationships that could be construed as a potential conflict of interest.

REFERENCES

1. Agren, R., Otero, J. M., and Nielsen, J. (2013). Genome-scale modeling enables metabolic engineering of *Saccharomyces cerevisiae* for succinic acid production. *J. Ind. Microbiol. Biotechnol.* 40, 735–747. doi: 10.1007/s10295-013-1269-3
2. Asadollahi, M. A., Maury, J., Patil, K. R., Schalk, M., Clark, A., and Nielsen, J. (2009). Enhancing sesquiterpene production in*Saccharomyces cerevisiae* through in silico driven metabolic engineering. *Metab. Eng.* 11, 328–334. doi:10.1016/j.

ymben.2009.07.001

3. Atsumi, S., Higashide, W., and Liao, J. C. (2009). Direct photosynthetic recycling of carbon dioxide to isobutyraldehyde. *Nat. Biotechnol.* 27, 1177–1180. doi:10.1038/nbt.1586
4. Atsumi, S., Wu, T. Y., Machado, I. M. P., Huang, W. C., Chen, P. Y., Pellegrini, M., et al. (2010). Evolution, genomic analysis, and reconstruction of isobutanol tolerance in *Escherichia coli*. *Mol. Syst. Biol.* 6, 449. doi:10.1038/msb.2010.98
5. Cabanelas, I. T., Ruiz, J., Arbib, Z., Chinalia, F. A., Garrido-Perez, C., Rogalla, F., et al. (2013). Comparing the use of different domestic wastewaters for coupling microalgal production and nutrient removal. *Bioresour. Technol.* 131, 429–436. doi:10.1016/j.biortech.2012.12.152
6. Cai, F., Axen, S. D., and Kerfeld, C. A. (2013). Evidence for the widespread distribution of CRISPR-Cas system in the phylum cyanobacteria. *RNA Biol.* 10, 687–693. doi:10.4161/rna.24571
7. Deng, M.-D., and Coleman, J. R. (1999). Ethanol synthesis by genetic engineering in cyanobacteria. *Appl. Environ. Microbiol.* 65, 523–528.
8. Dexter, J., and Fu, P. (2009). Metabolic engineering of cyanobacteria for ethanol production. *Energy Environ. Sci.* 2, 857. doi:10.1039/b811937f
9. Dismukes, G. C., Carrieri, D., Bennette, N., Ananyev, G. M., and Posewitz, M. C. (2008). Aquatic phototrophs: efficient alternatives to land-based crops for biofuels. *Curr. Opin. Biotechnol.* 19, 235–240. doi:10.1016/j.copbio.2008.05.007
10. Frigaard, N.-U., Sakuragi, Y., and Bryant, D. (2004). "Gene inactivation in the cyanobacterium *Synechococcus* sp. PCC 7002 and the green sulfur bacterium *Chlorobium tepidum* using in vitro-made DNA constructs and natural transformation," in *Photosynthesis Research Protocols*, ed. R. Carpentier (Totowa: Humana Press), 325–340.
11. Gao, Z. X., Zhao, H., Li, Z. M., Tan, X. M., and Lu, X. F. (2012). Photosynthetic production of ethanol from carbon dioxide in genetically engineered cyanobacteria. *Energy Environ. Sci.* 5, 9857–9865. doi:10.1038/nbt.1586
12. Georg, J., and Hess, W. R. (2011). cis-Antisense RNA, another level of gene regulation in bacteria. *Microbiol. Mol. Biol. Rev.* 75, 286–300. doi:10.1128/MMBR.00032-10
13. Golden, J. W., Robinson, S. J., and Haselkorn, R. (1985). Rearrangement of nitrogen fixation genes during heterocyst differentiation in the cyanobacterium *Anabaena*. *Nature* 314, 419–423. doi:10.1038/314419a0
14. Heidorn, T., Camsund, D., Huang, H. H., Lindberg, P., Oliveira, P., Stensjo, K., et al. (2011). Synthetic biology in cyanobacteria engineering and analyzing novel functions. *Meth. Enzymol.* 497, 539–579. doi:10.1016/B978-0-12-385075-1.00024-X
15. Holtman, C. K., Chen, Y., Sandoval, P., Gonzales, A., Nalty, M. S., Thomas, T. L., et al. (2005). High-throughput functional analysis of the*Synechococcus elongatus* PCC 7942 genome. *DNA Res.* 12, 103–115. doi:10.1093/dnares/12.2.103

16. Hu, B., Zhou, W., Min, M., Du, Z., Chen, P., Ma, X., et al. (2013). Development of an effective acidogenically digested swine manure-based algal system for improved wastewater treatment and biofuel and feed production. *Appl. Energy* 107, 255–263. doi:10.1016/j.apenergy.2013.02.033
17. Huang, H. H., Camsund, D., Lindblad, P., and Heidorn, T. (2010). Design and characterization of molecular tools for a Synthetic Biology approach towards developing cyanobacterial biotechnology. *Nucleic Acids Res.* 38, 2577–2593. doi:10.1093/nar/gkq164
18. Huffer, S., Roche, C. M., Blanch, H. W., and Clark, D. S. (2012). *Escherichia coli* for biofuel production: bridging the gap from promise to practice. *Trends Biotechnol.* 30, 538–545. doi:10.1016/j.tibtech.2012.07.002
19. Huo, Y.-X., Wernick, D. G., and Liao, J. C. (2012). Toward nitrogen neutral biofuel production. *Curr. Opin. Biotechnol.* 23, 406–413.
20. Imamura, S., and Asayama, M. (2009). Sigma factors for cyanobacterial transcription. *Gene Regul. Syst Biol.* 3, 65–87.
21. Inokuma, K., Liao, J. C., Okamoto, M., and Hanai, T. (2010). Improvement of isopropanol production by metabolically engineered*Escherichia coli* using gas stripping. *J. Biosci. Bioeng.* 110, 696–701. doi:10.1016/j.jbiosc.2010.07.010
22. Iwaki, T., Haranoh, K., Inoue, N., Kojima, K., Satoh, R., Nishino, T., et al. (2006). Expression of foreign type I ribulose-1,5-bisphosphate carboxylase/oxygenase (EC 4.1.1.39) stimulates photosynthesis in cyanobacterium *Synechococcus* PCC7942 cells. *Photosyn. Res.* 88, 287–297. doi:10.1007/s11120-006-9048-x
23. Lan, E. I., and Liao, J. C. (2011). Metabolic engineering of cyanobacteria for 1-butanol production from carbon dioxide. *Metab. Eng.* 13, 353–363. doi:10.1016/j.ymben.2011.04.004
24. Lan, E. I., and Liao, J. C. (2012). ATP drives direct photosynthetic production of 1-butanol in cyanobacteria. *Proc. Natl. Acad. Sci. U.S.A.*109, 6018–6023. doi:10.1073/pnas.1200074109
25. Lan, E. I., and Liao, J. C. (2013). Microbial synthesis of n-butanol, isobutanol, and other higher alcohols from diverse resources.*Bioresour. Technol.* 135, 339–349. doi:10.1016/j.biortech.2012.09.104
26. Lindberg, P., Park, S., and Melis, A. (2010). Engineering a platform for photosynthetic isoprene production in cyanobacteria, using*Synechocystis* as the model organism. *Metab. Eng.* 12, 70–79. doi:10.1016/j.ymben.2009.10.001
27. Liu, X., Sheng, J., and Curtiss, R. III (2011). Fatty acid production in genetically modified cyanobacteria. *Proc. Natl. Acad. Sci. U.S.A.*108, 6899–6904. doi:10.1073/pnas.1103014108
28. Ma, J., Campbell, A., and Karlin, S. (2002). Correlations between Shine-Dalgarno sequences and gene features such as predicted expression levels and operon structures. *J. Bacteriol.* 184, 5733–5745. doi:10.1128/JB.184.20.5733-5745.2002
29. Machado, I. M., and Atsumi, S. (2012). Cyanobacterial biofuel production. *J. Biotechnol.* 162, 50–56. doi:10.1016/j.jbiotec.2012.03.005

30. McEwen, J. T., Machado, I. M. P., Connor, M. R., and Atsumi, S. (2013). Engineering *Synechococcus elongatus* PCC 7942 for continuous growth under diurnal conditions. *Appl. Environ. Microbiol.* 79, 1668–1675. doi:10.1128/AEM.03326-12

31. Misra, A., Conway, M. F., Johnnie, J., Qureshi, T. M., Derrick, A. M., Agbo, E. C., et al. (2013). Metabolic analyses elucidate nontrivial gene targets for amplifying dihydroartemisinic acid production in yeast. *Front. Microbiol.* 4:200. doi:10.3389/fmicb.2013.00200

32. Ninomiya, N., Ashida, H., and Yokota, A. (2008). "Improvement of cyanobacterial Rubisco by introducing the latch structure involved in high affinity for CO_2 in red algal Rubisco," in *Photosynthesis, Energy from the Sun*, eds J. Allen, E. Gantt, J. Golbeck, and B. Osmond (Dordrecht: Springer), 868–870.

33. Oliver, J. W. K., Machado, I. M. P., Yoneda, H., and Atsumi, S. (2013). Cyanobacterial conversion of carbon dioxide to 2,3-butanediol.*Proc. Natl. Acad. Sci. U.S.A.* 110, 1249–1254. doi:10.1073/pnas.1213024110

34. Onai, K., Morishita, M., Kaneko, T., Tabata, S., and Ishiura, M. (2004). Natural transformation of the thermophilic cyanobacterium*Thermosynechococcus elongatus* BP-1: a simple and efficient method for gene transfer. *Mol. Genet. Genomics* 271, 50–59. doi:10.1007/s00438-003-0953-9

35. Pate, R., Klise, G., and Wu, B. (2011). Resource demand implications for US algae biofuels production scale-up. *Appl. Energy* 88, 3377–3388. doi:10.1016/j.apenergy.2011.04.023

36. Pratt, C., Parsons, S. A., Soares, A., and Martin, B. D. (2012). Biologically and chemically mediated adsorption and precipitation of phosphorus from wastewater. *Curr. Opin. Biotechnol.* 23, 890–896. doi:10.1016/j.copbio.2012.07.003

37. Price, G. D. (2011). Inorganic carbon transporters of the cyanobacterial CO_2 concentrating mechanism. *Photosyn. Res.* 109, 47–57. doi:10.1007/s11120-010-9608-y

38. Qi, L. S., Larson, M. H., Gilbert, L. A., Doudna, J. A., Weissman, J. S., Arkin, A. P., et al. (2013). Repurposing CRISPR as an RNA-guided platform for sequence-specific control of gene expression. *Cell* 152, 1173–1183. doi:10.1016/j.cell.2013.02.022

39. Qiang, H., Zarmi, Y., and Richmond, A. (1998). Combined effects of light intensity, light-path and culture density on output rate of*Spirulina platensis* (Cyanobacteria). *Eur. J. Phycol.* 33, 165–171. doi:10.1080/09670269810001736663

40. Radakovits, R., Jinkerson, R. E., Darzins, A., and Posewitz, M. C. (2010). Genetic engineering of algae for enhanced biofuel production.*Eukaryotic Cell* 9, 486–501. doi:10.1128/EC.00364-09

41. Robertson, D. E., Jacobson, S. A., Morgan, F., Berry, D., Church, G. M., and Afeyan, N. B. (2011). A new dawn for industrial photosynthesis. *Photosyn. Res.* 107, 269–277. doi:10.1007/s11120-011-9631-7

42. Rodriguez, G. M., and Atsumi, S. (2012). Isobutyraldehyde production from *Escherichia coli* by removing aldehyde reductase activity.*Microb. Cell Fact.* 11, 90. doi:10.1186/1475-2859-11-90
43. Sanderson, K. (2011). Lignocellulose: a chewy problem. *Nature* 474, S12–S14. doi:10.1038/474S012a
44. Savir, Y., Noor, E., Milo, R., and Tlusty, T. (2010). Cross-species analysis traces adaptation of Rubisco toward optimality in a low-dimensional landscape. *Proc. Natl. Acad. Sci. U.S.A.* 107, 3475–3480. doi:10.1073/pnas.0911663107
45. Sheehan, J., Dunahay, T., Benemann, J., and Reossler, P. (1998). *A Look Back at the U.S. Department of Energy's Aquatic Species Program – Biodiesel from Algae.* Golden, CO: U.S. Department of Energy, National Renewable Energy Laboratory.
46. Shen, C. R., Lan, E. I., Dekishima, Y., Baez, A., Cho, K. M., and Liao, J. C. (2011). Driving forces enable high-titer anaerobic 1-butanol synthesis in *Escherichia coli. Appl. Environ. Microbiol.* 77, 2905–2915. doi:10.1128/AEM.03034-10
47. Shen, C. R., and Liao, J. C. (2012). Photosynthetic production of 2-methyl-1-butanol from CO_2 in cyanobacterium *Synechococcus elongatus* PCC7942 and characterization of the native acetohydroxyacid synthase. *Energy Environ. Sci.* 5, 9574–9583. doi:10.1039/c2ee23148d
48. Steinberg, N. A., and Meeks, J. C. (1991). Physiological sources of reductant for nitrogen fixation activity in *Nostoc* sp. strain UCD 7801 in symbiotic association with *Anthoceros punctatus. J. Bacteriol.* 173, 7324–7329.
49. Suzuki, E., Ohkawa, H., Moriya, K., Matsubara, T., Nagaike, Y., Iwasaki, I., et al. (2010). Carbohydrate metabolism in mutants of the cyanobacterium *Synechococcus elongatus* PCC 7942 defective in glycogen synthesis. *Appl. Environ. Microbiol.* 76, 3153–3159. doi:10.1128/AEM.00397-08
50. Takahama, K., Matsuoka, M., Nagahama, K., and Ogawa, T. (2003). Construction and analysis of a recombinant cyanobacterium expressing a chromosomally inserted gene for an ethylene-forming enzyme at the *psbAI* locus. *J. Biosci. Bioeng.* 95, 302–305. doi:10.1263/jbb.95.302
51. Tcherkez, G. G. B., Farquhar, G. D., and Andrews, T. J. (2006). Despite slow catalysis and confused substrate specificity, all ribulose bisphosphate carboxylases may be nearly perfectly optimized. *Proc. Natl. Acad. Sci. U.S.A.* 103, 7246–7251. doi:10.1073/pnas.0600605103
52. Ungerer, J., Tao, L., Davis, M., Ghirardi, M., Maness, P.-C., and Yu, J. (2012). Sustained photosynthetic conversion of CO_2 to ethylene in recombinant cyanobacterium *Synechocystis* 6803. *Energy Environ. Sci.* 5, 8998. doi:10.1039/c2ee22555g
53. Witcover, J., Yeh, S., and Sperling, D. (2013). Policy options to address global land use change from biofuels. *Energy Policy* 56, 63–74. doi:10.1016/j.enpol.2012.08.030
54. Wondraczek, L., Batentschuk, M., Schmidt, M. A., Borchardt, R., Scheiner,

S., Seemann, B., et al. (2013). Solar spectral conversion for improving the photosynthetic activity in algae reactors. *Nat. Commun.* 4, 2047. doi:10.1038/ncomms3047

55. Yuan, Z., Pratt, S., and Batstone, D. J. (2012). Phosphorus recovery from wastewater through microbial processes. *Curr. Opin. Biotechnol.* 23, 878–883. doi:10.1016/j.copbio.2012.08.001

56. Zhang, S., and Bryant, D. A. (2011). The tricarboxylic acid cycle in cyanobacteria. *Science* 334, 1551–1553. doi:10.1126/science.1210858

57. Zhou, J., Zhang, H., Zhang, Y., Li, Y., and Ma, Y. (2012). Designing and creating a modularized synthetic pathway in cyanobacterium*Synechocystis* enables production of acetone from carbon dioxide. *Metab. Eng.* 14, 394–400. doi:10.1016/j.ymben.2012.03.005

CHAPTER 18

BIODIESEL PRODUCTION BY ASPERGILLUS NIGER LIPASE IMMOBILIZED ON BARIUM FERRITE MAGNETIC NANOPARTICLES

Ahmed I. El-Batal, Ayman A. Farrag, Mohamed A. Elsayed and Ahmed M. El-Khawaga

Keywords: Biodiesel, Aspergillus niger, lipase immobilization, barium ferrite magnetic nanoparticles, fatty acid methyl ester

INTRODUCTION

Biodiesel is defined as the fatty acid alkyl monoesters derived from renewable feed stocks such as vegetable oils and animal fats [1]. Biodiesel is an efficient, clean and 100% natural energy alternative to petroleum-based fuels. Biodiesel fuel has many advantages; it is safe for use in all conventional diesel engines, offers the same performance and engine durability as petroleum diesel fuel and is non-flammable and non-toxic. In addition. It reduces tailpipe emissions, visible smoke, noxious fumes, and odors [2]. Biodiesel is better than diesel fuel in terms of sulfur content, flash point, aromatic content and biodegradability [3]. The simple reaction to convert vegetable oil to biodiesel is called transesterification, in which an alcohol and a catalyst are mixed with oil in order to "crack" the oil into esters and glycerol. During this process, the catalyst allows the alcohol to react successively with triglyceride to produce esters and glycerol, as shown in Equation (1). Where, the heavier portion of the reaction medium, glycerol, falls out of the mixture, leaving methyl esters. On the other hand, the methyl esters are purified by distillation. The distilled product, methyl esters of fatty acids, is known as the biodiesel [4]. There are three steps involved in the transesterification of triglyceride (TG) into methyl esters (ME), with the formation of intermediates diglyceride (DG) and monoglyceride (MG), resulting in the production of three moles

Citation: Ahmed I. El-Batal, Ayman A. Farrag, Mohamed A. Elsayed and Ahmed M. El-Khawaga, Biodiesel Production by Aspergillus niger Lipase Immobilized on Barium Ferrite Magnetic Nanoparticles, doi:10.3390/bioengineering3020014.

of ester and one mole of glycerol, as shown in stepwise reactions Equations (2)–(4) [5].

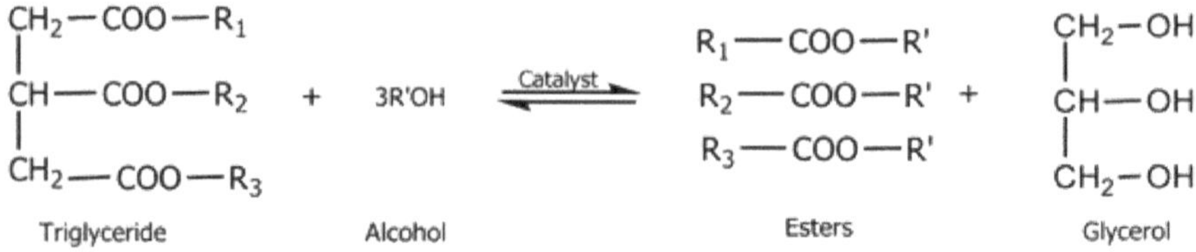

(1)

$$\text{Triglyceride} + \text{ROH} \rightleftharpoons \text{Diglyceride} + \text{RCOOR} \quad (2)$$

$$\text{Diglyceride} + \text{ROH} \rightleftharpoons \text{Monoglyceride} + \text{RCOOR} \quad (3)$$

$$\text{Monoglyceride} + \text{ROH} \rightleftharpoons \text{Glycerol} + \text{RCOOR} \quad (4)$$

A catalyst is usually used to improve the reaction rate and yield. Because the reaction is reversible, excess alcohol is used to shift the equilibrium to the products side. Lipases can catalyze this reaction [6].

Lipases (triacylglycerol acyl hydrolases, EC 3.1.1.3) are largely used as biocatalysts in biotechnology and modern chemistry [7]. These enzymes are also catalyzing several reactions like esterification [8], transesterification, acidolysis, interesterification, alcoholysis, aminolysis, oximolysis, thiotransesterification and ammoniolysis in anhydrous organic solvents [9]. Lipase is widely found in animals, plants and microorganisms [10]. Nowadays, most lipases produced commercially are currently obtained from fungi and yeasts. Fungal lipases have received attention because of their potential use in food processing, pharmaceuticals, cosmetics, oils/fats degradation, detergents and the leather industry [11]. Industrial applications of lipase are limited because it has poor stability, is easily inactivated, and is difficult to separate from the reaction system for reuse. In order to use lipase more economically and efficiently in reaction systems, its activity and operational stability need to be improved by an appropriate choice of immobilization process [12]. Immobilization of enzymes is a well reported technology that allows application of enzymes in many biocatalyzed processes, like in lipase-mediated biodiesel production. This process provides significant advantages, such as reuse of the biocatalyst, easier product recovery, and it frequently enhances the enzyme resistance against inactivation by different denaturants, providing more stable catalysts [13]. Besides, the enzyme immobilization onto magnetic supports such as nanosized magnetite particles allows an additional characteristic compared to other conventional support materials, such as the selective and secure enzyme recovery from the medium under the magnetic force. Hence, there is no need for expensive liquid chromatography systems, centrifuges, filters or other equipment [14]. In this study, the lipase from *Aspergillus nigerADM110* was immobilized onto the magnetic Barium Ferrite Nanoparticles (BFN) under different experimental conditions and characterized. The biodiesel production was carried out and analyzed by GC-MS.

MATERIALS AND METHODS

Chemicals

All the media components were purchased from Oxoid and Difco. Chemicals and reagents, including olive oil used, were purchased from Sigma-Aldrich (St Louis, MO, USA), were of analytical and HPLC grade, and were used without further purification. *Aspergillus niger ADM110* strain was from Drug Radiation Research Department (NCRRT) [15].

Lipase Production and Purification

Extracellular lipase was obtained from irradiated *Aspergillus niger ADM110* by submerged production using the optimized medium containing olive oil 5% as the most efficient carbon source and yeast extract 5.0% as the most suitable nitrogen source for the lipase biosynthesis. The fermentation was carried out in 100 mL of sterile production broth seeded with 1.0 mL (4.60×10^7) of spore inoculum and incubated at 25 °C, pH 7, 200 rpm agitation speed and for 72 h. *Aspergillus nigerADM110* was subjected to 0.14 kGy of gamma radiation to improve its lipolytic potential [15]. Crude lipase was obtained by centrifuging the culture broth at 10,000 rpm for 10 min at 4 °C. The lipase purification was carried out by ammonium sulfate precipitation followed by dialysis against 0.05 M sodium phosphate buffer solution (pH 7.2). Extracellular lipase activity was estimated by photometric assay [16].

Synthesis of Hexagonal Magnetic Barium Ferrite Nanoparticles (BNF)

Barium ferrite nanoparticles were prepared by the citrate sol-gel auto-combustion method [17,18]. Barium nitrate $Ba(NO_3)_2$, ferric nitrate $Fe(NO_3)_3 \cdot 9H_2O$ and citric acid were taken as starting materials. The nitrates were dissolved in the minimum amount of de-ionized water to get a clear solution in the molar ratio 1:10. An aqueous solution containing 12.5 moles of citric acid was mixed with both nitrate solutions (metals: citric acid, 1:3). After complete dissolving of all starting materials, an appropriate amount of ammonia solution was added dropwise with agitation until the pH of the solution reaches 7.0 giving a clear dark-green solution. The resulting solution was then heated in a drying oven at 85 °C for 3 h followed by heating at 110 °C until the transparent solution turned to viscous gel. The viscous gel was then heated at 150 °C until foaming occurred. The foamy gel was maintained at 150 °C until spontaneous ignition occurred. The combustion reaction was completed within a few minutes, and brown ash was formed. The fine powder was calcined (pre-sintered) in the calcination oven at 450 °C for 3 h to remove carbonic materials and then the temperature was increased to 850 °C for 4 h for the final formation of barium ferrite nanoparticles.

Immobilization of Lipase on BFN Particles

For the immobilization of lipase, 200 mg of BFN particles were added to 0.85% (*w/v*) sodium chloride solution containing lipase. The mixture was incubated for 4 h using an overhead stirrer. After washing twice with 0.85% (*w*/*v*) sodium chloride solution, the immobilized lipase was separated by magnetic decantation of the supernatants and stored at 4 °C. The amount of protein binding to the BFN particles was determined by measuring the protein concentration of the lipase solution and the supernatant by the Lowry method [19].

Assay of Enzyme Activity

The assay was modified from that described by Pencreac'h *et al.* [20]. The assay mixture contained 90 μL of 8.25 mM *p*-nitrophenyl palmitate in isopropanol and 810 μL of 50 mM Tris-HCl, pH 8.0, with 0.5% (*w*/*v*) Triton X-100 and 0.12% (*w*/*v*) Arabic gum. The mixture was then preheated to 40 °C. To initiate the reaction, 100 μL of lipase solution or suspension of immobilized lipase diluted to the appropriate concentration with 1% (*w*/*v*) bovine serum albumin was added. The change in absorbance at 410 nm was monitored for 5 min at 40 °C using a thermostated spectrophotometer (UV-1800, Shimadzu, Kyoto, Japan). The activity was calculated from the difference in absorbance between 2 and 5 min with a standard curve for the hydrolysis product, *p*-nitrophenol. One activity unit was defined as the production of 1 μmol of *p*-nitrophenol per min at 40 °C. Measurements were performed in triplicate.

After the reaction, BFN particles were separated magnetically and recycled. The specific activity of the lipase was defined in this study as the enzyme activity (unit) divided by the protein content and expressed as U/mg protein. Relative specific activity was calculated by dividing the specific activity of the immobilized lipase by that of the free lipase [21].

Biodiesel Production Using the Transestrification Process

Transesterification is the reaction of vegetable oil or animal fat with an alcohol, in most cases methanol, to form esters and glycerol. However, before entering the transesterification reactor, the FFA (Free Fatty Acids) content and humidity must be removed, to avoid the production of soap. The transesterification reaction is affected by (molar ratio of glycerides to alcohol, the amount of catalyst, reaction temperature, reaction time and shaking speed) [22].

The yield of the transesterification processes was calculated as a sum of the weight of FAME (fatty acid methyl ester) produced to the weight of cooking oil used, multiplied by 100. The formula is given as:

$$\text{Yield of FAME} = \frac{Weight\ of\ fatty\ acid\ methylester}{Weight\ of\ fat\ used} \times 100\%$$

Gas Chromatography Analysis of WCO (Waste Cooking Oil)

GC analysis of waste cooking oil was carried out on a GC system Agilent Technologies 7890A (Santa Clara, USA) equipped with FID, split/splitless injector and Agilent 7693

A automated liquid sampler. Column: HP INNOWAX, 30 m × 0.32 mm ID, 0.25 μm film thickness. Temperature program of the oven: initial temperature 210 °C for 9 min, rate 20 °C/min to 230 °C, 10 min. Detector temperature: 300 °C, injector temperature: 250 °C. Carrier gas: He, column flow 1.5 mL/min, split ratio 1:80. Hydrogen flow 40 mL/min, air flow 400 mL/min, make-up gas (nitrogen) 40 mL/min. Injection volume 1 μL. ChemStation for GC was used for instrument control, data acquisition and data analysis [23].

Fatty Acid Methyl Esters (FAMEs) Analysis (Biodiesel Products)

Five hundred milliliters of the reaction mixture were mixed with 1.0 mL isooctane for two min. Following centrifugal separation, the upper organic layer was collected and washed twice with distilled water and dried over anhydrous Na_2SO_4. The solvent was dried under N_2 steam and dissolved in 0.25 mL of CH_2Cl_2. The previous GC condition of WCO analysis was applied. The prepared FAMEs were then analyzed using particular fatty acid methyl ester standards (methyl palmitate, methyl stearate, methyl oleate, methyl linoleate, and methyl linolenate; Sigma-Aldrich).

Analytical Methods

The size and morphology of the magnetic nanoparticles were assessed by transmission electron microscopy (TEM) (JEOL, Peabody, MA, USA). The X-ray diffraction (XRD) (Rigaku Corporation, Austin, TX, USA) was performed to check the crystallinity of the magnetic nanoparticles. SEM/EDAX analysis (JEOL, Peabody, MA, USA), and TEM were performed for characterization of the magnetic nanoparticles.

Statistical Analysis

The analysis of data was carried out according to [24]. Means were compared using the least significant difference (LSD at the 5% level) and Duncan's multiple range tests at the significance $P = 0.05$.

RESULTS AND DISCUSSION

Characterization of BFN Particles

The result shows the production of the hexagonal phase with a high overall agreement between the entry database and the sample diffraction pattern. The XRD pattern illustrates the formation of 92.7% weight percent hexagonal barium ferrite and 7.3% some other phases, like $BaFe_2O_4$ (cubic phase), BaO and Fe_2O_3. TEM analysis of the prepared barium ferrite shows the formation of spherical nanoparticles with average particle size diameter ranging from 8 to 25 nm with some unidentified amorphous phases. According to the structure of hexagonal barium ferrite, it has exact element weight ratios of (Ba: Fe: O) equal to (12.3: 60.4: 27.3). By comparing this value with the prepared one, the result was found to be approximately the same by EDAX analysis using SEM.

The prepared $BaFe_{12}O_{19}$ hexaferrite particles were characterized via Fourier transformed Infrared spectra (FTIR) Shimadzu FTIR-8400S. The room temperature infrared spectra of prepared samples was recorded in mid-IR range, 4000 cm^{-1} to 400 cm^{-1}. A few milligrams of $BaFe_{12}O_{19}$ hexaferrite particles were mixed with anhydrous KBr powder and made in the form of a pellet for the measurements.

Figure 1a shows FTIR spectra of $BaFe_{12}O_{19}$ hexaferrite particles. The main absorption bands at 3440.4 cm^{-1} are attributed to the O–H stretching, while the characteristic band at 1631.5 cm^{-1} results from the anti-symmetrical and symmetrical stretching vibration bands of COO^- related to citric acid [25]. The absorption bands at 2925.5 cm^{-1} were due to OH vibrations. The other bands are at 1457, 1430, 1385.6 and 858.17 cm^{-1}, corresponding to the stretching and bending vibrations of C=O, H–C–H, C–H and C–C respectively. The characteristic absorption bands between 586.25 and 450.3 $cm^{-1}$are assigned to the vibration of the bond between the oxygen atom and the metal ions (F–O), confirming the formation of hexaferrite and corresponding to vibrations of the tetrahedral and octahedral sites for $BaFe_{12}O_{19}$. The Fe–O stretching vibration band of the bulk magnetite is usually at 570 cm^{-1} and the band shifted to high wave numbers because of the finite size of the nanoparticles. The bands located at 1351 cm^{-1} and 858.17 cm^{-1} are associated with the N–O stretching vibration and bending vibration of NO_3^- [26]. The notable bands at about 1385 and 1430 cm^{-1} are attributed to nitrate ion and barium carbonate, respectively.

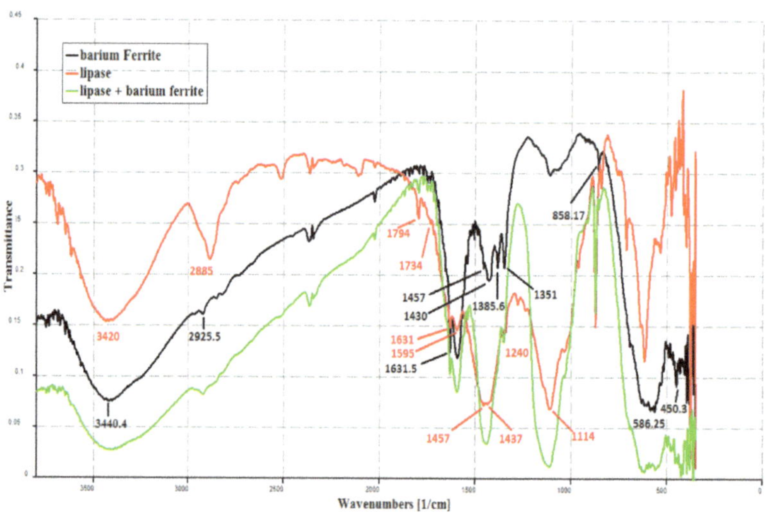

Figure 1: FTIR spectra of: (a) free *Aspergillus niger ADM110* lipase enzyme; (b) Barium ferrite magnetic nanoparticles; (**c**) Immobilized lipase enzyme on barium ferrite magnetic nanoparticles.

Figure 1b shows the FTIR spectrum of lipase from *Aspergillus nigerADM110*. There are many signals characteristic of different functional groups of the enzyme. They include a typical band at 2885 cm^{-1} assigned to the stretching C–H vibrations of –CH2 and –CH3 groups. A broad and intense band at 3420 cm^{-1} was assigned to the stretching vibrations of –OH group, and a band of the –N–H stretching vibrations, masked by the former one [27]. The characteristic signals coming from the stretching vibrations of carbonyl groups around 1734 cm-1 and stretching vibrations of ≡C–O– appear in the spectrum at 1240 cm^{-1}.

Figure 1c shows the FTIR spectrum of immobilized lipase on barium ferrite magnetic nanoparticles. It was evident that the characteristic bands of protein (*i.e.*, lipase) at 1794 for Amide I and 1457–1437 cm^{-1} for Amide II with characteristic band 1114 cm^{-1} for coil alpha helix. Furthermore, 1631, 1595 cm^{-1} were present in pure lipase and the lipase-bound (barium ferrite nano) Fe_3O_4 nanoparticles, confirming the binding of lipase to $BaFe_{12}O_{19}$ nanoparticles by covalent immobilization. The strong characteristic bands of proteins for the lipase-bound $BaFe_{12}O_{19}$ should be owing to the high enzyme loading [28]. In addition, it is noted that a characteristic band of 1385.6 cm^{-1} was observed in naked Fe_3O_4 nanoparticles. After binding of lipase, this characteristic band disappeared in lipase binding barium ferrite nano. Also, bands at 2885, 2515 and 2111.0 $cm^{-1}$of lipase disappeared in binding lipase on nanoparticles. Thus, it was suggested that the binding was accomplished via the reaction between the amine group of BaFerrite nanoparticles and the carboxyl group of lipase and confirmed the enzyme immobilization.

The Activity of the Lipase Immobilized on BFN Particles

It is expected that the binding has been taking place between the hydrophobic particle of barium ferrite and the hydrophobic area of the lipase via interfacial activation.

Various initial lipase concentrations (0.2–2 mg/mL) were tested for immobilization experiments for determining the optimum enzyme loading. As shown in Table 1, the amounts of lipase immobilized increased significantly with increasing the initial lipase concentration, and the activities attained a maximum value at an initial lipase concentration of 1.0 mg/mL. The lipase activity is, however, slowly decreased when the initial lipase concentration was above 1.0 mg/mL. The excessive enzyme loading is known to hinder the substrate conversion due to the increased protein–protein interaction [29]. In the rest of the experiments, the initial lipase concentration was maintained at 1.0 mg/mL.

Table 1: Activity of the lipase immobilized on BFN (barium ferrite nanoparticles) particles

Initial Lipase Concentration (mg/mL)	Activity of Immobilized Lipase (U/mL)	Protein Immobilized (mg/g Support)	Specific Activity (U/mg Protein)
00.2	4.8a ± 0.56	9.0a ± 0.70	6.15a ± 0.10
00.4	12.5b ± 0.35	15.7b ± 0.49	7.30b ± 0.21
00.6	23.9c ± 0.63	24.8c ± 0.42	8.82c ± 0.57
00.8	27.0d ± 0.56	36.5d ± 1.06	9.44de ± 0.39
01.0	30.5f ± 0.77	49.0e ± 0.91	10.10e ± 0.61
01.4	28.6e ± 0.77	57.8g ± 0.56	8.92cd ± 0.26
01.8	28.4e ± 0.98	52.6f ± 0.91	9.75de ± 0.53
02.0	28.5e ± 0.35	52.5f ± 0.56	9.60de ± 0.35
LSD	01.70	03.25	1.01

Note: Different letters indicate significant differences between treatments (Duncan test, $P \leqslant 0.05$). Means in each column followed by the same letter are not significantly different.

Activities of free and immobilized lipase were measured at various pH and temperatures values. The pH of the free and the immobilized lipase activities was compared and shown in Figure 2. The optimum pH of the immobilized lipase was 8.0, whereas that of the free one was 7.0. Also, the immobilized lipase showed higher activity than the free one, especially at pHs higher than 7.0.

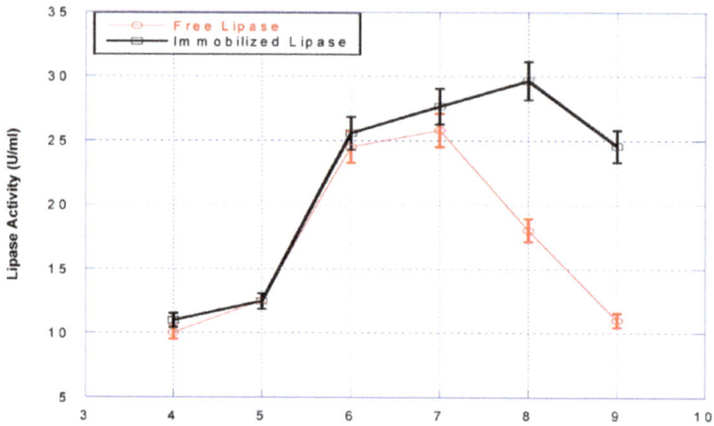

Figure 2: Effect of pH on the activity of free (red line) and immobilized (black line) lipases.

The optimum pH value of free lipase shifted one unit to the alkaline region after binding on the support. It would therefore appear that lipase active sites may well be occluded in some of the composites. Also, the BFN to which the lipase is immobilized retards the denaturing effect of increased pH and/or temperature, which is exhibited by the shift in the optimal pH/temperature for activity. Previous studies [30] have suggested that upon immobilization, the active site becomes more exposed to solvent than that in the folded-dissolved lipase form. Activities of free and immobilized lipase were measured at various temperatures and the results are shown in Figure 3.

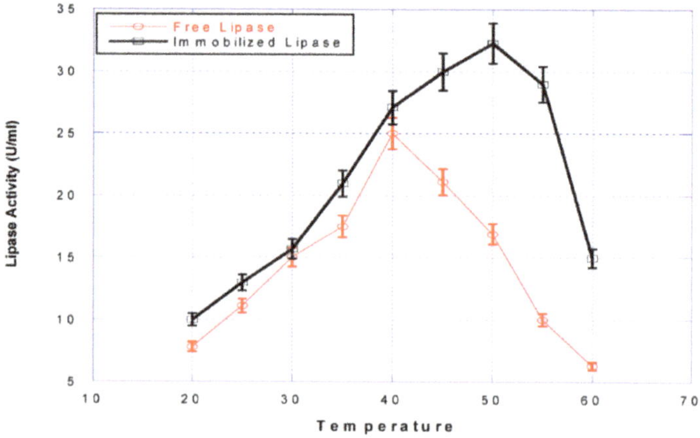

Figure 3: Effect of temperature (°C) on the activity of free (red line) and immobilized (black line) lipases at pH 8.0.

The optimum temperature of the immobilized lipase was 50 °C, whereas that of the free one was 40 °C. It can be concluded that the immobilization using BFN particles enhanced the thermal stability of lipase, which might be caused by multipoint attachment of the lipase to the support and/or by the hydrophobic interaction [31].

Recyclability of BFN-Lipase

After the reaction was complete, the immobilized lipase can be easily separated by a magnet. The results indicate that BFN-Lipase (5%) can be reused in biodiesel production without any treatment with 17% loss of activity after 5 cycles and a 66% loss in activity in the sixth cycle, with the activity of 29, 26, 25, 25 and 24 U/mL around the five cycles, respectively. Then the activity was decreased to 10 U/mL after the 6th cycle.

Therefore, no appreciable inhibition due to oil, glycerol or product was detected. Importantly, no aggregation of the particle was observed. The behavior of the prepared sample indicates that BFN particles prevent the undesirable hydrophilic interactions (glycerol and methanol adsorption, protein aggregation, particle aggregation) which are likely to occur in the hydrophobic oils. The results presented in Table 2 show the fatty acid profile of WCO and its biodiesel fatty acid methyl ester.

Table 2: Fatty acid profile of WCO and its biodiesel fatty acid methyl ester

Fatty Acids	Formula	Common Acronym	Methyl Esters	% Composition by Mass
Oleic acid	$C_{17}H_{33}COOH$	C18: 0	Methyl oleate	46.5d ± 0.91
Palmitic acid	$C_{15}H_{31}COOH$	C16: 0	Methyl palmitate	30.9c ± 0.77
Stearic acid	$C_{17}H_{35}COOH$	C18: 0	Methyl strearate	09.0b ± 0.56
Linoleic acid	$C_{17}H_{31}COOH$	C18: 2	Methyl linoleate	08.5b ± 0.35
Linolenic acid	$C_{17}H_{29}COOH$	C18: 3	Methyl linolenate	05.1a ± 0.28
LSD				02.95

Note: Different letters indicate significant differences between treatments (Duncan test, $P \leqslant 0.05$). Means in each column followed by the same letter are not significantly different.

Production of Biodiesel Using the Transesterification Process

One liter sample size of waste cooking oil was heated to 60 °C to remove any free water and allowed to settle for 24 h before reacting with methanol.

Effect of Methanol/Waste Cooking Oil Molar Ratio on Biodiesel Production

Stoichiometrically, three moles of methanol are required for each mole of triglyceride, but in practice, a higher molar ratio is needed to drive the reaction towards completion and produce more fatty acid methyl esters (FAMEs) as products.

In this study, biodiesel was obtained under transesterification conditions as follows: reaction temperature, 45 °C; catalyst amount, 5.0 wt %; reaction time, 4 h. The effect of methanol: oil molar ratio increases from 1:1 to 4:1, as listed in Table 3, in which the biodiesel yield increases as the molar ratio increases from 1:1 to 4:1. The maximum biodiesel yield of 90% is obtained when the molar ratio is very close to 4:1. However, beyond the molar ratio of 5:1, the excessively added methanol has no significant effect on the production yield. In contrast, when the amount of methanol is over 4:1, glycerol separation becomes more difficult, thus decreasing the biodiesel yield. Based on this, the optimum molar ratio of methanol to oil is 4:1.

Table 3: Factors affecting biodiesel production using transesterification process

Factors Affecting Biodiesel Production		Biodiesel Yield (%)
Methanol/oil ratio (mole/mole)	1:1	42a ± 1.41
	2:1	65b ± 2.12
	3:1	87d ± 0.707
	4:1	**90e ± 1.76**
	5:1	76c ± 0.707
LSD		03.75
Enzyme concentration (%)	3	69a ± 0.707
	5	**89b ± 1.06**
	10	91bc ± 1.41
	15	94c ± 0.707
	20	97d ± 1.909
LSD		02.25
Reaction temperature (°C)	15	55a ± 0.494
	25	73b ± 1.41
	35	81c ± 0.636
	45	**91d ± 1.41**
	55	75b ± 0.707
LSD		05.95
Reaction time (h)	2	50a ± 0.707
	4	**88d ± 1.06**
	6	88d ± 1.41
	8	61c ± 0.848
	10	58b ± 0.707
LSD		03.10
Shaking speed (rpm)	100	43a ± 1.41
	200	52b ± 1.48
	300	71c ± 1.41
	400	**88d ± 0.636**
	500	69c ± 1.13
LSD		09.05

Note: Different letters indicate significant differences between treatments (Duncan test, $P \leqslant 0.05$). Means in each column followed by the same letter are not significantly different.

Effect of Enzyme Concentration Percentage on Biodiesel Production

The effect of catalyst dosage was investigated with the mass ratio of immobilized lipase catalyst to waste cooking oil varying within the range of 3.0%–20.0%, under otherwise identical conditions as reaction temperature, 45 °C; methanol/oil, 3:1; reaction time, 4 h. The biodiesel yield was found to increase with increasing catalyst dosage, and the maximum was obtained at the dosage of 20% with the value being 93% at 4 h Table 3. It should be noted that we could not continue increasing catalyst concentration over 20%

due to the high cost of immobilized lipase. So, we can deduce that 89% of biodiesel obtained at 5% enzyme concentration is the superior result.

Effect of Reaction Temperature on Biodiesel Production

In this part of the experiments, the reaction temperature was varied within a range of 15–55 °C. Transesterification conditions: methanol/oil, 3:1; catalyst amount, 5.0 wt % (of the feed mass of waste cooking oil, similarly from now on); reaction time (4 h). The results listed in Table 3 indicated that the reaction rate was slow at low temperatures and the biodiesel yield was only 55% at 15 °C after 4 h. The biodiesel yield increased with the increase of the reaction temperature to nearly 91% at 45 °C, but at higher temperatures ($T > 55$ °C), the methanol was vaporized and formed a large number of bubbles in the interface, which inhibited the increase of biodiesel yield, then the yield of biodiesel decreased significantly. Thus, the optimum reaction temperature was 45 °C.

Effect of the Reaction Time on Biodiesel Production

The reaction time tells the fastness of the transesterification process of a particular feedstock. The results in Table 3indicated that the ester content increased with reaction time from 2 h onward and reached a maximum at a reaction time of 4 h at reaction temperature, 45 °C; methanol/oil, 3:1; reaction time, 4 h; catalyst amount, 5.0 wt % of the feed mass of waste cooking oil, and then remained relatively constant with increasing further the reaction time. An extension of the reaction time from 4 to 6 h had no significant effect on the conversion of triglycerides but led to a reduction in the product yield. Because longer reaction enhanced the hydrolysis of esters (reverse reaction of transesterification), this resulted in the loss of esters.

Effect of Shaking Speed on Biodiesel Production

The agitation rate improves the mixing during the transesterification process. It increases the intact area between oils and immobilized lipase enzyme methanol solution and facilitates the initiation of the reaction.

Transesterification conditions: methanol/oil, 3:1; catalyst amount, 5.0 wt % (of the feed mass of waste cooking oil, similarly hereinafter); reaction time, 4 h and at 45 °C. In methanolysis conducted with different rates of stirring, such as 100, 200, 300, 400 and 500 revolutions per minute (rpm), it was observed that the reaction of methanolysis was practically incomplete at 100 rpm and only exhibited a yield of 43%, as in Table 3. The yield was increased when the mixing intensity was accelerated up to 400 rpm.

Physicochemical Properties of the Used Cooking Oil and Its Corresponding Production of Biodiesel

Kinematic Viscosity

Viscosity refers to a fluid's resistance to flow at a given temperature. Fuel that is too viscous can hinder the operation of an engine. Kinematic viscosity measures the ease with which a fluid will flow under force. It is different from absolute viscosity, also called dynamic viscosity. Kinematic viscosity is obtained by dividing the dynamic viscosity by the density of the fluid [32]. Kinematic viscosity allows comparison between the engine performances of different fuels, independent of the density of the fuels. Two fuels with the same kinematic viscosity should have the same hydraulic fuel properties, even though one fuel may be denser than the other.

The kinematic viscosity of the used waste cooking oil was 60.0 cSt and its corresponding biodiesel was 5.83 cSt (Table 4).

Table 4: Physicochemical properties of the produced biodiesel

No.	Characteristics	Result	Unit	Test Method
1	Kinematic viscosity at 40 °C	5.83	$mm^2 \cdot s^{-1}$	ASTM D445
2	Density at 15.5 °C	0.850	$g \cdot cm^{-3}$	ASTM D1298
3	Calorific value	43.1	MJ/Kg	ASTM D-224
4	Total sulfur content	0.050	mass%	ASTM D4294
5	Flash point	188	°C	ASTM D92
6	Pour point	−9	°C	ASTM D97
7	Cloud point	−3	°C	ASTM D2500
8	Cetane number	59.5	—	ASTM D613
9	Water content	0.091	vol%	ASTM D6304
10	Acid number	0.182	mg KOH g^{-1}	ASTM D664
11	Distillation temperature (DT)	95% Recovery at 340	°C	ASTM D86
12	Iodine number	102	mg I_2/100 g oil	ASTM D4737
13	Saponification value	206	mg KOH/g oil	ASTM D 5558

Density at 15 °C

The density of biodiesel is used to judge the homogeneity of biodiesel. This property is important, mainly in airless combustion systems because it influences the efficiency of atomization of the fuel [33]. The result obtained (Table 4) showed that the methyl ester produced in this study had a density of 0.850 g/mL, which falls in the range 0.82–0.87 g/mL, specified according to Egyptian diesel oil.

Distillation at Atmospheric Pressure

Distillation is used to determine the boiling range of the biodiesel product quantitatively. Even though distillation at the atmospheric pressure provides some clues or information about the properties of methyl esters such as the boiling range of the biodiesel product, distillation at the reduced pressure (vacuum distillation) is required because the biodiesel will thermally decompose using atmospheric distillation. The plot pattern of the volume of distillate recovered *versus*temperature in Figure 4 indicates this fact. The decrease in temperature during the distillation process shows the decomposition of methyl ester which results in the formation of low boiling molecular substances.

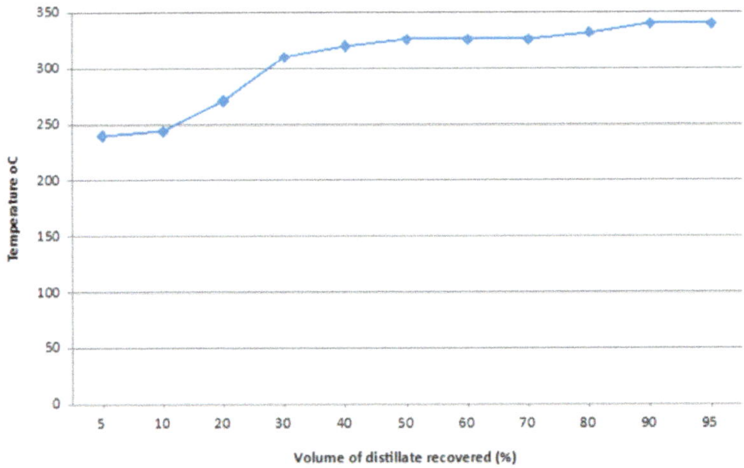

Figure 4: Relationship between volume of distillate recovered and temperature °C.

Flash Point (FP)

The flash point temperature is the measure of the fuel to form a flammable mixture with air. It is only one of many properties which must be considered in assessing flammability hazard of material. For biodiesel, a flash point of below 130 °C is found to be out of specification (ASTM D 6751, 2009). The measured flash point of this biodiesel was 188 °C (Table 4), indicating very small or negligible methanol levels in the biodiesel. This high flash point can prevent auto ignition and fire hazard at a high temperatures during transportation and storage periods.

Heat of Combustion/Calorific Value

Gross heat of combustion (HG) is a property proving the suitability of using fatty compounds as diesel fuel. The calorific value of the obtained biodiesel; 43.1 MJ/Kg is an acceptable value (Table 4). Although it is lower than the Egyptian standards for petrodiesel (44.3 MJ/Kg), it is higher than that of the European standard for biodiesel (32.9 MJ/Kg).

The Cetane Number

The cetane number (CN) is a dimensionless descriptor of the ignition quality of a diesel fuel (DF) [34]. It is a prime indicator of DF quality. It is a measure of how easily the fuel will ignite in the engine. The CN is related to the time that passes between injection of the fuel into the cylinder and the start of ignition. Because of the higher oxygen content, biodiesel has a higher cetane number compared to petroleum diesel. The cetane index of waste cooking oil from the experiment was found to be 59.5 (Table 4). The cetane number of methyl esters of rapeseed oil, soybean oil, palm oil, lard and beef tallow were found to be 58, 53, 65, 65 and 75, respectively [35]. Among these biodiesel feed stocks, beef tallow has the highest cetane number. The higher cetane number indicates, the higher engine performance of beef tallow compared to other fuels, resulting in the lower emission of all pollutants other than oxides of nitrogen (NO_x). As beef tallow has the higher amount of saturated fatty acids, the increase in the saturated fatty acids content positively enhanced the cetane number of biodiesel. The obtained data revealed the higher cetane number, 59.5 compared to Egyptian petrodiesel standards of 55, but within the recommended universal biodiesel standards (min 47).

Cloud Point (CP) and Pour Point

The cloud and pour points are also important properties of biodiesel fuel. The cloud point is the temperature at which crystals first appear in the fuel when cooled [36]. At temperatures below CP, larger crystals fuse together and form large agglomerates that can restrict or cut off flow through fuel lines and filters and cause start-up and performance problems the next morning [37]. The temperature at which crystal agglomeration is extensive enough to prevent free pouring of fluid is determined by measurement of its pour point [38]. These properties are related to the use of biodiesel in cold temperatures. The cloud and pour points are (−3 and −9 °C), respectively (Table 4). So the produced biodiesel would be more suitable to cold conditions as compared to petrodiesel.

Water and Sulfur Content

Biodiesel is sulfur free, but this test is an indicator of contamination of protein material and/or carryover catalyst material or neutralization material from the production process (ASTM D4294). Sulfur reduces the function of catalysts and causes SO_x emissions as in diesel engines and has an adverse effect with the formation of black smoke. Hence, a low level of sulfur, or no sulfur, is beneficial to the performance of the diesel engine due to the lower emissions and the decrease in the levels of corrosive sulfuric acid accumulating in the engine crankcase oil. Sulfur content of biodiesel is from 0.031 to 0.05. The synthesized kind is found to be in this range.

Water can cause corrosion of tanks and equipment, and if detergent is present, the water can cause emulsions or a hazy appearance. Water supports microbiological growth at the fuel/water interfaces in fuel systems. Biodiesel can contain as much as 1500 parts per million of dissolved water [39]. The produced biodiesel is characterized by low water and sulfur content, 0.091% and 0.050% respectively (Table 4), compared with the Egyptian petrodiesel standards, $<0.15\%$ and 1.2%, respectively.

Iodine Number

The iodine value is an important measure for the determination of the unsaturation in fatty acids, which is only dependent on the vegetable oil. This property greatly influences fuel oxidation and the deposits formed in the injector of diesel engines [40]. With the increasing iodine value of unsaturated fatty acids, the effect of polymerization is stronger. In this study, the iodine value of the WCO used was 125 mg I_2/100 g oil, and 102 mg I_2/100 g oil for the corresponding biodiesel (Table 4). According to EN 14214, the biodiesel must have an iodine value <120 mg I_2/100 g oil in the sample.

Acid Number

The acid number is the quantity of base, expressed as milligrams of KOH per gram of sample, required to titrate a sample to a specified end point. Acid number determination is an important test to assess the quality of a particular biodiesel. It can indicate the degree of hydrolysis of the methyl ester, a particularly important aspect when considering storage and transportation, as large quantities of free fatty acids can cause corrosion in tanks [41]. The acid value of feedstock and produced methyl esters was 1.90 and 0.182 (mg KOH/g oil), respectively (Table 4). The average percentage decrease of acid value from WCO to the produced biodiesel was about 90.4%, indicating a good transesterification process. This result meets the EN 14214 and D-6751 standards, but it was higher than that of Egyptian petrodiesel standards.

Saponification Value (mg KOH/g Oil)

Saponification value is the quantity of base, expressed as milligrams of KOH per gram of sample, required to saponify one gram of fat or oil. The obtained result (Table 4) indicated that the methyl esters produced had higher saponification value 206 (mg KOH/g oil) than the corresponding oils 201 (mg KOH/g oil).

CONCLUSIONS

Biodiesel production technology is competitive in terms of it being a low-cost and alternative source of energy, which should be not only sustainable but also environmentally friendly. Catalyst immobilization addresses several issues: repetitive and continuous use, localization of the interaction, prevention of product contamination, reduction of effluent problems and material handling, and effective control of the reaction parameters. In this study, we developed novel hydrophobic magnetic nanoparticles (barium ferrite nanoparticles) for lipase immobilization. This allows additional characteristics compared to other conventional support materials, such as selective and easy enzyme recovery from the medium under the magnetic force. The second advantage is that we can reuse the BFN-Lipase without any rinsing treatment for five cycles, with an activity of 29, 26, 25, 25 and 24 U/mL during the five cycles. The activities of free and immobilized lipase were measured at various pH and temperatures values. The optimum pH of the immobilized lipase was 8.0, whereas that of the free one was 7.0, and the optimum temperature of the immobilized lipase was 50 °C, whereas that of the free one was 40 °C. The fatty acid profile of collected waste cooking oil as feedstock for lipase production was determined using GC/MS and showed the presence of oleic, palmitic, stearic, linoleic and linolenic acids. The enzymatic conversion of waste cooking oil to biodiesel (transesterification) was carried out using methyl alcohol. Different factors affecting transesterification reaction, such as methanol/oil molar ratio, reaction temperature, shaking, reaction time and enzyme concentration, were studied. The previous results showed that the use of immobilized lipase enzyme on barium ferrite nanoparticles had high efficiency as a catalyst in the process of biodiesel production from waste cooking oil. Tests also demonstrated that the properties of biodiesel attained were fit as a substitute for diesel in addition to being a friend of the environment.

ACKNOWLEDGMENTS

The authors would like to thank the Nanotechnology Research Unit (Principal Investigator. Ahmed El-Batal), Drug Radiation Research Department, National Center for Radiation Research and Technology (NCRRT), Egypt, for financing and supporting this study under the project Nutraceuticals and Functional Foods Production by using Nano/Biotechnological and Irradiation Processes.

AUTHOR CONTRIBUTIONS

Ahmed I. El-Batal and Ayman A. Farrag conceived and designed the experiments; Ahmed M. El-Khawaga performed the experiments; Ahmed I. El-Batal and Mohamed A. Elsayed analyzed the data; and contributed reagents/materials/analysis tools; Ahmed I. El-Batal and Ahmed M. El-Khawaga wrote the paper. All authors read and approved the final manuscript.

REFERENCES

1. Yu, C.Y.; Huang, L.Y.; Kuan, I.; Lee, S.L. Optimized Production of Biodiesel from Waste Cooking Oil by Lipase Immobilized on Magnetic Nanoparticles. *Int. J. Mol. Sci.* 2013, *14*, 24074–24086.
2. Demirbas, A. Biodiesel production via non-catalytic SCF method and biodiesel fuel characteristics. *Energy Convers. Manag.* 2006, *47*, 2271–2282.
3. Bala, B.K. Studies on biodiesels from transformation of vegetable oils for diesel engines. *Energy Educ. Sci. Technol.*2005, *15*, 1–45.
4. Pighinelli, A.L.; Ferrari, R.A.; Miguel, A.M.; Park, K.J. High oleic sunflower biodiesel: Quality control and different purification methods. *Grasas Aceites* 2011, *62*, 171–180.
5. Pogaku, R.; Raman, J.K.; Ravikumar, G. Evaluation of Activation Energy and Thermodynamic Properties of Enzyme-Catalysed Transesterification Reactions. *Adv. Chem. Eng. Sci.* 2012, *2*, 150–154.
6. Ahmia, A.; Danane, F.; Bessah, R.; Boumesbah, I. Raw material for biodiesel production. Valorization of used edible oil. *Rev. Energies Renouv.* 2014, *17*, 335–343.
7. Gupta, R.; Kumari, A.; Syal, P.; Singh, Y. Molecular and functional diversity of yeast and fungal lipases: Their role in biotechnology and cellular physiology. *Prog. Lipid Res.* 2015, *57*, 40–54.
8. Babaei, M.; Karimi, A.; Hejazi, M.A. Use of mesoporous MnO_2 as a support for immobilization of lipase from *Candida rugosa*. *Chem. Ind. Chem. Eng. Q.* 2014, *20*, 371–378.

9. Villeneuve, P.; Muderhwa, J.M.; Graille, J.; Haas, M.J. Customizing lipases for biocatalysis: A survey of chemical, physical and molecular biological approaches. *J. Mol. Catal. B Enzym.* 2000, *9*, 113–148.
10. Metin, A.Ü. Immobilization studies and biochemical properties of free and immobilized *Candida rugosa* lipase onto hydrophobic group carrying polymeric support. *Macromol. Res.* 2013, *21*, 176–183.
11. Mendes, A.A.; Castro, H.F.D.; Pereira, E.B.; Furigo Júnio, F. Application of lipases for wastewater treatment containing high levels of lipids. *Quím. Nova* 2005, *28*, 296–305.
12. Turinayo, Y.K.; Kalanzi, F.; Mudoma, J.M.; Kiwuso, P.; Asiimwe, G.M.; Esegu, J.P.O.; Balitta, P.; Mwanja, C. Physicochemical Characterization of Jatropha curcas Linn Oil for Biodiesel Production in Nebbi and Mokono Districts in Uganda. *J. Sustain. Bioenergy Syst.* 2015, *5*, 104–113.
13. Cesarini, S.; Infanzón, B.; Pastor, F.I.; Diza, P. Fast and economic immobilization methods described for non-commercial Pseudomonas lipases. *BMC Biotechnol.* 2014, *14*, 1071–1075.
14. El-Hadi, A.A.; Saleh, H.I.; Moustafa, S.A.; Ahmed, H.M. Immobilization of Mucor racemosus NRRL 3631 lipase and characterization of silica-coated magnetite (Fe3O4) nanoparticles. *Egypt. Pharm. J.* 2013, *12*, 28–35.
15. El-Batal, A.I.; Farrag Ahmed, A.; Elsayed, M.A.; Soltan, A.M.; El-Khawaga, A.M. Enhancement of Lipase Biosynthesis by *Aspergillus nigerADM110* using Gamma Radiation. *Egypt. J. Med. Microbiol.* 2015, *24*, 87–94.
16. Xu, J.; Sun, J.; Wang, Y.; Sheng, J.; Wang, F.; Sun, M. Application of iron magnetic nanoparticles in protein immobilization. *Molecules* 2014, *19*, 11465–11486.
17. Bahadur, D.; Rajakumar, S.; Kumar, A. Influence of fuel ratios on auto combustion synthesis of barium ferrite nano particles. *J. Chem. Sci.* 2006, *118*, 15–21.
18. Abedini Khorrami, S.; Islampour, R.; Bakhtiari, H.; Sadr, M.N.Q. The effect of molar ratio on structural and magnetic properties of $BaFe_{12}O_{19}$ nanoparticles prepared by sol-gel auto-combustion method. *Int. J. Nano Dimens.* 2013, *3*, 191–197.
19. Lowry, O.H.; Rosebrough, N.J.; Farr, A.L.; Randall, R.J. Protein measurement with the Folin phenol reagent. *J. Boil. Chem.* 1951, *193*, 265–275.
20. Pencreac'h, G.; Baratti, J.C. Hydrolysis of *p*-nitrophenyl palmitate in *n*-heptane by the *Pseudomonas cepacia* lipase: A simple test for the determination of lipase activity in organic media. *Enzym. Microb. Technol.* 1996, *18*, 417–422.
21. Liu, X.; Guan, Y.; Shen, R.; Liu, H. Immobilization of lipase onto micron-size magnetic beads. *J. Chromatogr. B* 2005,*822*, 91–97.
22. Xu, Q.-Q.; Li, Q.; Yin, J.-Z.; Guo, D.; Qiao, B.-Q. Continuous production of biodiesel from soybean flakes by extraction coupling with transesterification under supercritical conditions. *Fuel Process. Technol.* 2016, *144*, 37–41.
23. Milina, R.; Mustafa, Z. Gas chromatographic investigations of compositional profiles of biodiesel from different origin. *Pet. Coal* 2013, *55*, 12–19.

24. Snedecor, G.; Cochran, W. *Statistical Methods*, 8th ed.; Iowa State University Press: Ames, IA, USA, 1989.
25. Kaur, T.; Srivastava, A. Effect of pH on Magnetic Properties of Doped Barium Hexaferrite. *Int. J. Res. Mech. Eng. Technol.* 2013, *3*, 171–173.
26. Chauhan, C.; Jotania, R.; Jotania, K. Structural properties of cobalt substituted barium hexaferrite nanoparticles prepared by a thermal treatment method. *J. Nanosyst. Phys. Chem. Math.* 2013, *4*, 363–369.
27. Wang, J.; Meng, G.; Tao, K.; Feng, M.; Zhao, X.; Li, Z.; Xi, H.; Xia, D.; Lu, J.R. Immobilization of lipases on alkyl silane modified magnetic nanoparticles: Effect of alkyl chain length on enzyme activity. *PLoS ONE* 2012, *7*, e43478.
28. Rani, K.; Goyal, S.; Chauhan, C. Novel approach of alkaline protease mediated biodegradation analysis of mustard oil driven emulsified bovine serum albumin nanospheres for controlled release of entrapped Pennisetum glaucum (Pearl Millet) amylase. *Am. J. Adv. Drug Deliv.* 2015, *3*, 135–148.
29. Lee, D.-G.; Ponvel, K.M.; Kim, M.; Hwang, S.; Ahn, I.S.; Lee, C.H. Immobilization of lipase on hydrophobic nano-sized magnetite particles. *J. Mol. Catal. B Enzym.* 2009, *57*, 62–66.
30. Ting, W.-J.; Tung, K.-Y.; Giridhar, R.; Wu, W.T. Application of binary immobilized *Candida rugosa* lipase for hydrolysis of soybean oil. *J. Mol. Catal. B Enzym.* 2006, *42*, 32–38.
31. Ferrario, V.; Veny, H.; De Angelis, E.; Navarini, L.; Ebert, C.; Gardossi, L. Lipases immobilization for effective synthesis of biodiesel starting from coffee waste oils. *Biomolecules* 2013, *3*, 514–534.
32. Koria, L.; Nithya, G. Analysis of *Datura stramonium* Linn. biodiesel by gas chromatography-mass spectrometry (gc-ms) and influence of fatty acid composition on the fuel related characteristics. *J. Phytol.* 2012, *4*, 6–9.
33. Felizardo, P.; Correia, M.J.N.; Raposo, I.; Mendes, J.F.; Rui, B.; Bordado, J.M. Production of biodiesel from waste frying oils. *Waste Manag.* 2006, *26*, 487–494.
34. Chhetri, A.B.; Watts, K.C.; Islam, M.R. Waste cooking oil as an alternate feedstock for biodiesel production. *Energies*2008, *1*, 3–18.
35. Hilber, T.; Ahn, E.; Mittelbach, M.; Schmitd, E. Animal fats perform well in biodiesel. *Render Magazine*, February 2006; 16–18.
36. Shrestha, D.; Van Gerpen, J.; Thompson, J. Effectiveness of cold flow additives on various biodiesels, diesel, and their blends. *Trans. ASABE* 2008, *51*, 1365–1370.
37. Dunn, R.O. Cold flow properties of biodiesel: A guide to getting an accurate analysis. *Biofuels* 2015, *6*, 115–128.
38. Ibiari, N.N.; El-Enin, S.A.A.; Attia, N.K.; El-Diwani, G. Ultrasonic comparative assessment for biodiesel production from rapeseed. *J. Am. Sci.* 2010, *6*, 937–943.
39. Brown, E.K.; Palmquist, M.; Luning Prak, D.J.; Mueller, S.S.; Bowen, L.L.; Sweely, K.; Ruiz, O.N.; Trulove, P.C. Interaction of Selected Fuels with Water: Impact on Physical Properties and Microbial Growth. *J. Pet. Environ. Biotechnol.* 2015, *6*.

40. Cancela, Á.; Maceiras, R.; Alfonsín, V.; Sánchez, Á. Transesterification of waste frying oil under ultrasonic irradiation.*Eur. J. Sustain. Dev.* 2015, *4*, 401–406.

41. Akanawa, T.T.; Moges, H.G.; Babu, R.; Bisrat, D.; Akanawa, T.T.; Babu, R.; Bisrat, D. Castor Seed from Melkasa Agricultural Research Centre, East Showa, Ethiopia and it's biodiesel performance in Four Stroke Diesel Engine. *Int. J. Renew. Energy Dev.* 2014, *3*, 99–105.

INDEX

A

Accelerating medicine partnership (AMP) 7
Alkaline phosphatase (ALP) 67, 71
Ambulatory blood pressure (ABP) 227
Ambulatory blood pressure measurement (ABPM) 228
Armed Forces Institute of Regenerative Medicine (AFIRM) 7
Atomic force microscopy (AFM) 26
Average real variability (ARV) 227

B

Basilar artery (BA) 254
Bilateral vestibular loss (BVL) 137
Biomaterial-associated infection (BAI) 64
Blood pressure (BP) 227
Blood pressure variability (BPV) 227

C

Citrate phosphate dextrose (CPD) 52
Clinical and Translational Science Awards (CTSA) 4
Common carotid artery (CCA) 173
Computational fluid dynamic (CFD) 254
Computed tomography angiography (CTA) 254
Computed Tomography (CT) 120, 125
Coronary artery bypass graft (CABG) 171

D

Defense Advanced Research Projects Agency's (DARPA) 7
Diamond-Like –Carbon (DLC) 111
Dip pen nanolithography (DPN) 26

E

Electron beam lithography (EBL) 28
Extracellular matrix (ECM) 12, 21

F

Focal adhesion kinase (FAK) 25
Focal adhesions (FAs) 24
Fractional flow reserve (FFR) 254

I

Internal carotid artery (ICA) 254
Internal diameter (ID) 192
International Council for Laboratory Animal Science (ICLAS) 176
Intima-media thickness (IMT) 228

L

Left ventricular (LV) 119
Long-term depression (LTD) 142

M

Magnetic Resonance Angiography (MRA) 243

Magnetic Resonance Imaging (MRI) 119
Major histocompatibility complex (MHC) 23
Mesenchymal stem cell (MSC) 23
Mesenchymal stem cells (MSCs) 65
Middle cerebral artery (MCA) 245
Mitogen-activated protein kinase (MAPK) 25

N

National Institutes of Health (NIH) 4

O

Outer diameter (OD) 188

P

Percutaneous transluminal coronary angioplasty (PTCA) 171
Phosphate-buffered saline (PBS) 65, 188
Phosphate Buffered Saline (PBS) 175
Platelet rich plasma (PRP) 189
Polyglycolic acid (PGA) 22
Polymer pen nanolithography (PPL) 27
Pressure gradient (PG) 256
Pressure ratio (PR) 254
Pulse amplitude modulation (PAM) 138
Pulse rate modulation (PRM) 138

S

Scanning electron microscopy (SEM) 189
Semicircular canals (SCCs) 137
Standard deviation (SD) 161, 227
Stratum corneum (SC) 85
Systolic blood pressure variability (SBPV) 230

T

Tissue engineering (TE) 21
Total Hip Arosthroplasty (THA) 97
Total Hip Replacement (THR) 97
Translational Centre for Regenerative Medicine (TRM) 4

U

Ultra High Molecular Weight Polyethylene (UHMWPE) 109

V

Vascular smooth muscle cells (VSMC) 172